Pediatric and Neonatal Critical Care Certification Review

Pediatric and Neonatal Critical Care Certification Review

M.K. Gaedeke, RN, MSN, CCRN, CS

Clinical Nurse Specialist
Nurse Practitioner
Pediatric Critical Care

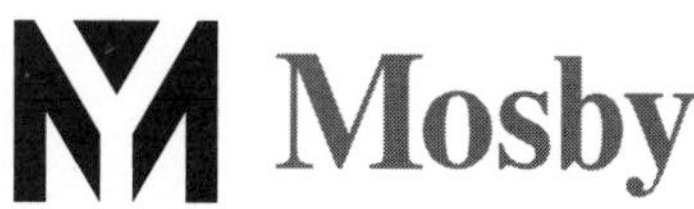

St. Louis Baltimore Boston Carlsbad Chicago Naples New York Philadelphia Portland
London Madrid Mexico City Singapore Sydney Tokyo Toronto Wiesbaden

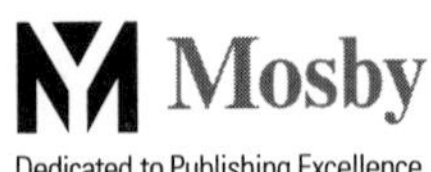

Dedicated to Publishing Excellence

Publisher: Nancy L. Coon
Senior Editor: Sally Schrefer
Associate Developmental Editor: Michele D. Hayden
Project Manager: Mark Spann
Production Editor: Jennifer Doll
Designer: Judi Lang
Cover Art: Judi Lang

A NOTE TO THE READER:
The author and publisher have made every attempt to check dosages and nursing content for accuracy. Because the science of pharmacology is continually advancing, our knowledge base continues to expand. Therefore we recommend that the reader always check product information for changes in dosage or administration before administering any medication. This is particularly important with new or rarely used drugs.

1st EDITION

Printed in the United States of America

Composition by Shepherd, Inc.
Printing and binding by R.R. Donnelley and Sons Co.

Mosby–Year Book, Inc.
11830 Westline Industrial Drive
St. Louis, Missouri 63146

Library of Congress Cataloging-in-Publication Data

Gaedeke, M. K.
Pediatric and neonatal critical care certification review / M.K. Gaedeke.—1st ed.
p. cm.
Includes bibliographical references and index.
ISBN 0-8151-3455-X
1. Pediatric intensive care—Examinations, questions, etc. 2. Pediatric nursing—Examinations, questions, etc. 3. Neonatal intensive care—Examinations, questions, etc. 4. Pediatric intensive care—Outlines, syllabi, etc. 5. Pediatric nursing—Outlines, syllabi, etc. 6. Neonatal intensive care—Outlines, syllabi, etc. I. Title.
[DNLM: 1. Pediatric Nursing—examination questions. 2. Neonatal Nursing—examination questions. 3. Critical Care—examination questions. 4. Licensure, Nursing—examination questions. WY 18.2 G127p 1996]
RJ370.G34 1996
618.92′0028′076—dc20
DNLM/DLC
for Library of Congress 95-39931
CIP

96 97 98 99 00 / 9 8 7 6 5 4 3 2 1

Reviewers

Margaret-Ann Carno, RN, MS, MBA, CCRN
Staff Nurse Specialist
University Hospital
State University of New York
Health Science Center at Syracuse;
Clinical Instructor
College of Nursing
Syracuse University
Syracuse, New York

Ellen M. Chiocca, RNC, MSN
Instructor
Department of Maternal-Child Health
Loyola University
Chicago, Illinois

Mary K. Cousins, RN, BSN, CCRN
Staff Nurse
Department of Pediatric Critical Care;
Assistant Coordinator, ECMO Program
Children's Hospital of Buffalo
Buffalo, New York

Catherine L. Headrick, RN, MS
Clinical Nurse Specialist
Pediatric Intensive Care Unit
Children's Medical Center of Dallas
Dallas, Texas

Anita Mitchell, RN, MSN, CCRN
Associate Professor
Department of Nursing
Northeast Louisiana University
Monroe, Louisiana

Marisa G. Mize, RN, MSN, CCRN, PNP
Clinical Nurse Specialist
Pediatric Critical Care
Walter Reed Army Medical Center
Washington, D.C.

Jean-Michel A. Roland, MD
Pediatric Cardiologist
Children's Hospital of Buffalo
Buffalo, New York

Debbie Gearner Thompson, RN, MS, CCRN
Neonatal Clinical Specialist
The North Carolina Baptist Hospitals, Inc.
Winston-Salem, North Carolina

Preface

This book was conceived more than 3 years ago as I began to prepare for the first pediatric CCRN examination. The fact that there were no study materials available for this examination made preparation difficult and frankly intimidating. I was already certified in adult critical care nursing and found the availability of study materials to be invaluable. Out of necessity and opportunity, this book was developed.

Pediatric and Neonatal Critical Care Certification Review is a unique review book for busy nurses who need a concise yet thorough reference to study for pediatric and/or neonatal certification. The content is based on recommended study guidelines for all the major critical care examinations in both pediatric and neonatal critical care nursing. The book is simply designed to help busy nurses study either entire chapters or small sections of content as time allows. Only essential material has been included to help separate the "nice to know" from the "need to know."

The first eight chapters cover the various body systems. Each chapter is divided into three main sections:

Passkeys—brief, bulleted, and essential key points to studying for certification.

Questions—multiple-choice practice questions that test more basic information, as well as higher-level knowledge encountered on the examinations.

Answers—to the questions, including rationales for both correct and incorrect responses.

The last chapters focus on successfully passing the examination itself. A chapter on test-taking strategies helps address and overcome test anxiety and offers tips on eliminating wrong answers and selecting correct answers to increase test scores. The last chapters contain 200-item practice examinations for both pediatric and neonatal certification, the correct answers, and a key for analyzing test scores.

It is my hope that this book will help many neonatal and pediatric critical care nurses successfully achieve certification. Through achieving certification, nurses can better make their optimal contribution to patient- and family-centered care.

M.K. Gaedeke

Acknowledgements

I'd like to express my gratitude and thanks for the support many people offered me in producing this project. First, I'd like to acknowledge the expertise shared with me by the neonatal and pediatric critical care nurses at Children's Hospital of Buffalo who have mentored and supported me in my practice. Thanks also to David Steinhorn, Michele Papo, Lynn Hernan, Brad Fuhrman, Chris Foley, Tara Smith, and Scott Penfil, the intensivists who have so freely shared their expertise. Finally, thanks to Shelly Hayden and Sally Schrefer who believed in this project and made it a joy to accomplish.

DEDICATION

- Jessica, to you I always will be grateful for more than I can ever express, more than you knew. I miss you.
- Thanks, Jeff and Adam, for the privilege of being your mom. I love you always.
- Ma grenouille, mon prince. Je t'ai aimé un mille fois. Je vais t'aimé un mille fois de plus.

Contents

Pediatric and Neonatal Critical Care Certification Review

CHAPTER 1

Cardiovascular Care Problems

Passkeys

GENERAL PRINCIPLES OF CARDIOLOGY

- Cardiac output (CO)—the amount of blood ejected by the heart—is determined by the stroke volume (SV) multiplied by the heart rate (HR) and commonly expressed as liters/minute (l/min):

$$CO = SV \times HR.$$

- Cardiac output is influenced by arterial blood pressure (afterload), heart rate, ventricular filling (preload), ventricular compliance (stretching), and contractility of the myocardium. Figure 1-1 represents the normal conduction system.

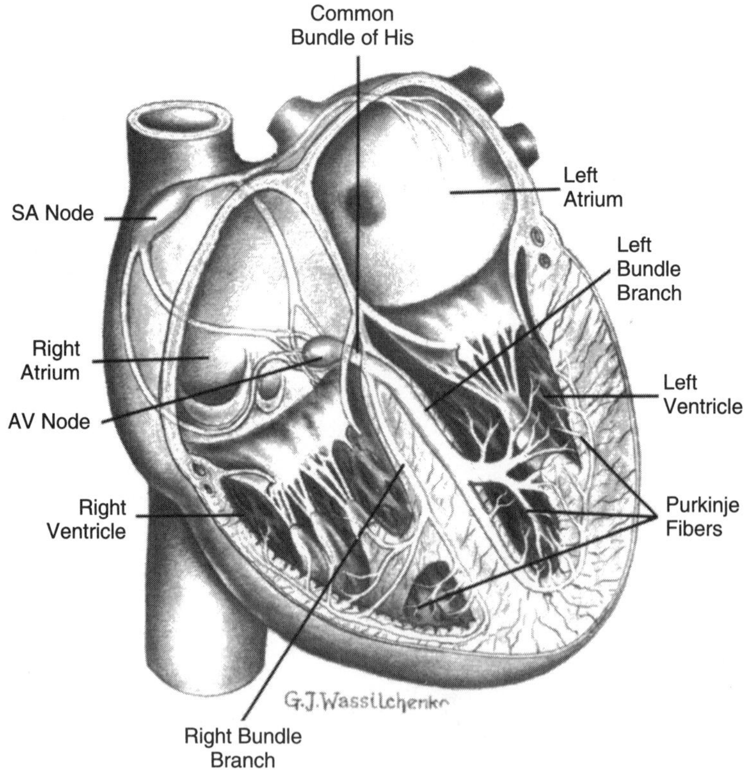

Fig. 1-1 The normal conduction pathway. The electrical impulse begins in the SA node and is transmitted to the AV node, bundle of His, bundle branches, and Purkinje fiber network. (From Grauer K: A practical guide to ECG interpretation, St Louis, 1992, Mosby.)

Normal cardiac output:
Neonates 200 ml/kg/min
Infants and Children 150 ml/kg/min
Adolescents 100 ml/kg/min

- Cardiac index is an expression of the cardiac output per square meter of body surface area. Normal cardiac index: 3.5 to 4.5 l/min/m^2

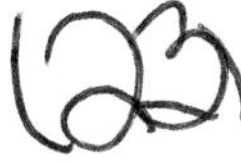

The estimated amount of circulating blood volume is as follows:
Neonates 85 to 90 ml/kg
Infants 75 to 80 ml/kg
Children 70 to 75 ml/kg
Adolescents 65 to 70 ml/kg

- Stroke volume—the output of each ventricle at every contraction—is in relation to the size of the child: the smaller the child the lower the volume.

- Contractility is impaired by acidosis, electrolyte imbalances, hypoxia, and hypoglycemia. Contractility is measured or assessed by the ejection fraction.

- Oxygen demand and, therefore, cardiac output is highest at birth, rapidly decreasing in the first 8 weeks (to half of demand and output at birth) and then tapering more gradually.

- Right ventricular end-diastolic pressure (RVEDP) = right atrial pressure (RAP) = central venous pressure (CVP) in patients with normal cardiac anatomy.

- Left ventricular end-diastolic pressure (LVEDP) = left atrial pressure (LAP) = pulmonary artery occlusion pressure (PAOP) or pulmonary artery wedge pressure (PAWP) in patients with normal cardiac anatomy.

- Ventricular end-diastolic pressures (VEDP) = filling pressures. Extreme tachycardia increases VEDP because the ventricles do not have time to empty well. (See Table 1-1 for further pressure and volume information.)

- Stimulation of the sympathetic nervous system, which prepares the body for "fight or flight," results in increased heart rate, stroke volume, cardiac output, and blood pressure. Beta-adrenergic and anticholinergic drugs also produce these effects. The sympathetic nervous system is immature at birth and does not fully mature until 1 to 2 years of age.

- Stimulation of the parasympathetic nervous system, which allows the body to "slow down" from an emergency, results in decreased heart rate, stroke volume, cardiac output, and blood pressure. Beta-blockers and cholinergic drugs also produce these effects.

Table 1-1
Pressure and Volume Results during Cardiac Catheterization

Pressure/Volume	Normal Values: Adults	Normal Values: Pediatric and Neonatal
Systemic arterial pressure	90-140/60-90 mm Hg	90-125/50-80 mm Hg (2 years to adolescense) 60-90/20-60 mm Hg (birth to 5 days)
Right atrial pressure	0-5 mm Hg	3 mm Hg
Right ventricular pressure	25/0-5 mm Hg	30/3 mm Hg
Pulmonary artery pressure	25/20 mm Hg	30/10 mm Hg
Pulmonary artery occlusive pressure	5-10 mm Hg	6-10 mm Hg
Left atrial pressure	5-10 mm Hg	8 mm Hg
Left ventricular pressure	120/0-5 mm Hg	100/6 mm Hg
Aortic pressure	90-140/60-90 mm Hg	100/60 mm Hg
Cardiac index	3.5-5.5 L/min/m^2	3.5-4.5 L/min/m^2 3.5-5.5 L/min/m^2

- Alveolar hypoxia promotes pulmonary vasoconstriction that leads to decreased pulmonary blood flow and consequently more hypoxemia. Appropriate use of oxygen therapy is important to prevent pulmonary hypertension.

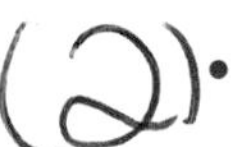

- Pediatric and neonatal cardiac arrests usually result from primary respiratory or shock problems not cardiac causes.
- Intubation for respiratory distress should be done earlier in infants and children than in adults. Respiratory distress and subsequent arrest can be more sudden and is more frequent in young patients.
- Metabolic acidosis is best treated by increasing perfusion and oxygenation.

Fetal Circulation

- Fetal cardiac development occurs between the fourth and seventh week of gestation.

- Fetal cardiac output is so high that even with oxygen saturations of only 60% to 70%, tissue hypoxia does not occur because delivery to tissues is adequate.

- Fetal pulmonary vascular resistance (PVR) is high. Within 24 hours after birth, PVR has fallen to one-half systemic vascular resistance (SVR). It is normally the same as adult levels within weeks after birth.

- The ductus arteriosus shunts blood away from the lungs in the fetus by directing blood flow from the pulmonary artery to the aorta. This is possible because of fetal pulmonary hypertension, which makes the blood flow more easily from the higher-pressure right side to the lower-pressure left side.

- The ductus arteriosus normally closes within 10 to 24 hours after birth.

- The foramen ovale is a one-way flap opening in the atrial septal wall. In the fetus, the high-pressure right side of the heart allows shunting of blood directly to the left atrium to the systemic circulation. Once again, blood bypasses the lungs because of the high right-sided pressures of the pulmonary circulation. Some blood, though a small amount, does circulate through the lungs. (See Fig. 1-2 for changes in circulation at birth.)

Assessment Factors

- Fatigue, poor nutritional consumption, and weight loss can be indicative of poor cardiac output or hypoxemia. Weight gain (wet vs. dry) can indicate fluid retention rather than growth in children with heart defects.

- Cyanosis that worsens with crying often indicates a cardiac problem. Cyanosis that improves with crying often indicates a pulmonary problem.

- Gray, pale, or mottled coloring indicates poor cardiac output, not necessarily hypoxemia.

- Strong upper-extremity pulses with weak or absent lower-extremity pulses usually indicate coarctation of the aorta or interrupted aortic arch.

- Bounding pulses may indicate high-volume state such as a ventricular septal defect or patent ductus arteriosus.

- A palpable thrill can indicate valvular disease, septal defects, or obstructions to normal flow.

Review of heart sounds

S_1

- Occurs with closure of mitral and tricuspid valves during systole.
- Failure to close will result in pansystolic or regurgitant murmurs.
- Heard best at 4th intercostal space, midclavicular line.

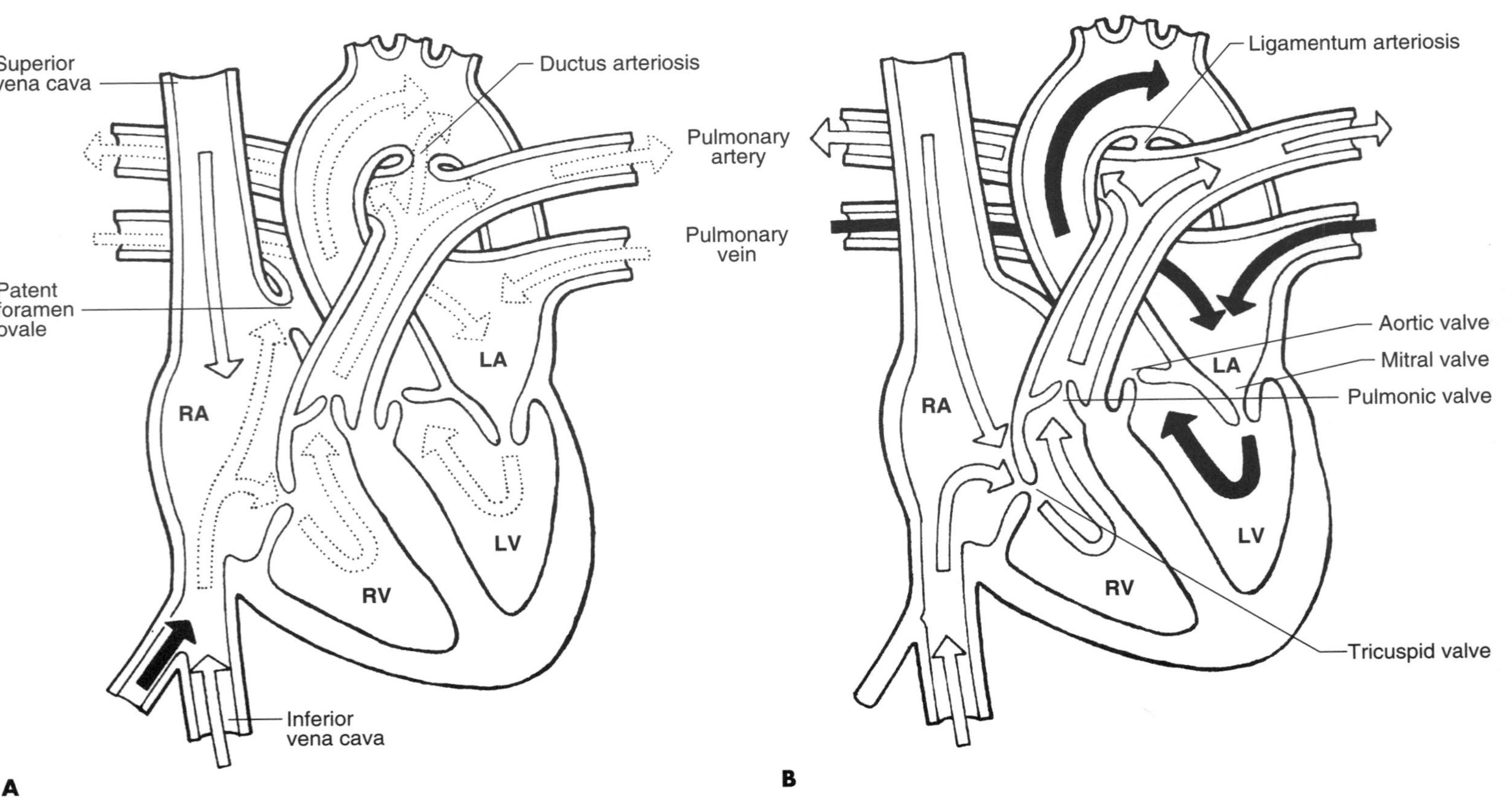

Fig. 1-2 Changes in circulation at birth. **A,** Prenatal circulation. **B,** Postnatal circulation. (Arrows indicate direction of blood flow.)

S_2

- Occurs with closure of aortic and pulmonic valves during diastole.
- Failure to close will result in diastolic or regurgitant murmurs.
- This heart sound is typically split in the neonate due to initial high pulmonary pressures. Absence of a split second heart sound at birth can sometimes indicate pulmonary or tricuspid atresia.
- Split second heart sounds can be a normal finding in infants and children, especially during inspiration.
- Heard best at 2nd intercostal space, midclavicular line.

S_3

- May be a normal finding in children; also may indicate a ventricular gallop, in which the ventricle is overly stretched from failure.
- Heard early in diastole.
- Heard best with the bell of the stethoscope.

S_4

- May be a normal finding in children, or may indicate ventricular overload and failure.
- Also called an atrial gallop because the atrium has trouble filling a poorly functioning ventricle.
- Heard late in diastole.
- Heard best with the bell of the stethoscope.

Review of murmurs

- Murmurs of stenosis occur because valves are not opening properly. Mitral stenosis and tricuspid stenosis are types of diastolic murmurs; aortic and pulmonic stenosis are types of systolic murmurs. These murmurs are usually harsh.
- Murmurs of regurgitation or insufficiency occur because valves are not closing properly. Mitral and tricuspid insufficiency are types of systolic murmurs; aortic and pulmonic insufficiency are types of diastolic murmurs.
- Systolic murmurs occur commonly with fever and anemia, even in the absence of structural heart disease.
- Ventricular septal defect murmurs may not be heard at birth or until 4 to 6 weeks of life as a result of persistently increased pulmonary vascular resistance that limits or prevents shunting. When present, this murmur is harsh and systolic, but the intensity is not necessarily well correlated to the size of the defect.

- The bell of the stethoscope hears low-pitched sounds best, whereas the diaphragm hears high-pitched sounds best.

CONGENITAL HEART DEFECTS

- Classification of congenital heart defects is often done as lesions which increase pulmonary blood flow, decrease pulmonary blood flow, obstruct blood flow, or mix blood flow. (The following boxes summarize this information.)

Defects with Increased Pulmonary Blood Flow

Atrial Septal Defect (ASD)

Description: Abnormal opening between the atria, allowing blood from the higher-pressure left atrium to flow into the lower-pressure right atrium. There are three types:

Ostium primum (ASD 1°)—Opening at lower end of septum; may be associated with mitral valve abnormalities

Ostium secundum (ASD 2°)—Opening near center of septum

Sinus venosus defect—Opening near junction of superior vena cava and right atrium; may be associated with partial anomalous pulmonary venous connection

Pathophysiology: Because left atrial pressure slightly exceeds right atrial pressure, blood flows from the left to the right atrium, causing an increased flow of oxygenated blood into the right side of the heart. Despite the low pressure difference, a high rate of flow can still occur because of low pulmonary vascular resistance and the greater distensibility of the right atrium, which further reduces flow resistance. This volume is well tolerated by the right ventricle because it is delivered under much lower pressure than in a ventricular septal defect. Although there is right atrial and ventricular enlargement, cardiac failure is unusual in an uncomplicated atrial septal defect. Pulmonary vascular changes usually occur only after several decades if the defect is unrepaired.

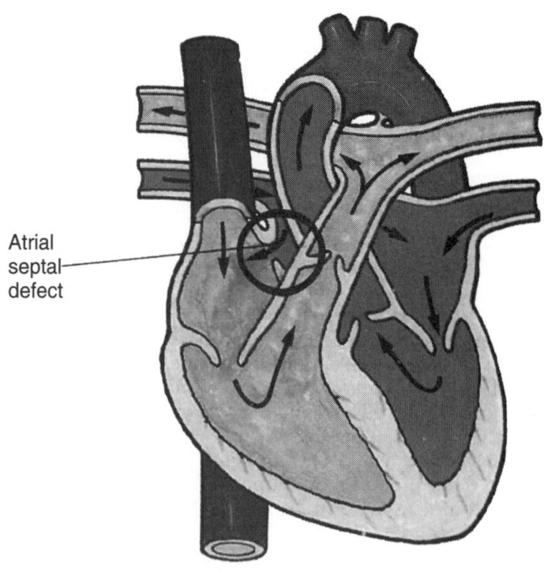

Defects with Increased Pulmonary Blood Flow—cont'd

Clinical manifestations: Patients may be asymptomatic. They may develop congestive heart failure. There is a characteristic murmur. Patients are at risk for atrial dysrhythmias (probably caused by atrial enlargement and stretching of conduction fibers) and pulmonary vascular obstructive disease and emboli formation later in life from chronic increased pulmonary blood flow.

Surgical treatment: Surgical Dacron patch closure of moderate to large defects similar to closure of ventricular septal defects. Open repair with cardiopulmonary bypass is usually performed before school age. In addition, the sinus venosus defect requires patch placement, so the anomalous right pulmonary venous return is directed to the left atrium with a baffle. The ASD 1° may require repair or, rarely, replacement of the mitral valve.

Nonsurgical treatment: ASD 2° may also be closed using devices during cardiac catheterization. This technique is in clinical trials in some centers.

Prognosis: Very low operative mortality, less than 1%.

Ventricular Septal Defect (VSD)

Description: Abnormal opening between the right and left ventricles. May be classified according to location: membranous (accounting for 80%) or muscular. May vary in size from a small pinhole to absence of the septum, resulting in a common ventricle. Frequently associated with other defects, such as pulmonary stenosis, transposition of the great vessels, patent ductus arteriosus, atrial defects, and coarctation of the aorta. Many VSDs (20% to 60%) are thought to close spontaneously. Spontaneous closure is most likely to occur during the first year of life in children having small or moderate defects. A left-to-right shunt is caused by the flow of blood from the higher-pressure left ventricle to the lower-pressure right ventricle.

Pathophysiology: Because of the higher pressure within the left ventricle and because the systemic arterial circulation offers more resistance than the pulmonary circulation, blood flows through the defect into the pulmonary artery. The increased blood volume is pumped into the lungs, which may eventually result in increased pulmonary vascular resistance. Increased pressure in the right ventricle as a result of left-to-right shunting and pulmonary resistance causes the muscle to hypertrophy. If the right ventricle is unable to accommodate the increased workload, the right atrium may also enlarge as it attempts to overcome the resistance offered by incomplete right ventricular emptying. In severe defects Eisenmenger syndrome may develop.

Clinical manifestations: Congestive heart failure is common. There is a characteristic murmur. Patients are at risk for bacterial endocarditis and pulmonary vascular obstructive disease. In severe defects, Eisenmenger syndrome may develop.

Continued.

Defects with Increased Pulmonary Blood Flow—cont'd

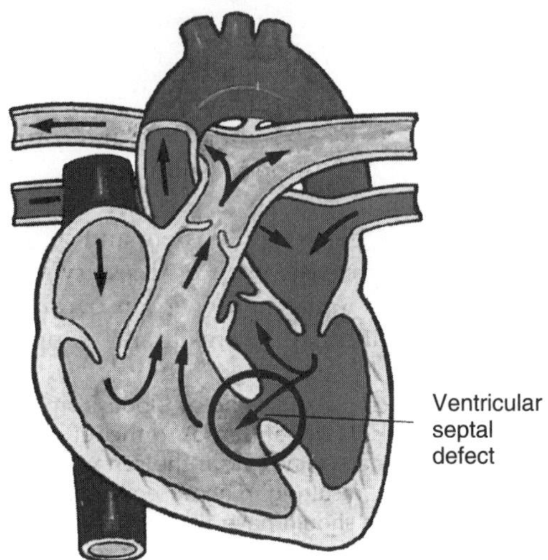

Surgical treatment:

Palliative: Pulmonary banding in symptomatic infants who cannot be well managed with diuretics and digoxin. Although palliation using a pulmonary artery band is used in some institutions, data suggest that complete primary repair can be performed without an increased risk during the first year of life. Age alone has little influence on the outcome of the repair, although younger infants are frequently sicker in the postoperative period.

Complete repair: Small defects are repaired with a purse-string approach. Large defects usually require a knitted Dacron patch sewn over the opening. Both procedures are performed via cardiopulmonary bypass. The repair is generally approached through the right atrium and the tricuspid valve. Postoperative complications include residual VSD and conduction disturbances.

Nonsurgical treatment: Device closure during cardiac catheterization is under clinical trials in some centers for closure of muscular defects that carry a high operative risk.

Prognosis: Risks depend on the location of the defect, number of defects, and other associated cardiac defects. Single membranous defects have a low mortality (less than 5%); multiple muscular defects can have a risk of more than 20%.

Defects with Increased Pulmonary Blood Flow—cont'd

Atrioventricular Canal (AVC) Defect

Description: Incomplete fusion of endocardial cushions. Consists of a low atrial septal defect that is continuous with a high ventricular septal defect and clefts of the mitral and tricuspid valves, creating a large central atrioventricular valve that allows blood to flow between all four chambers of the heart. The directions and pathways of flow are determined by pulmonary and systemic resistance, left and right ventricular pressures, and the compliance of each chamber, although flow is generally from left to right. It is the most common cardiac defect in children with Down syndrome.

Pathophysiology: The alterations in the hemodynamics depend on the defect's severity and the child's pulmonary vascular resistance. Immediately after birth, while the newborn's pulmonary vascular resistance is high, there is minimum shunting of blood through the defect. Once this resistance falls, left-to-right shunting occurs and pulmonary blood flow increases. The resultant pulmonary vascular engorgement predisposes to development of CHF.

Clinical manifestations: Patients usually have moderate to severe congestive heart failure. There is a characteristic murmur. There may be mild cyanosis that increases with crying. Patients are at high risk for developing pulmonary vascular obstructive disease.

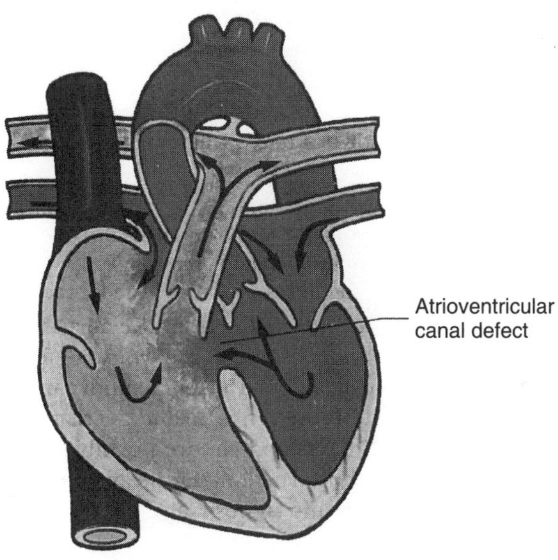

Continued.

Defects with Increased Pulmonary Blood Flow—cont'd

Surgical treatment:

Palliative: Pulmonary artery banding for infants with severe symptoms that are caused by increased pulmonary blood flow in some centers. Other centers believe complete repair can be performed in infants.

Complete repair: Surgical repair consists of patch closure of the septal defects and reconstruction of the AV valve tissue (either repair of the mitral valve cleft or fashioning two AV valves). If the mitral valve defect is severe, a valve replacement may be needed. Postoperative complications include heart block, CHF, mitral regurgitation, dysrhythmias, and pulmonary hypertension.

Prognosis: Operative mortality is about 10%. Potential later problem is mitral regurgitation, which may require valve replacement.

Patent Ductus Arteriosus (PDA)

Description: Failure of the fetal ductus arteriosus (artery connecting the aorta and pulmonary artery) to close within the first weeks of life. The continued patency of this vessel allows blood to flow from the higher-pressure aorta to the lower-pressure pulmonary artery, causing a left-to-right shunt.

Pathophysiology: The hemodynamic consequences of PDA depend on the size of the ductus and the pulmonary vascular resistance. At birth the resistance in the pulmonary and systemic circulations is almost identical, thus, equalizing the resistance in the aorta and pulmonary artery. As the systemic pressure exceeds the pulmonary pressure, blood begins to shunt from the aorta, across the duct, to the pulmonary artery (left-to-right shunt).

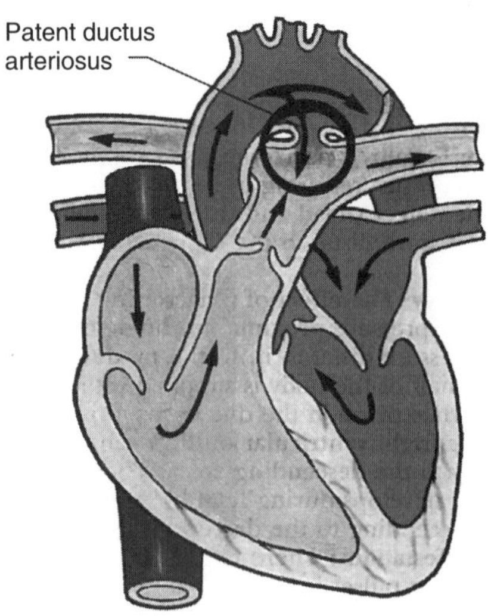

Defects with Increased Pulmonary Blood Flow—cont'd

The additional blood is recirculated through the lungs and returned to the left atrium and left ventricle. The effect of this altered circulation is increased workload on the left side of the heart, increased pulmonary vascular congestion and possibly resistance, and potentially increased right ventricular pressure and hypertrophy.

Clinical manifestations: Patients may be asymptomatic or show signs of congestive heart failure. There is a characteristic machinerylike murmur. A widened pulse pressure and bounding pulses result from runoff of blood from the aorta to the pulmonary artery. Patients are at risk for bacterial endocarditis and pulmonary vascular obstructive disease in later life from chronic excessive pulmonary blood flow.

Medical management: Administration of indomethacin (prostaglandin inhibitor) has proved successful in closing a patent ductus in premature infants and some newborns.

Surgical treatment: Surgical division or ligation of the patent vessel via a left thoracotomy. A newer technique, visual assisted thoracoscopic surgery (VATS), uses a thoracoscope and instruments placed through three small incisions on the left side of the chest to place a clip on the ductus. It is used in some centers and eliminates the need for a thoracotomy, thereby speeding postoperative recovery.

Nonsurgical treatment: Closure with placement of an occluder device during cardiac catheterization is done in some institutions.

Prognosis: Both procedures can be done at low operative risk with less than 1% mortality.

From Wong DL: Whaley and Wong's nursing care of infants and children, ed 5, St Louis, 1995, Mosby.

Obstructive Defects

Coarctation of the Aorta (COA)

Description: Localized narrowing near the insertion of the ductus arteriosus, resulting in increased pressure proximal to the defect (head and upper extremities) and decreased pressure distal to the obstruction (body and lower extremities).

Pathophysiology: The effect of a narrowing within the aorta is increased pressure proximal to the defect and decreased pressure distal to it. In the preductal type of COA the lower half of the body is supplied with blood by the right ventricle through the ductus arteriosus. In the postductal type, right ventricular outflow cannot maintain blood flow to the descending aorta. Therefore, collateral

Continued.

Obstructive Defects—cont'd

circulation develops during fetal life to maintain flow from the ascending to the descending aorta.

Clinical manifestations: There may be high blood pressure and bounding pulses in arms, weak or absent femoral pulses, and cool lower extremities with lower blood pressure. There are signs of congestive heart failure in infants. Often these patients' hemodynamic condition deteriorates rapidly, and they are admitted to the intensive care unit near death, usually severely acidotic and hypotensive. Mechanical ventilation and inotropic support are often necessary before surgery. Older children may experience dizziness, headaches, fainting, and epistaxis resulting form hypertension. Patients are at risk for hypertension, ruptured aorta, aortic aneurysm, or stroke.

Surgical treatment: Either resection of the coarcted portion with an end-to-end anastomosis of the aorta or enlargement of the constricted section using a graft of prosthetic material or a portion of the left subclavian artery. Because this defect is outside the heart and pericardium, cardiopulmonary bypass is not required and a thoracotomy incision is used. Postoperative hypertension (greater than 160 mm Hg) is treated with intravenous sodium nitroprusside or amrinone, followed by oral medications, such as captopril, hydralazine, and/or propranolol. Residual permanent hypertension after repair of COA seems to be related to age and time of repair. To prevent both hypertension at rest and exercise-provoked systemic hypertension after repair, elective surgery for COA is advised within the first 2 years of life. There is a 5% to 10% risk of recurrent narrowing in patients who underwent surgical repair as infants. Percutaneous balloon angioplasty techniques have proved very effective in relieving residual postoperative coarctation gradients.

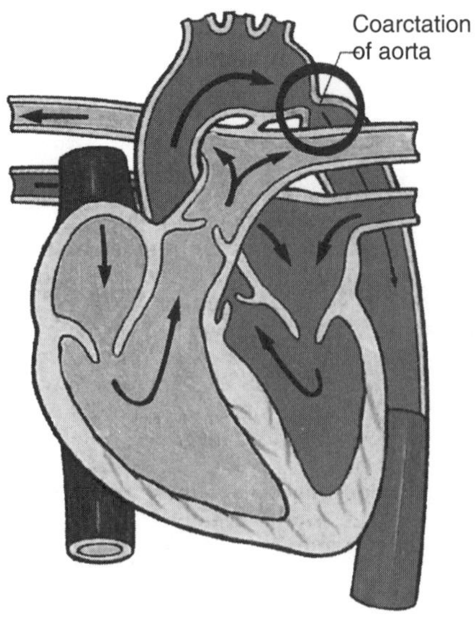

Obstructive Defects—cont'd

Nonsurgical treatment: Balloon angioplasty as a primary intervention for COA is being performed in some centers, but concerns about inadequate relief of gradients, risk of aneurysm formation, and restenosis have limited its widespread use. More clinical experience and longer follow-up are needed.

Prognosis: Less than 5% mortality in patients with isolated coarctation; increased risk in infants with other complex cardiac defects.

Aortic Stenosis (AS)

Description: Narrowing or stricture of the aortic valve, causing resistance to blood flow in the left ventricle, decreased cardiac output, left ventricular hypertrophy, and pulmonary vascular congestion. The prominent anatomic consequence of AS is the hypertrophy of the left ventricular wall, which eventually will lead to increased end-diastolic pressure, resulting in pulmonary venous and pulmonary arterial hypertension. Left ventricular hypertrophy also interferes with coronary artery perfusion and may result in myocardial infarction or scarring of the papillary muscles of the left ventricle, causing mitral insufficiency. ***Valvular stenosis***, the most common type, is usually caused by malformed cusps resulting in a bicuspid rather than tricuspid valve or fusion of the cusps. ***Subvalvular stenosis*** is a stricture caused by a fibrous ring below a normal valve; ***supravalvular stenosis*** occurs infrequently. Valvular AS is a serious defect for the following reasons: (1) the obstruction tends to be progressive; (2) sudden episodes of myocardial ischemia, or low cardiac output, can result in sudden death; and (3) surgical repair rarely results in a normal valve. This is one of the rare instances in which strenuous physical activity may be curtailed because of the cardiac condition.

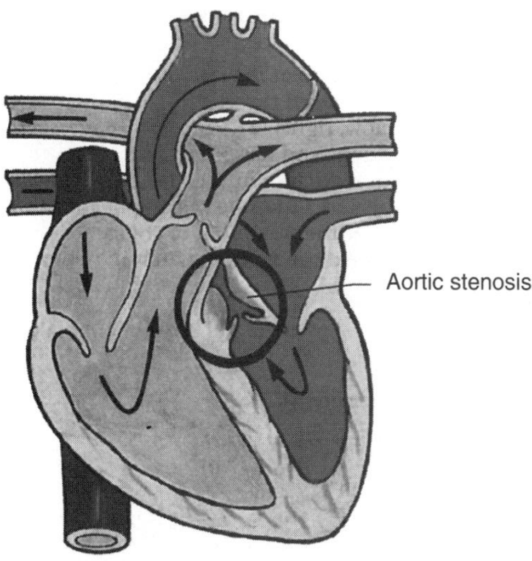

Continued.

Obstructive Defects—cont'd

Pathophysiology: A stricture in the aortic outflow tract causes resistance to ejection of blood from the left ventricle. The extra workload on the left ventricle causes hypertrophy. If left ventricular failure develops, left atrial pressure will increase; this causes increased pressure in the pulmonary veins, resulting in pulmonary vascular congestion (pulmonary edema).

Clinical manifestations: Infants with severe defects demonstrate signs of decreased cardiac output with faint pulses, hypotension, tachycardia, and poor feeding. Children show signs of exercise intolerance, chest pain, and dizziness when standing for long periods. There is a characteristic murmur. Patients are at risk for bacterial endocarditis, coronary insufficiency, and ventricular dysfunction.

Valvular Aortic Stenosis

Surgical treatment: Aortic valvotomy under inflow occlusion.

Prognosis: Aortic valvotomy in critically ill neonates and infants still carries a mortality of 10% to 20% in major medical centers. Results of aortic valvotomy in older children are very good, with mortality close to 0%. However, aortic valvotomy remains a palliative procedure, and approximately 25% of patients require additional surgery within 10 years for recurrent stenosis. A valve replacement may be required at the second procedure.

Nonsurgical treatment: Dilating narrowed valve with balloon angioplasty in the catheterization laboratory.

Prognosis: The incidence of side effects and complications, including aortic insufficiency or valvular regurgitation, tearing of the valve leaflets, loss of pulse in the catheterized limb, or serious dysrhythmias, is about 40%. In critically ill neonates the mortality rate is similar to that of surgery, approximately 15% to 30%.

Subvalvular Aortic Stenosis

Surgical treatment: May involve incising a membrane, if one exists, or cutting the fibromuscular ring. If the obstruction results from narrowing of the left ventricular outflow tract and a small aortic valve annulus, a patch may be required to enlarge the entire left ventricular outflow tract and annulus and replace the aortic valve, an approach known as the ***Konno*** procedure. An aortic homograft with a valve may also be used (***extended aortic root replacement***), or the pulmonary valve may be moved to the aortic position and replaced with a homograft valve (***Ross*** procedure).

Prognosis: Mortality from surgical repairs of subvalvular AS is less than 2% in major centers; however, about 10% of these patients develop recurrent

Obstructive Defects—cont'd

subaortic stenosis and require additional surgery. All operations to replace the aortic root and enlarge the left ventricular outflow tract require further evaluation.

Pulmonic Stenosis (PS)

Description: Narrowing at the entrance to the pulmonary artery. Resistance to blood flow causes right ventricular hypertrophy and decreased pulmonary blood flow. ***Pulmonary atresia*** is the extreme form of PS in that there is total fusion of the commissures and no blood flows to the lungs. The right ventricle may be hypoplastic.

Pathophysiology: When PS is present, resistance to blood flow causes right ventricular hypertrophy. If right ventricular failure develops, right atrial pressure will increase and this may result in reopening of the foramen ovale, shunting of unoxygenated blood into the left atrium, and systemic cyanosis. If PS is severe, CHF occurs, and systemic venous engorgement will be noted. An associated defect such as a PDA partially compensates for the obstruction by shunting blood from the aorta to the pulmonary artery and into the lungs.

Clinical manifestations: Patients may be asymptomatic; some have mild cyanosis or congestive heart failure. Newborns with severe narrowing will be cyanotic. There is a characteristic murmur. Cardiomegaly is evident on chest x-ray film. Patients are at risk for bacterial endocarditis, with progressive narrowing causing increased symptoms.

Surgical treatment: In infants, transventricular (closed) valvotomy (***Brock***) procedure. In children, pulmonary valvotomy with cardiopulmonary bypass.

Nonsurgical treatment: Balloon angioplasty in the cardiac catheterization laboratory to dilate valve. A catheter is inserted across the stenotic pulmonic valve into the pulmonary artery, and a balloon at the end of the catheter is inflated and rapidly passed through the narrowed opening (see bottom figure on p. 18). The procedure is associated with few complications and has proved highly effective, with a 50% to 75% reduction in pressure gradient across the pulmonic valve and a low rate of complications. It is the treatment of choice for discrete PS in most centers and can be done safely in neonates.

Prognosis: Low risk for both procedures; less than 2% mortality. Both balloon dilation and surgical valvotomy leave the pulmonic valve incompetent because they involve opening the fused valve leaflets; however, these patients are clinically asymptomatic. Long-term problems with restenosis or valve incompetence may occur.

Continued.

Obstructive Defects—cont'd

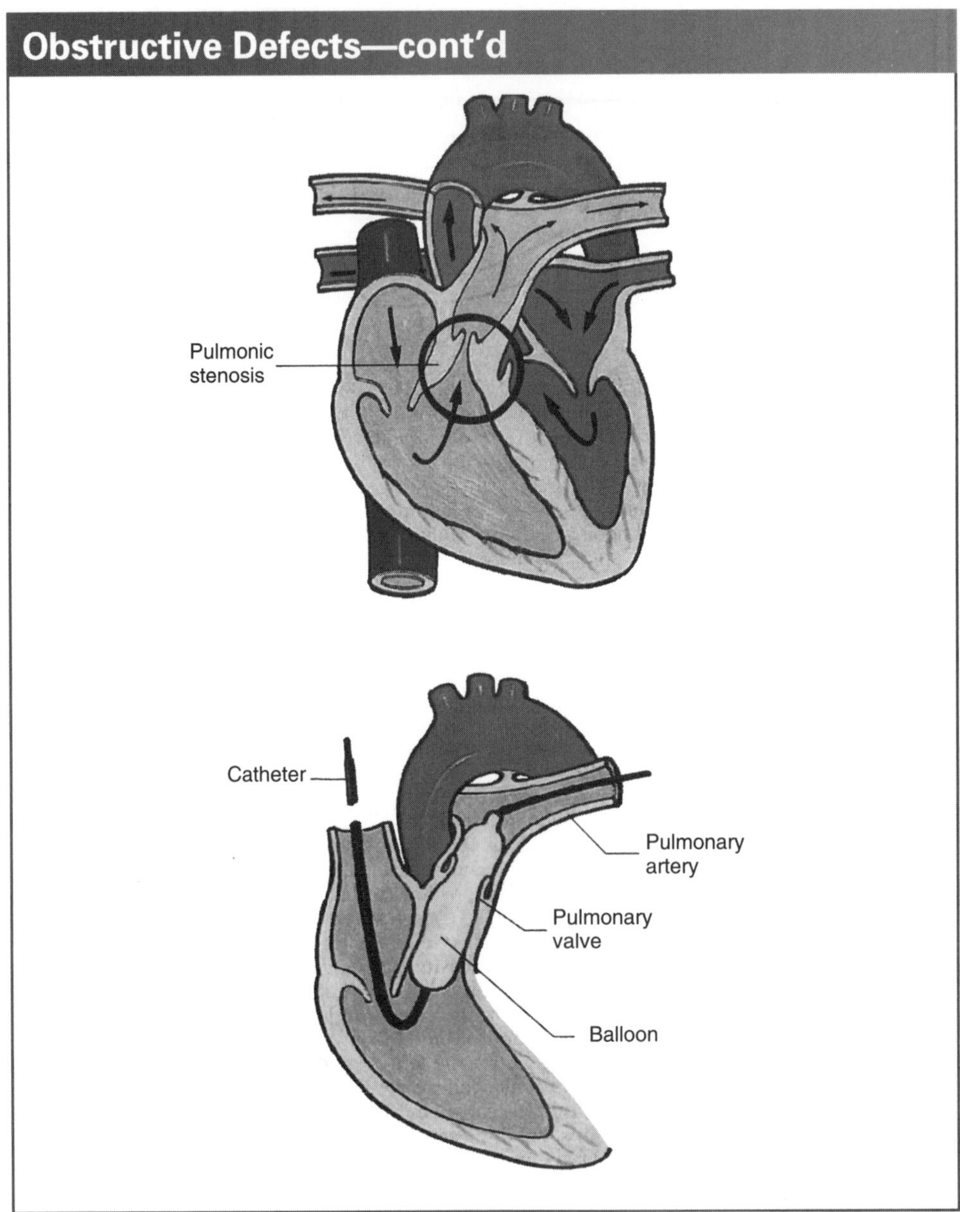

From Wong DL: Whaley and Wong's nursing care of infants and children, ed 5, St Louis, 1995, Mosby.

Defects with Decreased Pulmonary Blood Flow

Tetralogy of Fallot (TOF)

Description: The classic form includes four defects: (1) ventricular septal defect, (2) pulmonic stenosis, (3) over-riding aorta, and (4) right ventricular hypertrophy.

Pathophysiology: The altered hemodynamics vary widely, depending primarily on the degree of pulmonary stenosis, but also on the size of the VSD and the pulmonary and systemic resistance to flow. Because the VSD is usually large, pressures may be equal in the right and left ventricles. Therefore, the shunt direction depends on the difference between pulmonary and systemic vascular resistance. If pulmonary vascular resistance is higher than systemic resistance, the shunt is from right to left. If systemic resistance is higher than pulmonary resistance, the shunt is from left to right. Pulmonic stenosis decreases blood flow to the lungs and, consequently, the amount of oxygenated blood that returns to the left heart. Depending on the position of the aorta, blood from both ventricles may be distributed systemically.

Clinical manifestations:

Infants: Some infants may be acutely cyanotic at birth; others have mild cyanosis that progresses over the first year of life as the pulmonic stenosis worsens. There is a characteristic murmur. There are acute episodes of cyanosis and hypoxia, called blue spells or tet spells. Anoxic spells occur when the infant's oxygen requirements exceed the blood supply, usually during crying or after feeding.

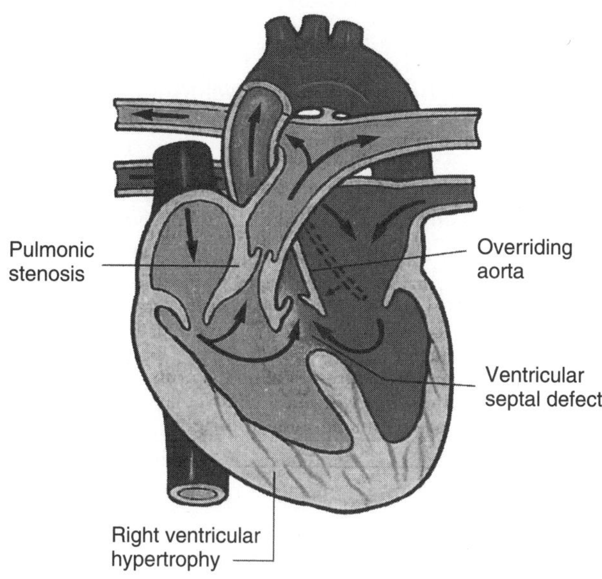

Continued.

Defects with Decreased Pulmonary Blood Flow—cont'd

Children: With increasing cyanosis, there may be clubbing of the fingers, squatting, and poor growth.

Patients are at risk for emboli, cerebrovascular disease, brain abscess, seizures, and loss of consciousness or sudden death following an anoxic spell.

Surgical treatment:

Palliative shunt: In infants who cannot undergo primary repair, a palliative procedure to increase pulmonary blood flow and increase oxygen saturation may be performed. The preferred procedure is the ***Blalock-Taussig*** or ***modified Blalock-Taussig shunt***, which provides blood flow to the pulmonary arteries from the left or right subclavian artery. In general, however, shunts are avoided because they may result in pulmonary artery distortion.

Complete repair: Elective repair is usually performed in the first year of life. Indications for repair include increasing cyanosis and the development of hypercyanotic spells. Complete repair involves closure of the VSD and resection of the infundibular stenosis, with a pericardial patch to enlarge the right ventricular outflow tract. The procedure requires a median sternotomy and the use of cardiopulmonary bypass.

Prognosis: The operative mortality for total correction of TOF is less than 5%. With improved surgical techniques there is a lower incidence of dysrhythmias and sudden death; surgical heart block is rare. CHF may occur postoperatively.

Tricuspid Atresia

Description: Failure of the tricuspid valve to develop, consequently no communication from right atrium to right ventricle. Blood flows through an atrial septal defect or a patent foramen ovale to the left side of the heart and through a ventricular septal defect to the right ventricle and out to the lungs. It is often associated with pulmonic stenosis and transposition of the great arteries. There is complete mixing of unoxygenated and oxygenated blood in the left side of the heart, resulting in systemic desaturation and varying amounts of pulmonary obstruction, causing decreased pulmonary blood flow.

Pathophysiology: At birth the presence of a patent foramen ovale (or other atrial septal opening) is required to permit blood flow across the septum into the left atrium; the PDA allows blood flow to the pulmonary artery into the lungs for oxygenation. A VSD allows a modest amount of blood to enter the right ventricle and pulmonary artery for oxygenation. Pulmonary blood flow usually is diminished.

Clinical manifestations: Cyanosis is usually seen in the newborn period. There may be tachycardia and dyspnea. Older children have signs of chronic

Defects with Decreased Pulmonary Blood Flow—cont'd

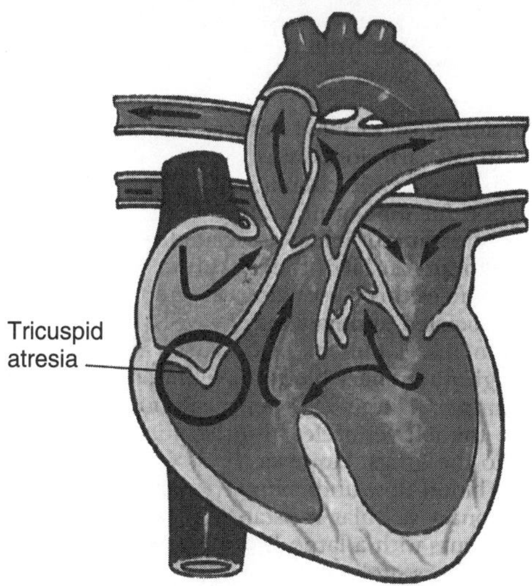

hypoxemia with clubbing. Patients are at risk for bacterial endocarditis, brain abscess, and stroke.

Therapeutic management: For the neonate whose pulmonary blood flow depends on the patency of the ductus arteriosus, a continuous infusion of prostaglandin E_1 is started at 0.1 mg/kg of body weight/min until surgical intervention can be arranged.

Surgical treatment: *Palliative* treatment is the placement of a shunt (***pulmonary-to-systemic artery anastomosis***) to increase blood flow to the lungs. If the ASD is small, an atrial septostomy is done during cardiac catheterization. Some children have increased pulmonary blood flow and require ***pulmonary artery banding*** to lessen the volume of blood to the lungs. A ***bidirectional Glenn shunt*** (cardiopulmonary anastomosis) may be performed at 6 to 9 months as a second stage.

Modified Fontan procedure—Systemic venous return is directed to the lungs without a ventricular pump through surgical connections between the right atrium and the pulmonary artery. A fenestration (opening) in the right atrial baffle is sometimes done to relieve pressure. Patient must have normal ventricular function and a low pulmonary vascular resistance for the procedure to be successful. The modified Fontan procedure separates oxygenated and unoxygenated blood inside the heart and eliminates the excess volume load on the ventricle, but does not restore normal anatomy or hemodynamics.

Continued.

Defects with Decreased Pulmonary Blood Flow—cont'd

Prognosis: Surgical mortality is greater than 10%. Postoperative complications include dysrhythmias, systemic venous hypertension, pleural and pericardial effusion, elevated pulmonary vascular resistance, and ventricular dysfunction. While initial results have been encouraging, long-term survival and morbidity must await future studies.

From Wong DL: Whaley and Wong's nursing care of infants and children, ed 5, St Louis, 1995, Mosby.

Mixed Defects

Transposition of the Great Arteries (TGA) or Transposition of the Great Vessels (TGV)

Description: The pulmonary artery leaves the left ventricle, and the aorta exits from the right ventricle, with no communication between the systemic and pulmonary circulations.

Pathophysiology: Associated defects such as septal defects or patent ductus arteriosus must be present to permit blood to enter the systemic circulation and/or the pulmonary circulation for mixing of saturated and desaturated blood. The most common defect associated with TGA is a patent foramen ovale. At birth there is also a PDA, although in most instances this closes after the neonatal period. Another associated anomaly may be VSD. Presence of these defects increases the risk of CHF, since they often produce high pulmonary blood flow under high pressure. For example, a large VSD permits blood to flow from the right to the left ventricle, into the pulmonary artery, and finally to the lungs. However, it also produces high pulmonary blood flow under high pressure, which can result in pulmonary vascular resistance. The same series of events occurs with a large PDA, since blood directly from the aorta flows under high pressure into the pulmonary artery and lungs.

Clinical manifestations: Depend on the type and size of the associated defects. Children with minimum communication are severely cyanotic and depressed at birth. Those with large septal defects or a patent ductus arteriosus may be less severely cyanotic but may have symptoms of congestive heart failure. Heart sounds vary according to the type of defect present. Cardiomegaly is usually evident a few weeks after birth.

Therapeutic management:

To provide intracardiac mixing: The administration of intravenous prostaglandin E_1 may be initiated to temporarily increase blood mixing if

Mixed Defects—cont'd

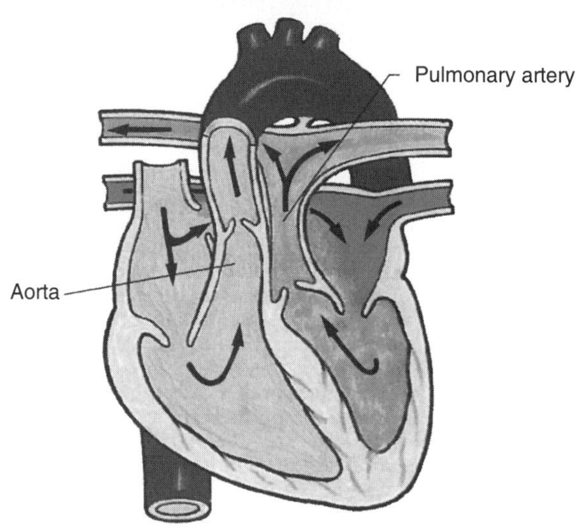

systemic and pulmonary mixing is inadequate to provide an oxygen saturation of 75% or to maintain cardiac output. During cardiac catheterization a balloon atrial septostomy (***Rashkind procedure***) may also be performed to increase mixing and maintain cardiac output over a longer period.

Surgical treatment:

Arterial switch procedure: Procedure of choice performed in first weeks of life. Involves transecting the great arteries and anastomosing the main pulmonary artery to the proximal aorta (just above the aortic valve) and anastomosing the ascending aorta to the proximal pulmonary artery. The coronary arteries are switched from the proximal aorta to the proximal pulmonary artery, creating a new aorta. Reimplantation of the coronary arteries is critical to the infant's survival, and they must be reattached without torsion or kinking to provide the heart with its supply of oxygen. The advantage of the arterial switch procedure is the reestablishment of normal circulation, with the left ventricle acting as the systemic pump. Potential complications of the arterial switch include narrowing at the great artery anastomoses or coronary artery insufficiency.

Creation of an intraatrial baffle to divert venous blood to the mitral valve and pulmonary venous blood to the tricuspid valve using the patient's atrial septum (***Senning procedure***) or a prosthetic material (***Mustard procedure***). Performed in first year of life. A disadvantage is the continuing role of the right ventricle as the systemic pump and the late development of right ventricular failure and rhythm disturbances. Other potential postoperative

Continued.

Mixed Defects—cont'd

complications include loss of normal sinus rhythm, baffle leaks, and ventricular dysfunction.

Rastelli procedure: Operative choice in infants with TGA, VSD, and severe PS. It involves closure of the VSD with a baffle, directing left ventricular blood through the VSD into the aorta. The pulmonic valve is then closed, and a conduit is placed from the right ventricle to the pulmonary artery, creating a physiologically normal circulation. Unfortunately, this procedure requires multiple conduit replacements as the child grows.

Prognosis: Operative mortality is about 5% to 10% with all procedures; with atrial level repairs there is a later risk of dysrhythmias and ventricular dysfunction.

Total Anomalous Pulmonary Venous Connection (TAPVC)

Description: Rare defect characterized by failure of the pulmonary veins to join the left atrium. Instead, the pulmonary veins are abnormally connected to the systemic venous circuit via the right atrium or various veins draining toward the right atrium, such as the superior vena cava. The abnormal attachment results in mixed blood being returned to the right atrium and shunted from the right to the left through an ASD. The type of TAPVC is classified according to the pulmonary venous point of attachment as:

Suspracardiac—Attachment above the diaphragm, such as to the superior vena cava (most common form)

Cardiac—Direct attachment to the heart, such as to the right atrium or coronary sinus

Infracardiac—Attachment below the diaphragm, such as to the inferior vena cava (most severe form)

TAPVC is also called total anomalous pulmonary venous return (TAPVR) or total anomalous pulmonary venous drainage (TAPVD).

Pathophysiology: The right atrium receives all the blood that normally would flow into the left atrium. As a result, the right side of the heart hypertrophies, whereas the left side, especially the left atrium, may remain small. An associated ASD or patent foramen ovale allows systemic venous blood to shunt from the higher-pressure right atrium to the left atrium and into the left side of the heart. As a result, the oxygen saturation of the blood in both sides of the heart (and ultimately, in the systemic arterial circulation) is the same. If the pulmonary blood flow is large, pulmonary venous return is also large and the amount of saturated blood is relatively high. However, if there is obstruction to pulmonary venous drainage, pulmonary venous return is

Mixed Defects—cont'd

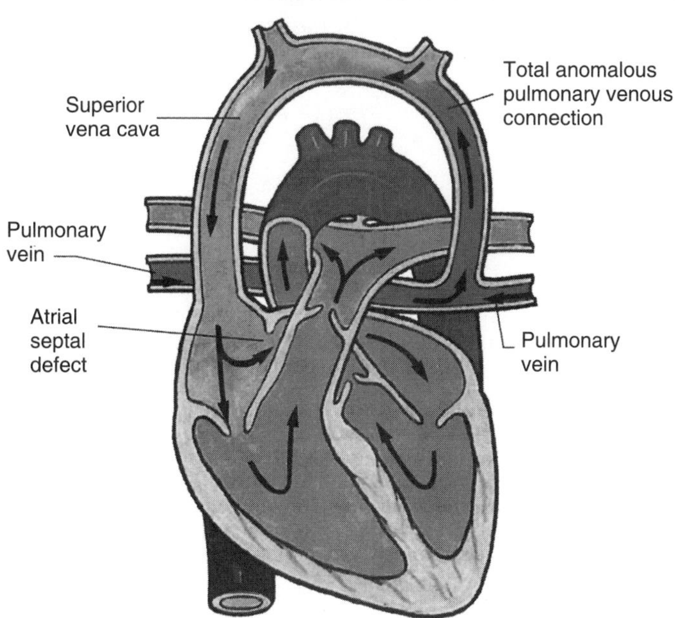

impeded, pulmonary venous pressure rises, and pulmonary interstitial edema develops and eventually contributes to CHF. Infracardiac TAPVC is often associated with obstruction to pulmonary venous drainage and is a surgical emergency.

Clinical manifestations: Most infants develop cyanosis early in life. The degree of cyanosis is inversely related to the amount of pulmonary blood flow—the more pulmonary blood, the less cyanosis. Children with unobstructed TAPVC may be asymptomatic until pulmonary vascular resistance decreases during infancy, increasing pulmonary blood flow, with resulting signs of CHF. Cyanosis becomes worse with pulmonary vein obstruction; once obstruction occurs, the infant's condition usually deteriorates rapidly. Without intervention, cardiac failure will progress to death.

Surgical treatment: Corrective repair in early infancy. The surgical approach varies with the anatomic defect. In general, however, the common pulmonary vein is anastomosed to the left atrium, the ASD is closed, and the anomalous pulmonary venous connection is ligated. The cardiac type is most easily repaired; the infracardiac type has the highest morbidity and mortality because of the higher incidence of pulmonary vein obstruction. Potential postoperative complications include reobstruction; bleeding; dysrhythmias, particularly heart block; pulmonary artery hypertension; and persistent heart failure.

Continued.

Mixed Defects—cont'd

Prognosis: The cardiac type has a surgical mortality of less than 5%; the incidence of morbidity is greater with the other types and increases with the presence of pulmonary vein obstruction.

Truncus Arteriosus (TA)

Description: Failure of normal septation and division of the embryonic bulbar trunk into the pulmonary artery and the aorta, resulting in a single vessel that overrides both ventricles. Blood from both ventricles mixes in the common great artery, causing desaturation and hypoxemia. Blood ejected from the heart flows preferentially to the lower-pressure pulmonary arteries, causing increased pulmonary blood flow and reduced systemic blood flow. There are three types:

Type I—A single pulmonary trunk arises near the base of the truncus and divides into the left and right pulmonary arteries.

Type II—The left and right pulmonary arteries arise separately from the posterior aspect of the truncus.

Type III—The pulmonary arteries arise independently from the lateral aspect of the truncus.

Pathophysiology: Blood ejected from the left and right ventricles enters the common trunk, mixing pulmonary and systemic circulations. Blood flow is distributed to the pulmonary and systemic circulations according to the relative resistances of each system. The amount of pulmonary blood flow depends on the size of the pulmonary arteries and the pulmonary vascular resistance.

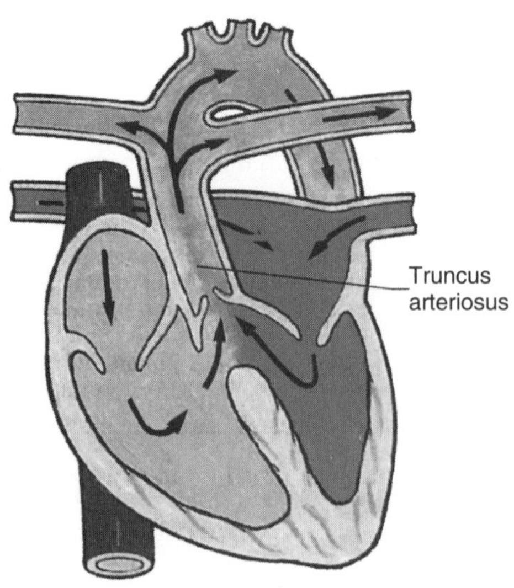

Mixed Defects—cont'd

Generally, resistance to pulmonary blood flow is less than systemic vascular resistance, resulting in preferential blood flow to the lungs. Pulmonary vascular disease develops at an early age in patients with truncus arteriosus.

Clinical manifestations: Most infants are symptomatic with moderate to severe congestive heart failure and variable cyanosis, poor growth, and activity intolerance. There is a characteristic murmur. Patients are at risk for brain abscess and bacterial endocarditis.

Surgical treatment: Early repair in the first few months of life. Corrective repair is a modified Rastelli procedure. It involves closing the VSD so that the truncus arteriosus receives the outflow from the left ventricle, excising the pulmonary arteries from the aorta, and attaching them to the right ventricle by means of a homograft. Currently, homografts (segments of cadaver aorta and pulmonary artery that are treated with antibiotics and cryopreserved) are preferred over synthetic conduits to establish continuity between the right ventricle and pulmonary artery. Homografts are more flexible and easier to use during the procedure and appear less prone to obstruction. Postoperative complications include persistent heart failure, bleeding, pulmonary artery hypertension, dysrhythmias, and residual VSD. These children require additional procedures to replace the conduit as its size becomes inadequate in relation to their growth.

Prognosis: Mortality is greater than 10%; future operations are required to replace the conduits.

Hypoplastic Left Heart Syndrome (HLHS)

Description: Underdevelopment of the left side of the heart, resulting in a hypoplastic left ventricle and aortic atresia. Most blood from the left atrium flows across the patent foramen ovale to the right atrium, to the right ventricle, and out the pulmonary artery. The descending aorta receives blood from the patent ductus arteriosus supplying systemic blood flow.

Pathophysiology: An ASD or patent foramen ovale allows saturated blood from the left atrium to mix with desaturated blood from the right atrium and to flow through the right ventricle and out into the pulmonary artery. From the pulmonary artery the blood flows to the lungs, then through the ductus arteriosus into the aorta and out to the body. The amount of blood flow to the pulmonary and systemic circulations depends on the relationship between the pulmonary and systemic vascular resistances. The coronary and cerebral vessels receive blood by retrograde flow through the hypoplastic ascending aorta.

Clinical manifestations: There is mild cyanosis and signs of congestive failure until the patent ductus arteriosus closes, then progressive deterioration with

Continued.

Mixed Defects—cont'd

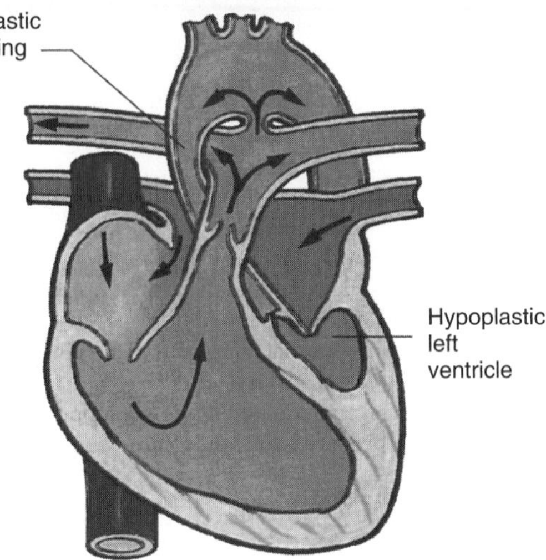

cyanosis and decreased cardiac output, leading to cardiovascular collapse. It is usually fatal in the first months of life without intervention.

Therapeutic management: Neonates require stabilization with mechanical ventilation and inotropic support preoperatively. A prostaglandin E_1 infusion is needed to maintain ductal patency, ensuring adequate systemic blood flow.

Surgical treatment: Several-staged approach: First stage is ***Norwood procedure***—anastomosis of the main pulmonary artery to the aorta to create a new aorta, shunting to provide pulmonary blood flow, and creation of a large atrial septal defect. Postoperative complications include imbalance of systemic and pulmonary blood flow, bleeding, low cardiac output, and persistent heart failure. Second stage is often a ***bidirectional Glenn shunt*** done at 6 to 9 months of age to relieve cyanosis and reduce the volume load on the right ventricle. The final repair is a ***modified Fontan procedure*** (see Tricuspid Atresia in box on p. 21).

Transplantation: Some programs believe that heart transplantation in the newborn period is the best option for these infants. Problems include the shortage of newborn organ donors, risk of rejection, long-term problems with chronic immunosuppression, and infection.

Prognosis: Mortality risks of more than 25% with both surgery and transplantion. Currently, only about half the patients survive to complete the last stage, the modified Fontan procedure. This may improve in the future. Because of the high-risk nature of both surgical palliation and neonatal heart transplantation, some cardiologists continue to recommend no treatment for this defect.

From Wong DL: Whaley and Wong's nursing care of infants and children, ed 5, St Louis, 1995, Mosby.

- Hallmark signs of serious congenital heart defects include respiratory distress, cyanosis, congestive heart failure, poor cardiac output, murmurs, failure to thrive, irregular cardiac rhythm, fatigue, lethargy, poor sucking or feeding, poor peripheral pulses, diaphoresis, and hepatomegaly.

- A left-to-right shunt occurs when oxygenated blood from the high-pressure left (systemic) side of the heart flows back to the right (pulmonary) side of the heart through a defect and not out to the body. Such defects are acyanotic because unoxygenated blood does not reach the body.

- A right-to-left shunt occurs when blood from the high-pressure right (pulmonary) side of the heart flows directly to the left side of the heart through a defect without ever passing through the lungs to be oxygenated. Such defects are cyanotic because unoxygenated blood *does* reach the body.

- Symptoms of left-to-right shunting from defects usually are not seen for 4 to 12 weeks after birth because such abnormal shunting prolongs the period of pulmonary hypertension, decreasing the amount of systemic-to-pulmonary shunting. For example, an infant with a large ventricular septal defect may not show symptoms of congestive heart failure, including any audible murmur, for 1 to 3 months.

- Most congenital heart defects (about 90%) result from multifactorial inheritance—a combination of genetic and environmental factors.

- Administering oxygen in a mild to moderate intracardiac shunt (using arterial O_2 saturations of 85% to 90%) usually is not helpful. However, administering oxygen in a severe shunt (using arterial O_2 saturations of 60% to 75%) may be helpful.

ACUTE CONGESTIVE HEART FAILURE (CHF)

- Acute congestive heart failure (CHF) may be related to high-output failure (such as left-to-right shunts in ventricular septal defects or patent ductus arteriosus) or low-output failure (such as in aortic stenosis, coarctation, or hypoplastic left heart syndrome).

- CHF is manifested by tachycardia, tachypnea, cardiomegaly, hepatomegaly, poor peripheral perfusion, edema, diaphoresis, poor activity tolerance, failure to thrive, and feeding problems. See Fig. 1-3 for a schemata of CHF.

- Hepatomegaly is an important, early, and sensitive sign of CHF in infants and children.

- CHF may result from hypervolemia, cardiomyopathy, arrhythmias, increased pulmonary blood flow, or obstruction to ventricular emptying (left-to-right shunts).

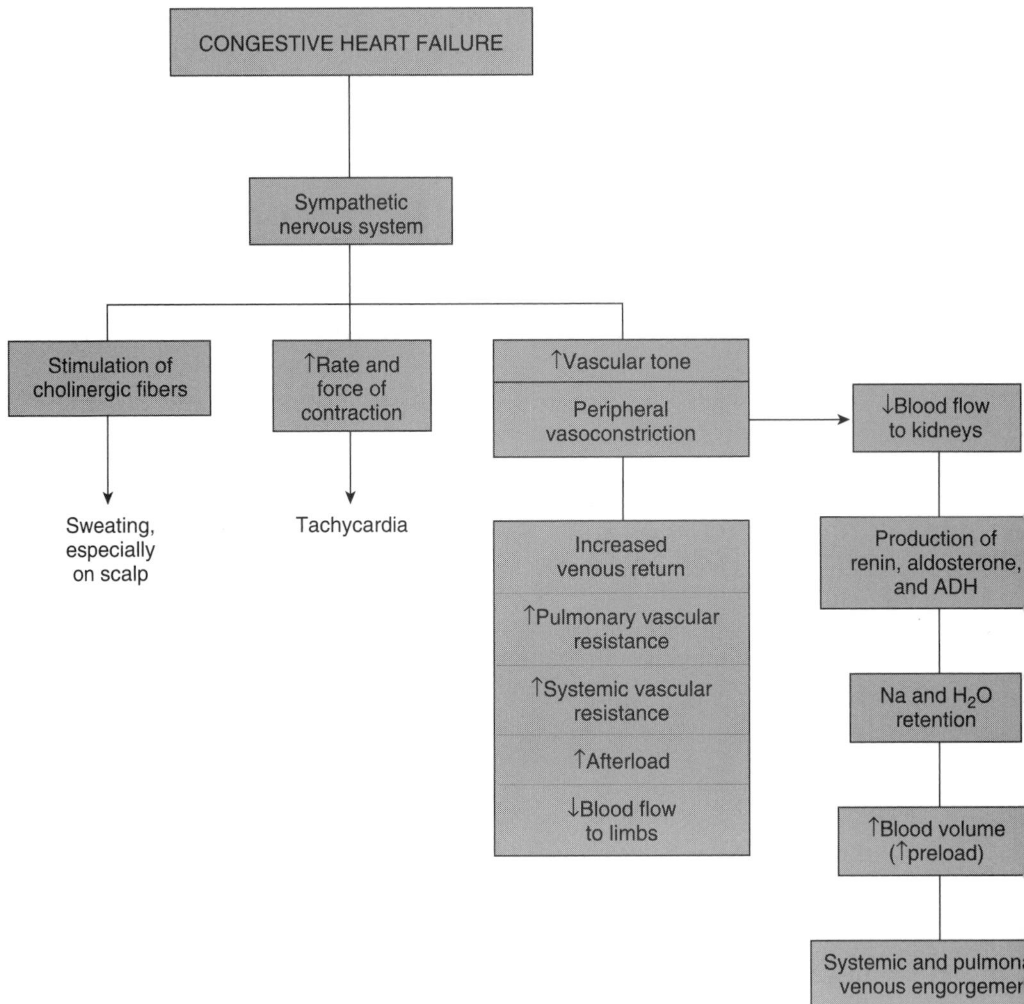

Fig. 1-3 Pathophysiology of congestive heart failure. (From Wong DL: Whaley and Wong's nursing care of infants and children, ed 5, St Louis, 1995, Mosby.)

- Management of CHF focuses on decreasing oxygen demands and increasing oxygen delivery.
- Pharmacologic management includes the use of digoxin and diuretics, such as furosemide (Lasix).
- For defects with increased pulmonary blood flow that cause intractable CHF, pulmonary artery banding may be required in very young, small, or high-risk infants before corrective cardiac surgery can be performed.

- An S_3 heart sound is audible before pulmonary rales develop as a result of congestive heart failure.

- For infants and young children with chronic CHF, weight gain is typically poor or absent.

CARDIOGENIC SHOCK

- Cardiogenic shock occurs when the cardiac output is impaired by myocardial dysfunction to the point that tissue oxygen needs are not adequately met.

- Cardiogenic shock may be primary from intrinsic cardiac disease, or secondary to such conditions as sepsis, acid-base imbalances, and electrolyte disturbances.

- Goals of treating shock are to decrease afterload, decrease oxygen demand, and increase oxygen delivery.

- Cardiogenic shock in infants and children is typically caused by cardiomyopathy, severe congestive heart failure, supraventricular tachycardia, congenital heart block, cardiac tamponade, or the effects of cardiac surgery. Myocardial infarcts are extremely rare in infants and children.

HYPOVOLEMIC SHOCK

- Hypovolemic shock, the most common form of shock in children, is often caused by blood loss, fluid and electrolyte loss, third-space fluid shifts, or redistribution of blood volume (as in vasodilation).

- Hemorrhagic hypovolemic shock produces severe symptoms with 20% to 25% blood loss.

- Dehydration will effect perfusion when only 5% to 7% of body weight is lost.

- Blood drawn for laboratory tests should always be counted as output on intake and output sheets.

- Hypotension is a *late* sign of shock in children. Tachycardia and signs of poor perfusion (pale, cool, mottled skin) are earlier and more reliable indicators than hypotension.

- Signs of hypovolemia include fluid loss in excess of intake, sunken fontanels (in infants), dry mucous membranes, poor skin turgor, rising blood urea nitrogen level, tachycardia, mottling, decreased renal perfusion, and high urine specific gravity.

- A normal hematocrit does not necessarily indicate adequate blood volume. It can take hours for a hematocrit to fall, consequently, blood loss may be significant.

FLUID RESUSCITATION

- Typically, a 4:1 ratio of crystalloids to colloids is recommended for fluid resuscitation in treating hypovolemic shock. Generally 10 to 20 cc/kg boluses are administered until a clinical response is achieved.
- Only about 25% of isotonic crystalloids administered remains in the vascular space. The other 75% moves into the intracellular and interstitial spaces.
- About 25% of colloids also remain in the vascular space; however, the colloids exert a greater oncotic (pulling) pressure, which draws other fluids into the vascular space.

PHARMACOLOGIC PRINCIPLES

Adenosine

- Adenosine is the first-line drug to treat supraventricular tachydysrhythmias. It works by slowing atrioventricular nodal conduction, and may actually interfere with abnormal accessory pathways.
- This drug has a very short half-life (10 seconds) so it must be administered by very rapid IV push.
- Side effects include bradycardia and hypotension.

Amrinone

- An inotropic and chronotropic agent as well as a vasodilator, amrinone is particularly useful in treating normotensive shock and congestive heart failure. The usual dosage is 3 to 5 mg/kg when given as a loading dose; 5 to 10 mcg/kg/min when given as a maintenance dose.
- Amrinone must be used cautiously with hypotension because it may further decrease blood pressure.
- Amrinone can cause thrombocytopenia. This effect can last for days after the drug is discontinued.

Atropine

- Atropine is used to treat bradycardias and works by increasing heart rate, sinus node automaticity, and atrioventricular conduction.

- The normal dose is 0.02 mg/kg IV push with a minimum dose of 0.1 mg and a maximum dose of 1.0 mg.
- Failure to administer the minimum dose of 0.1 mg may result in paradoxical bradycardia in infants.
- Atropine may be given intravenously or down an endotracheal tube.
- Give with caution to infants and children with either renal or liver disease.

Bretylium

- Bretylium is especially helpful in treating refractory ventricular fibrillation (VF) because it increases its threshold.
- Normal dosage is 5 mg/kg bolus given over 5 minutes. This dosage may be repeated every 6 hours.

Digoxin

- When using digoxin in very young children, it is more difficult to achieve therapeutic effects without toxicity. When effective, digoxin seems to help not by improving cardiac function, but rather by decreasing oxygen consumption.
- Oral digitalizing doses range from 25 to 50 mcg/kg/. Higher doses are administered to neonates and children under age 2 because they have more red blood cells available for binding sites.
- Cardioversion should not be performed on a patient with digoxin toxicity because ventricular tachycardia may lead to refractory ventricular fibrillation.
- Parents do not need to count a child's pulse rate before administering digoxin at home. Symptoms of digoxin toxicity (such as bradycardia) in a child are less related to heart rate and more to overall assessment.
- Therapeutic digoxin serum levels range from 1.1 to 2.2 ng/mL.
- Maintenance dose is usually 10 mcg/kg/day.
- Administer with caution to infants and children with renal impairment.

Dobutamine

- Dobutamine is not a drug of choice in treating hypotension associated with cardiogenic or septic shock because it may further lower systemic vascular resistance and blood pressure. Its best use may be with myocardial failure, cardiomyopathy, or shock—conditions not associated with hypotension.

- The dosage range for dobutamine is 1 to 20 mcg/kg/min.
- Dobutamine is an inotropic agent; tachydysrhythmias and hypotension are common side effects related to a decrease in systemic vascular resistance.

Dopamine

- Dopamine is an endogenous catecholamine and a precursor to norepinephrine.
- At low doses (1 to 2 mcg/kg/min), dopamine increases renal blood flow, urinary output, and perfusion of the heart, gut, and cerebrum.
- At moderate doses (2 to 10 mcg/kg/min), the same effects as low dose therapy are achieved in addition to an increase in rate, contractility, and conduction of the heart.
- At high doses (>8 to 20 mcg/kg/min), probably the only effects are vasoconstriction of both veins and arteries without beneficial effects on specific organ perfusion.
- Dopamine is not a drug of choice in hypotension associated with hypovolemia. It further increases systemic vascular resistance and afterload, thereby increasing the myocardial work load. The usual dosage range is 1 to 20 mcg/kg/min.
- Dopamine is not considered a drug of choice in treating hypovolemic shock because of its vasoconstrictive action. In hypovolemic shock, systemic vascular resistance and afterload are already increased; treatment focuses on increasing the intravascular volume. This is accomplished by raising the blood pressure and systemic perfusion by increasing intravascular volume and preload, not by increasing systemic vascular resistance with dopamine.

Epinephrine

- An endogenous catecholamine, epinephrine produces both alpha- and beta-adrenergic effects. In low doses (0.005 to 0.002 mcg/kg/min), beta effects such as tachycardia, increased conduction, and improved ventricular contraction occur. Alpha effects occur at doses greater than 0.3 mcg/kg/min resulting in vasoconstriction.
- Epinephrine is a drug of choice with shock, especially cardiogenic or septic shock where vasodilation and/or myocardial dysfunction are important factors.
- Epinephrine is also a drug of choice for both bradycardia and hypotension.
- Side effects of epinephrine include increased myocardial oxygen consumption, tachydysrhythmias, and decreased blood flow to the kidneys and gut.

Isoproterenol

- Isoproterenol (Isuprel) has pure beta-adrenergic effects and is therefore used to treat symptomatic bradycardia. Heart rate, ventricular contractility, and atrioventricular conduction are all enhanced by this drug.
- Negative side effects include profound tachycardia and a serious increase in myocardial oxygen demand.
- Isoproterenol is contraindicated for those with hypotension or tachycardia.
- The usual dosage range is 0.05 to 0.1 mcg/kg/min.

Lidocaine

- Lidocaine is a sodium channel blocker used to treat ventricular ectopy due to its specific effect on the ventricles.
- Normal dose is 1 mg/kg/dose with a maintenance infusion of 10 to 20 mcg/kg/min.
- Side effects include seizures and worsening of supraventricular tachycardia (SVT).
- Use with caution in infants and children with hepatic dysfunction.

Norepinephrine

- Norepinephrine is also an endogenous catecholamine used to treat only profound shock that has not responded to other treatments. Even at normal ranges of 0.05 to 1.0 mcg/kg/min, this drug produces renal vasoconstriction making it *not* a first-line drug in the treatment of shock in children.
- Negative side effects of norepinephrine include tachydysrhythmias, decreased circulation to the kidneys and gut, and increased myocardial oxygen consumption.

Prostaglandin E_1

- Prostaglandin E_1 is used to maintain patency in the ductus arteriosus for ductal-dependent lesions (such as pulmonary atresia, pulmonary stenosis, tricuspid atresia, tetralogy of Fallot, hypoplastic left-heart syndrome, transposition of the great arteries, coarctation of the aorta, and aortic atresia). The usual dosage range for this drug is 0.05 to 0.1 mcg/kg/min, but it may be given up to a maximum of 0.4 mcg/kg/min.
- Prostaglandin E_1 can cause apnea, fever, seizures, flushing, hypotension, and bradycardia.

Sodium Nitroprusside

- Sodium nitroprusside provides both arterial and venous vasodilation. It decreases afterload and systemic and pulmonary vascular resistance. The usual dosage range is 0.5 to 8 mcg/kg/min.

- Nitroprusside should be used cautiously in those with hypotension because it may exacerbate this condition.

- Nitroprusside has a short half-life and is metabolized into cyanide. Monitor for confusion, rash, decreased level of consciousness, seizures, and cardiac arrest. Monitor arterial blood gases every 4 hours for cyanide effects by noting an acidotic pH and decreased bicarbonate levels.

- Nitroprusside may cause thrombocytopenia.

SUPRAVENTRICULAR TACHYCARDIA (SVT)

- Supraventricular tachycardia (SVT) commonly manifests as congestive heart failure. The heart rate is usually regular; QRS complexes are narrow.

Usual heart rates in SVT:
Neonates 190 to 350 beats/min
Infants and children 150 to 250 beats/min

- Cardiac output is decreased in supraventricular tachycardia because of decreased filling time.

- Vagal maneuvers, such as applying ice to the face, bearing down, gagging, taking rectal temperatures, and coughing, may be effective in terminating SVT.

- Symptomatic SVT should be first treated with adenosine according to pediatric advanced life-support protocols. SVT may be also treated with verapamil or digoxin. Verapamil is not recommended for use in children under age 1 and needs to be used cautiously in those with congestive heart failure.

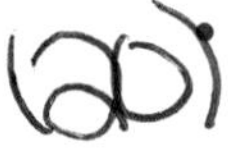

- Wolf-Parkinson-White syndrome must be ruled out before digoxin is used to treat SVT.

- Synchronized cardioversion at 1 to 2 joules/kg is indicated for SVT unresponsive to vagal maneuvers or pharmacologic therapy and in SVT with hemodynamic compromise.

- Overdrive pacing may also be used for supraventricular tachycardia.

HYPERCYANOTIC SPELLS (TET SPELLS)

- A hypercyanotic spell consists of severe right-to-left shunting, cyanosis, pulmonary hypertension, systemic hypotension, and acidosis which can progress to unconsciousness and even death.

- Hypercyanotic spells typically occur in the morning, with crying, and during feeding or defecation.

- Hypercyanotic spells begin with right-to-left shunting which is severe enough to cause acidosis and loss of left ventricular preload. Acidosis and hypoxemia probably contribute to a rise in pulmonary vascular resistance (relative pulmonary hypertension) and a decrease in systemic vascular resistance (relative systemic hypotension) which exacerbate the right-to-left shunting.

- Treatment is focused on raising systemic vascular resistance and lowering pulmonary vascular resistance. Morphine, oxygen, knee-chest positions, and even general anesthesia are common interventions.

PEDIATRIC-SPECIFIC PRINCIPLES

ACUTE INFLAMMATORY DISEASES

Myocarditis

- Myocarditis, inflammation of the myocardium, can occur from viral, bacterial, or other microbiological causes, as well as from systemic autoimmune disorders.

- Signs and symptoms of myocarditis are the same as those of congestive heart failure or shock. (See Table 1-2.)

- ST-segment changes may occur, indicating myocardial ischemia or necrosis.

- Treatment includes resolution of the infective agent and measures to control congestive heart failure and shock. Use of steroids is controversial.

Endocarditis

- Endocarditis may involve infection of the endocardium or heart valves. Bacteria, especially streptococci and staphylococci, are the most common causative agents. The mitral and tricuspid valves are commonly affected.

- Risk factors for endocarditis include congenital heart defects and valvular abnormalities.

- The congenital cardiac defects that are associated with the highest incidence of endocarditis include ventricular septal defect, aortic stenosis, tetralogy of Fallot, coarctation of the aorta, transposition of the aorta, and patent ductus arteriosus.

Table 1-2
Selected Cardiovascular Problems

This table reviews the major cardiovascular problems, assessment findings, and clinical manifestations associated with these defects, and common medical and surgical management.

Cardiovascular Problem	Assessment Findings	Usual Treatment
Dysrhythmias		
Bradydysrhythmias	Sinus bradycardia, first degree heart block, second degree heart block types I and II, and complete heart block. Poor peripheral pulses, altered mental status, loss of consciousness, hypotension, cold and clammy skin, decreased organ perfusion.	Support ventilation as needed and administer oxygen. Atropine, isoproterenol, pacemaker for refractory bradycardias and heart block.
Tachydysrhythmias	Supraventricular: Poor peripheral pulses, rapid and weak peripheral pulses, altered mental status, loss of consciousness, hypotension, cold and clammy skin, anxiety, decreased organ perfusion.	Supraventricular: Vagal maneuvers, adenosine, encainide, flecainide, propafenone, inderal, digoxin, verapamil (for those over 1 year of age). Synchronized cardioversion as needed for unstable rhythms.
	Ventricular: Weak or absent peripheral pulses, irregular pulse, cold and clammy skin, altered mental status, loss of consciousness, hypotension, anxiety.	Ventricular: Lidocaine, procainamide, bretylium, isopyramide, encainide, tocainide, synchronized cardioversion.
Lethal dysrhythmias	Absent pulses, loss of consciousness, no measurable systemic pressure, apnea.	Epinephrine, antidysrhythmics, defibrillation, synchronized cardioversion.
Cardiac trauma	Poor systemic perfusion, increased central venous pressure, cardiomegaly, hepatomegaly, respiratory distress, peripheral and pulmonary edema.	Maintain airway and ventilation, maximize oxygen delivery and minimize oxygen demand, administer IV fluids therapy to optimize preload, vasodilators to reduce afterload, inotropic agents.

Table 1-2
Selected Cardiovascular Problems—cont'd

Cardiovascular Problem	Assessment Findings	Usual Treatment
Cardiomyopathy	Congestive heart failure, poor systemic perfusion, chest pain, lethargy, exercise intolerance, sudden death.	Administration of calcium channel blockers for idiopathic hypertrophic subaortic stenosis, inotropic agents, vasodilators, prophylactic treatment for dysrhythmias.
Congestive heart failure	Poor perfusion, gallop rhythm, tachycardia, pale, mottled, and cold skin, decreased urine output, hepatomegaly, cardiomegaly, respiratory distress, activity intolerance, feeding difficulties, failure to thrive.	Administration of digoxin, diuretics, inotropic agents, oxygen, ventilatory management when indicated.
Endocarditis	Malaise, fever, positive blood cultures, symptoms of bacterial emboli.	Symptomatic support, antibiotic therapy.
Hypertensive crisis	Headache, papilledema, retinal hemorrhages, hemiplegia, coma, stupor, convulsions, visual disturbances.	Administration of calcium channel blockers, vasodilators, sympathetic blocking agents.
Hypovolemic shock	Fluid or blood loss, poor systemic perfusion, decreased hemodynamic and blood pressures, development of symptoms of shock with 5% to 7% fluid loss or with severe hemorrhage causing a 20% to 25% blood loss.	Administration of isotonic crystalloids, blood, or colloids. May require more fluids to be replaced than were lost.
Kawasaki's disease	High fever, skin rash, swollen hands and feet, conjunctivitis, swollen lymph nodes, coronary artery dilation, symptoms of congestive heart failure and myocarditis.	Administration of antiinflammatory medications. Monitoring of cardiac involvement.

Continued.

Table 1-2
Selected Cardiovascular Problems—cont'd

Cardiovascular Problem	Assessment Findings	Usual Treatment
Myocarditis	History of recent illness and fever, congestive heart failure, gallop rhythm, dysrhythmias, fatigue, dyspnea, exercise intolerance, congestive heart failure.	Reduction of fever, treatment for congestive failure and dysrhythmias.
Pericarditis	Epicardial friction rub, fever, leukocytosis, elevated erythrocyte sedimentation rate.	Drainage of clinically significant pericardial effusions. Administration of antiinflammatory medications.
Pulmonary edema	Tachypnea and dyspnea, retraction (suprasternal, intercostal, substernal) use of accessory muscles, expiratory grunting (in infants), crackles (typically not heard in infants due to shallow respirations).	Administration of digoxin, diuretics, inotropic agents, or oxygen. Ventilatory management when needed.

- Vegetative bacterial growth in the heart can break off and embolize to other parts of the body, which produces symptoms depending on the location of embolization.
- Prevention of bacterial endocarditis is the most effective treatment. Prophylaxis antibiotic administration before dental procedures and other surgery or invasive diagnostic tests is indicated.
- Treatment of bacterial endocarditis consists of at least 4 to 6 weeks of intravenous antibiotics.

Pericarditis

- Pericarditis, an inflammation of the heart that commonly follows open heart surgery, is associated with pericardial effusion leading to tamponade.
- Symptoms include those of decreased left and right cardiac output, including paradoxical rise of central venous pressure with inspiration (Kussmaul's sign), pulsus paradoxus, and hepatojugular reflux.

- ECG changes associated with pericarditis may include ST-segment elevation or depression along with T-wave inversion.

- Signs and symptoms of acute tamponade indicate pericardiocentesis.

Kawasaki's Disease

- Kawasaki's disease is characterized by inflammation of microvessels. This is best treated early with gamma globulin.

- Symptoms include high fever, rash, erythema of the hands, feet, conjunctiva, and mouth, and also cervical lymphadenopathy.

- Cardiac manifestations include coronary artery dilation (and resultant aneurysms), possibly leading to thrombosis and myocardial infarction. Treatment includes aspirin therapy or antithrombolytic therapy with acute occlusion.

Cardiomyopathy

- In dilated or congestive cardiomyopathy, ventricles enlarge and decrease functioning. This condition is treated with beta-adrenergic agents, digoxin, and inotropes or vasodilators to reduce afterload.

- Restrictive cardiomyopathy—an impingement of the ventricular cavity leading to inadequate cardiac output—is treated with vasodilators or other individualized therapy.

- Hypertrophic occlusive cardiomyopathy (also known as idiopathic hypertrophic subaortic stenosis) is characterized by hypertrophy of the ventricular septum, which impedes left ventricular volume and outflow. This condition should never be treated with digoxin, which may exacerbate outflow obstruction. Instead, treatment involves the use of propranolol or calcium channel blockers to decrease how dynamic, and therefore obstructive, the heart muscle is.

- Assessment for and treatment of all types of arrhythmias are critical in cardiomyopathy.

CARDIAC TRAUMA

- Cardiac enzymes (such as CPK-MB and LDH_5) are elevated with significant cardiac trauma.

- ST-segment changes help identify ischemia (depressed) or infarction (elevated).

- Cardiac trauma increases the risk of arrhythmias, tamponade, and ventricular or aortic aneurysms.

- Cardiac tamponade is evidenced by tachycardia, narrowing pulse pressure, tachypnea, dyspnea, increased central venous pressure, jugular vein distension, poor peripheral perfusion, and decreased urinary output.

ECG INTERPRETATION

- See Fig. 1-1 for normal conduction pathway.
- ST-segment depression indicates ischemia, whereas ST-segment elevation indicates myocardial damage or ventricular hypertrophy.
- The PR interval is prolonged in digoxin toxicity.

INTRAOSSEOUS INFUSIONS

- Intraosseous infusions are an excellent alternative when vascular access cannot be obtained. Fluids can be infused directly into the bone marrow for safe, rapid infusions.
- The preferred site for intraosseous infusions is the anterior tibia or lower portion of the femur.
- Bone marrow needles or #16-#18-guage IV needles may be used for intraosseous infusions.
- Crystalloids, colloids, blood products, and inotropes all can be infused through an intraosseous line.

NEONATAL-SPECIFIC PRINCIPLES

- In neonates, stroke volume may be increased with fluid therapy if the systemic vascular resistance and aortic pressures are not high and the ventricular function is adequate.
- Persistent hyperextension of the neck ("sniffing position") may indicate hypoxia related to respiratory problems.
- Infants with congenital heart defects, especially cyanotic defects, commonly become fatigued with feeding. They may not take in sufficient calories to ensure normal growth and development.
- Assess for fluid overload in the sacral, periorbital, and supraclavicular areas in infants.

- Grunting, a hallmark indication of respiratory distress in infants, serves to increase end-expiratory pressure, prolong exhalation, and improve gas exchange. When associated with cardiac disease, it often is related to congestive heart failure and pulmonary edema.
- Quick volume expansion, which causes a rapid rise in systolic blood pressure, has been associated with intraventricular hemorrhages in neonates.
- Isotonic solutions should be used for volume expansion to prevent acute changes in osmolarity, which may lead to intraventricular or intrapulmonary hemorrhages.

Questions

GENERAL CARDIAC CARE QUESTIONS

1. Cardiac output is a product of:
   A. Diastolic and systolic pressure
   B. Heart rate and end-diastolic pressure
   C. Heart rate and stroke volume
   D. Stroke volume and blood pressure

2. Which is the primary cause of cardiac arrest in infants and children?
   A. Congestive heart failure
   B. Cardiac arrhythmias
   C. Respiratory problems
   D. Trauma

3. Stimulation of the sympathetic nervous system has which effect on the cardiovascular system?
   A. Decreases stroke volume and increases blood pressure
   B. Increases stroke volume and decreases blood pressure
   C. Slows conduction through the atrioventricular node
   D. Increases stroke volume and heart rate

Case Study

An infant with coarctation of the aorta is admitted to the pediatric unit, where he undergoes a physical examination and diagnostic testing. Tests include echocardiography and cardiac catheterization. Questions 4 to 7 refer to this case study.

---

4. Which signs and symptoms of coarctation would most likely be seen during the physical examination?
   A. Bounding femoral pulses and weak brachial pulses
   B. Bounding femoral and brachial pulses
   C. Weak femoral pulses and absent brachial pulses
   D. Weak femoral pulses and strong brachial pulses

5. Before surgery, an infant with coarctation of the aorta is likely to be treated with which medication?
   A. Dopamine to increase systemic pressure
   B. Dobutamine to increase myocardial contraction
   C. Sodium bicarbonate to treat acidosis
   D. Diuretic therapy to treat congestive heart failure

(Not help)

6. Following a cardiac catheterization, the nurse should expect to observe for all of the following *except:*
   A. Seizures
   B. Decreased pulses distal to the venipuncture site
   C. Respiratory distress
   D. Hematoma at the venipuncture site

7. Poor cardiac output is indicated by:
   A. Cold, pale, and mottled extremities
   B. Cyanotic lips, gums, and nail beds
   C. Increased urinary output
   D. Cyanotic extremities

8. Which outcome indicates effective management of an infant with coarctation prior to surgical correction?
   A. Adequate hourly urinary output
   B. Active precordium
   C. Absence of pleural effusion
   D. Decrease in arterial pH level

9. The nurse is *least* likely to effectively assess for fluid overload in an infant in which area?
   A. Periorbital
   B. Sacral
   C. Supraclavicular
   D. Pedal

10. Right-to-left cardiac shunts are associated with which symptom?
   A. Pulmonary edema
   B. Clubbing of fingers and toes
   C. Mottled, gray coloring
   D. Hepatomegaly

11. In right-to-left cardiac shunts, the nursing diagnostic category Impaired Gas Exchange typically is related to:
   A. Increased pulmonary blood flow
   B. Decreased ventilation to perfusion
   C. Decreased pulmonary vascular pressures
   D. Decreased pulmonary blood flow

12. Which conditions increase pulmonary vascular resistance?
   A. Hypercapnia, acidosis, and hypoxemia
   B. Hyperthermia, alkalosis, and hypocapnia
   C. Hypothermia, hypocapnia, and hyperoxemia
   D. Sepsis, acidosis, and hypocapnia

13. Which heart sound is *not* normal in infants and children?
A. Fixed split of S_2
B. Physiologic split of S_2
C. Systolic murmur
D. An S_3 heart sound

14. Which statement about S_3 heart sounds in infants and children is *not* true?
A. May be a normal finding
B. May indicate aortic stenosis
C. May precede the development of rales
D. May indicate poor ventricular function

15. Heart sounds such as S_1 and S_2 are typically caused by:
A. Turbulent blood flow
B. The sound of shunting blood
C. Blood crossing valves
D. Closing of valves

16. Which treatment is used initially to control congestive heart failure from excessive pulmonary blood flow caused by lesions?
A. Diuretics and digoxin
B. Banding of the aorta
C. Corrective surgery
D. Antihypertensive medications

17. Which statement best describes a major difference between fetal and adult circulation?
A. The foramen ovale opens after birth to allow more blood flow to the lungs
B. Pulmonary vascular resistance is higher than systemic vascular resistance in the fetus
C. The ductus arteriosus becomes patent after birth to allow diversion of blood from high pulmonary pressure
D. The foramen ovale closes so that there is no blood mixing in the ventricles

18. Which symptom does *not* indicate supraventricular tachycardia (SVT)?
A. Restlessness
B. Poor feeding in infants
C. Bounding pulses
D. Tachypnea

19. To differentiate SVT from a normal increase in sinus rhythm, which criterion must be met?
A. Rate must be greater than 250 beats/min
B. The rhythm must be irregular
C. Aberrant conduction pathways must be identified
D. The rate must change little with varying activities

20. Which disorder must be ruled out before digoxin is used in treating SVT?
A. Seizure disorder
B. Bronchopulmonary dysplasia
C. Wolf-Parkinson-White syndrome
D. Premature ventricular beats

21. Beta-blockers, such as propranolol, should *not* be used to treat SVT accompanied by congestive heart failure because:
A. Beta-blockers may decrease cardiac output
B. Beta-blockers can increase circulating catecholamines
C. SVT is refractory to treatment with beta-blockers
D. Cardioversion is the only effective treatment

22. Which nursing diagnostic category is appropriate for the child with SVT?
A. High risk for infection
B. Altered tissue perfusion
C. Fluid volume deficit
D. Ineffective airway clearance

23. Cardiac index is determined by:
A. Multiplying the heart rate by stroke volume
B. Dividing the cardiac output by body surface area
C. Adding the cardiac output and systolic pressure
D. Taking ⅓ the diastolic pressure

24. Which compensatory mechanism is used by infants to increase cardiac output?
A. Increased stroke volume
B. Decreased afterload
C. Increased heart rate
D. Increased preload

25. Which statement about congenital heart block is *true*?
A. The atrial rate is slower than the ventricular rate
B. The atrial rate paces the ventricles too slowly
C. The atrioventricular node is the dominant pacemaker
D. The atria and ventricles beat independently

26. Symptomatic congenital heart block is treated by:
A. Digoxin to increase the pumping of the heart
B. Beta-blocking agents to block abnormal impulses
C. Temporary or permanent pacing
D. Electrocardioversion

27. Congenital heart block (CHB) is commonly associated with all of the following *except:*
A. Bronchopulmonary dysplasia
B. Maternal systemic lupus erythematosus (SLE)
C. Myocarditis in the infant
D. Endocardial fibroelastosis

Case Study

An infant female patient has critical aortic stenosis. During the past hour, she has developed tachycardia, urinary output of less than 0.5 ml/kg, mottling of the skin, elevation in central venous pressure, increased liver size, and barely palpable pulses.

Questions 28 to 32 refer to this case study.

---

28. Her symptoms are probably the result of:
A. Hypovolemic shock
B. Septic shock
C. Cardiogenic shock
D. Hemorrhagic shock

29. Which nursing diagnosis is most appropriate for this patient?
A. Ineffective thermoregulation associated with poor perfusion of temperature regulation centers
B. Impaired gas exchange related to decreased pulmonary flow
C. Decreased cardiac output related to myocardial dysfunction
D. Ineffective breathing pattern related to obstructed pulmonary flow

30. The physician may prescribe dopamine for this patient. This drug helps to improve cardiovascular function by:
A. Increasing systemic vascular resistance
B. Inotropic and chronotropic actions
C. Decreasing afterload
D. Improving renal perfusion

31. To decrease the workload on her heart and improve her cardiac output, the nurse would expect the physician to prescribe:
A. Nitroprusside
B. Propranolol
C. Digoxin
D. Captopril

32. Which would *not* be considered a positive outcome for her therapy?
A. Urinary output of 0.5 cc/kg/hr
B. Resolution of an S_3 heart sound
C. Warm, dry skin
D. A rise in arterial oxygen saturation

33. Pulmonary hypertension is identified by which hemodynamic readings?
A. Pulmonary artery pressure of 28/10 mm Hg; right ventricular pressure of 27/4 mm Hg; right atrial pressure of 4 mm Hg; pulmonary capillary wedge pressure of 11 mm Hg
B. Pulmonary artery pressure of 41/18 mm Hg; right ventricular pressure of 39/15 mm Hg; right atrial pressure of 11 mm Hg; pulmonary capillary wedge pressure of 5 mm Hg
C. Pulmonary artery pressure of 20/10 mm Hg; right ventricular pressure of 27/4 mm Hg; right atrial pressure of 4 mm Hg; pulmonary capillary wedge pressure of 18 mm Hg
D. Pulmonary artery pressure of 24/6 mm Hg; right ventricular pressure of 22/6 mm Hg; right atrial pressure of 5 mm Hg; pulmonary capillary wedge pressure of 10 mm Hg

34. At what point would pulmonary artery pressure readings be recorded?
A. At the end of inspiration
B. At the end of expiration
C. As inspiration begins
D. As expiration begins

35. If a pulmonary artery waveform becomes dampened, the nurse should suspect all of the following causes *except:*
A. Severe hypovolemia or hemorrhage
B. Faulty or wet transducer
C. Kinking or wedging of the catheter
D. Slippage of the tip into the ventricle

36. For patients with right-to-left shunts, a pulmonary artery balloon-tipped catheter should be inflated with:
A. Sterile water
B. Sterile saline solution
C. Air
D. Carbon dioxide

37. The atrioventricular node plays an important part in the cardiac conduction system by:
A. Delaying the impulse so the ventricles can fill
B. Serving as the pacemaker of the ventricles
C. Preventing supraventricular tachycardia
D. Speeding the impulse to the ventricles

38. Which of the following is *not* likely to cause dysrhythmias in infants and children?
A. Anesthesia
B. Sepsis
C. Acyanotic lesions
D. Intubation

Case Study

A 3-day-old male infant is transferred from the emergency room to the intensive care unit. He was brought in earlier by his parents, who stated that he became extremely blue when he awoke this morning and started crying. He is diagnosed with tetralogy of Fallot and as having had a hypercyanotic, or tet, spell. Questions 39 to 43 refer to this case study.

---

39. When assessing this baby, what area of the body is *best* for reliably assessing cyanosis?
A. Earlobes
B. Palms of hands
C. Soles of feet
D. Nail beds

40. If this patient were to remain cyanotic without surgical correction, which finding would the nurse expect to observe in future assessments?
A. Anemia
B. Clubbed fingers
C. Obesity
D. Thick, coarse hair

41. For cyanotic lesions such as tetralogy of Fallot that cause decreased pulmonary blood flow, an early palliative intervention before final correction may include:
A. Pulmonary artery banding
B. Systemic-to-pulmonary shunt
C. Aortoplasty
D. Intubation and oxygen therapy

42. A hypercyanotic, or tet, spell typically is characterized by:
A. Decreased pulmonary pressure and increased systemic pressure
B. Increased pulmonary pressure and increased systemic pressure
C. Decreased pulmonary pressure and decreased systemic pressure
D. Increased pulmonary pressure and decreased systemic pressure

43. All of the following could be used to treat hypercyanotic spells *except*:
A. Knee-chest position
B. Sodium bicarbonate
C. Morphine
D. Nitroprusside

44. Aortic stenosis would produce which type of sound?
A. Diastolic murmur heard best at the apex of the heart
B. Systolic murmur heard best at the base of the heart
C. Diastolic murmur heard best at the base of the heart
D. Systolic murmur heard best at the apex of the heart

45. A patent ductus arteriosus (PDA) produces which type of murmur?
A. Continuous murmur at the base of the heart
B. Pansystolic murmur at the apex of the heart
C. Diastolic murmur at the base of the heart
D. No audible murmur

46. The pathophysiology of cardiogenic shock is:
A. Inadequate pumping action of the heart
B. Decreased preload
C. Decreased afterload
D. Inadequate endogenous catecholamines

47. Chronotropic agents are used to:
A. Increase force of contraction
B. Increase blood pressure
C. Increase heart rate
D. Decrease afterload

48. An infant or child will show signs of hypovolemic shock when fluid loss approaches what percentage of body weight?
A. 15% to 20%
B. 7% to 10%
C. 25%
D. 30% to 40%

49. Positive patient outcomes in treating hypovolemic shock would *not* include:
A. Sunken fontanels
B. Central venous pressure of 8 mm Hg
C. Warm, dry skin
D. Pulmonary artery wedge pressure of 12 mm Hg

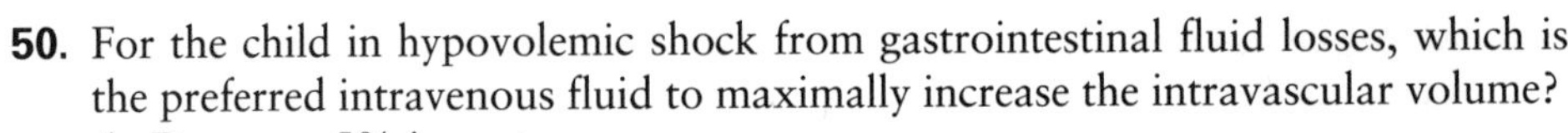

50. For the child in hypovolemic shock from gastrointestinal fluid losses, which is the preferred intravenous fluid to maximally increase the intravascular volume?
A. Dextrose 5% in water
B. 0.45% normal saline solution
C. 0.9% normal saline solution
D. 7% normal saline solution

51. For hypovolemic shock, which fluid therapy is usually most effective?
A. Crystalloids alone
B. Colloids alone
C. Crystalloids and colloids
D. Crystalloids and whole blood

52. What do all forms of shock have in common?
A. Decreased cardiac output
B. Insufficient tissue perfusion
C. Massive vasodilation
D. Decreased renal perfusion

53. Which electrolyte imbalance is most likely to develop following multiple transfusions to treat hemorrhagic shock?
A. Hypernatremia
B. Hypokalemia
C. Hypophosphatemia
D. Hypocalcemia

54. Parasympathetic stimulation of the cardiovascular system would produce which symptoms?
A. Tachycardia and vasoconstriction
B. Bradycardia and increased vascular resistance
C. Bradycardia and vasodilation
D. Tachycardia and decreased vascular resistance

55. Which factor does *not* affect arterial blood pressure?
A. Body surface area
B. Fear
C. Age
D. Tricuspid insufficiency

56. Mean arterial pressure is affected by:
A. Cardiac output and systemic vascular resistance
B. Cardiac output and systemic venous pressure
C. Venous return and pulmonary vascular resistance
D. Cardiac output and pulmonary venous pressure

57. Which of the following are important in obtaining a history of an infant or child with congenital cardiac disease?
A. Family history of coronary heart disease
B. Mother's cholesterol intake during pregnancy
C. Maternal allergies
D. Fetal exposure to medications or alcohol

58. What effect does inspiration have on cardiac physiology?
A. Increases ejection fraction
B. Increases venous return
C. Decreases preload
D. Decreases afterload

59. Which factors does *not* increase afterload and, therefore, cardiac work?
A. Aortic valvular stenosis
B. Use of vasodilating agents
C. Use of vasoconstricting agents
D. Polycythemia

60. Pulsus paradoxus is characterized by:
A. Alternating strong and weak pulses in all extremities
B. A fall in arterial pressure of greater than 10 mm Hg during inspiration
C. Weak pulses in the presence of normal or increased intravascular fluid volume
D. Weak pulses with high blood pressure

61. In assessing a patient with congestive heart failure, the nurse would use the bell of the stethoscope to best hear:
A. S_3 and S_4 heart sounds
B. High-pitched murmurs
C. Stenotic valves
D. An ejection click

62. To use the bell of the stethoscope, the nurse would:
A. Press firmly to avoid environmental noise
B. Press lightly to best hear low-pitched sounds
C. Hold the bell barely off the chest wall
D. Cushion the bell between the fingers

63. Which diagnostic test would be most helpful in documenting blood flow through a patent ductus arteriosus?
A. Chest x-ray
B. Magnetic resonance imaging
C. Doppler echocardiography
D. Electrocardiogram

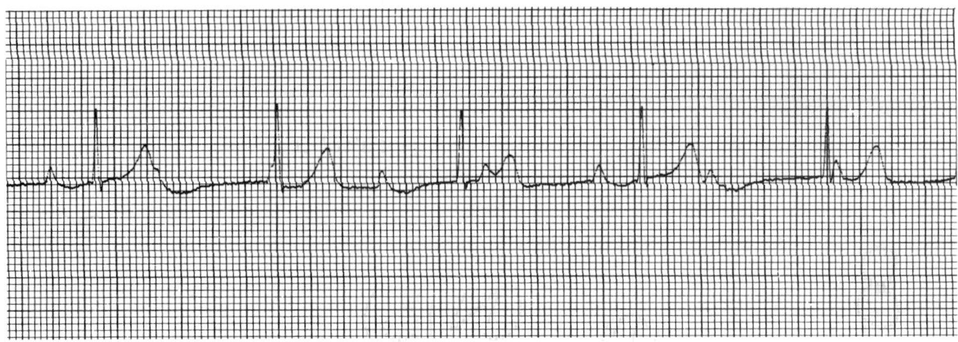

(From Hazinski, 1992.)

64. Your patient's monitor suddenly presents the rhythm shown above. Which treatment would the physician *most* likely prescribe?
A. Vagal maneuvers
B. Verapamil
C. Atropine
D. Isuprel

65. Mitral stenosis would produce which type of murmur?
A. Pansystolic
B. Diastolic
C. Holosystolic
D. Diastolic ejection

66. Which hemodynamic pressures would be increased in mitral stenosis?
A. Right atrial and central venous pressure
B. Left atrial and pulmonary capillary wedge
C. Left atrial and left ventricular
D. Systemic arterial and pulmonary capillary wedge

67. Which statement does *not* refer to an advantage of magnetic resonance imaging of the heart?
A. It is safe for pregnant women and children
B. There is no need for contrast dye
C. It is safe for patients with pacemakers
D. It provides a three-dimensional view of the heart

68. Prostaglandin E_1 therapy would most likely be helpful in treating which defect during the neonatal period?
A. Pulmonary atresia
B. Atrioventricular canal
C. Truncus arteriosus
D. Patent ductus arteriosus

69. Which components are common to all chest tube systems?
A. Bubble collector, suction-control chamber, ventilating bottle
B. Collection chamber, ventilating bottle, suction-control chamber
C. Water seal, collection chamber, ventilating bottle
D. Collection chamber, water seal, suction-control chamber

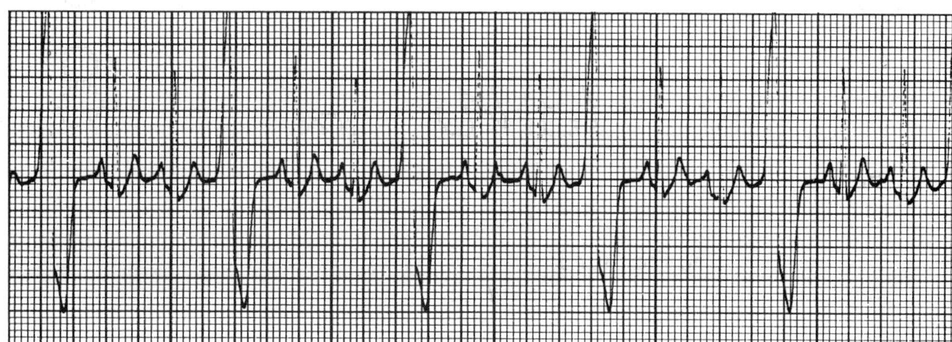

(From Hazinski, 1992.)

70. Which of the following are possible causes of this dysrhythmia in your patient?
A. Electrolyte imbalances, fever, pain
B. Increased atrial pressure, crying
C. Hypoglycemia, hypoxia
D. Increased parasympathetic tone

71. Which of the following is an indication for the use of an umbilical artery catheter?
A. Frequent blood gas level monitoring
B. Meconium aspiration
C. Surfactant deficiency
D. All of the above

72. An umbilical vein catheter can be used to monitor:
A. Arterial blood pressure
B. Central venous pressure
C. Left atrial pressure
D. Left ventricular filling pressure

73. In fetal circulation, the umbilical vein carries:
A. Oxygenated blood to the right atrium
B. Oxygenated blood to the left atrium
C. Deoxygenated blood to the right atrium
D. Deoxygenated blood to the left atrium

74. An umbilical artery line would measure systemic:
A. Arterial pressures
B. Venous pressures
C. Pulmonary pressures
D. Renal pressures (NIM)

75. Which nursing diagnostic categories are appropriate for a patient on prostaglandin E_1 therapy?
I. Ineffective breathing pattern
II. Ineffective thermoregulation
III. Altered tissue perfusion: peripheral
IV. High risk for ineffective airway clearance
A. I and II
B. II and III
C. II and IV
D. I and IV

Case Study

A full-term infant of a diabetic mother is admitted to your critical care unit with hyperbilirubinemia. She weighs 4.25 G. Questions 76 to 80 refer to this case study.

---

76. This patient's bilirubin level is elevated at 15 mg/dL. Which treatment is indicated?
A. Infusions of normal saline solution to hemodilute the bilirubin level
B. No treatment
C. Phototherapy
D. Exchange transfusion

77. What precautions must the nurse take while drawing blood samples for bilirubin levels during her phototherapy?
A. Discontinue the phototherapy lights for 1 hour before sampling
B. Discontinue the phototherapy lights during sampling
C. Draw a sample from an umbilical venous catheter only
D. Avoid drawing a sample for 1 hour after feeding

78. As her bilirubin levels continue to rise to 22 mg/dL, an exchange transfusion is ordered. In planning nursing interventions to avoid the most common problems during her exchange transfusion, the nurse plans to closely monitor:
A. Blood pressure and cardiac rhythm
B. Urinary output and blood pressure
C. Cardiac rhythm and urinary output
D. Neurologic and renal status

79. An appropriate nursing diagnosis related to the complications discussed above would be:
A. Potential for decreased cardiac output related to changes in intravascular volume and electrolytes
B. Potential for alterations in elimination related to rapid infusion of blood
C. Potential for hypothermia related to autonomic response associated with cardiovascular function
D. Impaired gas exchange related to decreased surfactant production

80. For this patient, the most appropriate expected outcome following exchange transfusion therapy would be:
A. Absence of Babinski reflex
B. Absence of extrusion reflex
C. Absence of opisthotonic posturing
D. Absence of Moro reflex

81. Patients experiencing respiratory distress related to increased pulmonary blood flow and elevated pulmonary pressures should be positioned with their head elevated to:
A. Increase peripheral perfusion
B. Increase vital capacity
C. Decrease the work of breathing (NOT)
D. Increase cardiac output

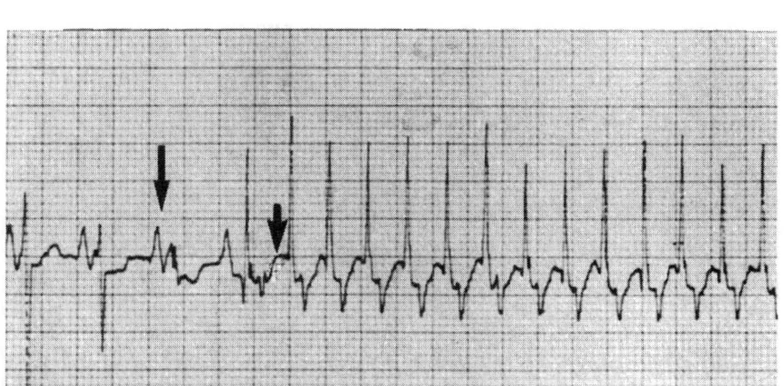

(From Hazinski, 1992.)

82. The strip above indicates:
A. Increased sinus rhythm
B. Accelerated junctional tachycardia
C. Supraventricular tachycardia
D. Ventricular tachycardia

83. An infant has been admitted to the critical care unit with a history of poor growth and feeding. Her current assessment findings include heart rate of 188 beats/min, respiratory rate of 76 breaths/min, nasal flaring, rales, and differential cyanosis. The most likely cause of these symptoms is:
A. Persistent pulmonary hypertension
B. Transient tachypnea of the newborn
C. Coarctation of the aorta
D. Diaphragmatic hernia

84. Which level is most likely to be a safe and effective therapeutic serum level of digoxin?
A. 2.6 mg/mL
B. 2.0 ng/mL
C. 0.6 mg/mL
D. 0.8 ng/mL

(NIE)

85. For the patient on prostaglandin E_1 with a ductal-dependent lesion, for which important assessment finding would the critical care nurse look to assume that therapy is effective?
A. Presence of peripheral pulses
B. Presence of fixed, split S_2
C. Continuous murmur at base of the heart
D. Continuous murmur at apex of the heart

86. Prostaglandin E_1 may be used to improve blood flow and oxygenation in:
I. Hypoplastic left heart syndrome
II. Pulmonary atresia
III. Atrioventricular canal
IV. Aortic insufficiency
A. II and III
B. I and II
C. II and III
D. I and IV

87. A postoperative open-heart patient has the following clinical findings: cardiac index of 2.8 liters/minute/m^2, systemic vascular resistance of 2780 dynes, a sodium level of 141 mEq/liter, and a total calcium level of 8.1 mg/dL. The most appropriate pharmacologic management would be:
A. Calcium chloride 10% at 20 mg/kg
B. Dobutamine at 0.5 mg/kg/min
C. Calcium gluconate at 100 mL/kg
D. Dopamine at 3 mcg/kg/min

88. A patient is diagnosed with tetralogy of Fallot and intubated for acute acidosis and hypoxemia. She is on room-air, pressure support, and a rate of 26 breaths/min. She also is started on prostaglandin E_1 at 0.1 mcg/kg/min. Her physical examination reveals clear, bilateral breath sounds. At the end of her assessment, the critical care nurse notices a sudden drop in the pulse oximeter from 85% to 78%. The most important *immediate* nursing action would be to:

A. Check the patency of the endotracheal tube
B. Increase the FiO_2 to 0.3
C. Suction aggressively for a mucous plug
D. Assess the patency of the prostaglandin E_1 infusion

89. The nurse documents the following vital signs for a postoperative open-heart patient whose extremities are cold, femoral pulses are weak, and pedal pulses are absent: blood pressure of 53/28 mm Hg, heart rate of 195 beats/min, urinary output of 0.03 ml/kg/hr, right atrium (RA) pressure of 8 mm Hg, and a pulmonary capillary wedge pressure of 15 mm Hg. The drug of choice for treating this patient would be:

A. Dobutamine at 20 mcg/kg/min
B. Epinephrine at 0.01 mcg/kg/min
C. Amrinone at 10 mcg/kg/min
D. Isuprel at 0.05 mcg/kg/min

PEDIATRIC-SPECIFIC QUESTIONS

Case Study

A patient has been transferred to the critical care unit following repair of a ventricular septal defect (VSD). Questions 90 to 92 refer to this case study.

---

90. Which finding does *not* indicate that this patient still has a leak in the patch repair?

A. Systolic murmur
B. Mottling
C. Congestive heart failure
D. Tachypnea

91. Which test would be *most* helpful in diagnosing a residual ventricular defect?

A. Electrocardiogram
B. Echocardiogram
C. Chest x-ray
D. Computed tomography scan

92. Over time, a ventricular septal defect will cause which finding?
A. Ventricular hypertrophy
B. Decreased pulmonary blood flow
C. Systemic hypertension
D. Arteriovenous malformations

Case Study

A young male patient has severe congestive heart failure related to a ventricular septal defect. Questions 93 to 95 refer to this case study.

---

93. The nurse would expect this patient to have all of the following signs and symptoms of congestive heart failure *except*:
A. Increased urinary output
B. Decreased cardiac output
C. Hepatomegaly
D. Cardiomegaly

94. An adrenergic response to congestive heart failure is typically manifested by:
A. Polyuria
B. Warm, dry skin
C. Tachycardia
D. Poor feeding

95. A positive outcome of this patient's care management would *not* include:
A. Decreased liver size
B. Urinary output of greater than 1 mL/kg/hr
C. Absence of adventitious breath sounds
D. Increased pulmonary pressures

Case Study

A patient was admitted to the critical care unit after being brought to the emergency department by her mother, who reported that her daughter demonstrated poor feeding for the past 36 hours, rapid breathing, decreased level of activity, and fewer wet diapers. Physical assessment showed moderate sinus tachycardia, increased liver size, rales, 2^+ peripheral pulses, and a gallop rhythm. Laboratory results showed decreased serum osmolarity and slightly decreased hematocrit and blood urea nitrogen levels. Questions 96 to 99 refer to this case study.

---

96. The most likely cause of her symptoms is:
A. Hypovolemic shock
B. Acute renal failure
C. Pneumonia
D. Congestive heart failure

97. The first action the nurse should take for this patient is to:
A. Begin oxygen therapy at ½ liter flow
B. Assess airway, adequacy of respirations, and peripheral pulses
C. Monitor cardiac rhythm
D. Draw blood for baseline arterial blood gas levels

98. Which diagnostic test would be most helpful in confirming her diagnosis?
A. Magnetic resonance imaging
B. Electrocardiogram
C. Echocardiogram
D. Stress testing

99. A desired outcome in treating this patient includes:
A. Liver palpable <2 to 3 cm below the costal margin
B. Increased arterial blood pressure
C. Negative cultures of pulmonary secretions
D. Normal serum creatinine levels

100. A patient is admitted to the critical care unit 2 weeks after repair of a ventricular septal defect with the following clinical findings: temperature of 38.6°C (103.8°F), white blood cell count of 14,500/cm^3, erythrocyte sedimentation rate (ESR) of 61 mm/hr, nasal flaring, pleural effusion, and decreased activity tolerance. The most likely cause of these symptoms is:
A. Viral pneumonia
B. Pericarditis
C. Postpericardiotomy syndrome
D. Respiratory syncytial virus

Case Study

An 8-year-old girl, Lindsay, who is now being admitted to the intensive care unit was diagnosed at birth with congenital heart block. Recently, she collapsed during play and was unable to maintain a pulse rate greater than 40 beats/min. She has a temporary pacemaker in place and is waiting for insertion of a permanent pacemaker. Questions 101 to 104 refer to this case study.

---

101. Where would this patient's pacing catheter be positioned if it were inserted percutaneously?
A. Left ventricle
B. Right ventricle
C. Touching the sinoatrial node
D. Distal to the atrioventricular node

102. Once her transvenous leads are placed, the critical care nurse needs to observe for all of the following complications *except:*
A. Hemorrhage
B. Cardiac perforation
C. Hiccups
D. Seizures

103. Lindsay's pacemaker is set on the demand mode, but it is failing to sense. Which problem may ensue?
A. Paced beats could fall on the T-wave of her own beats
B. The pacemaker could fail to generate any beats
C. The pacemaker could signal, but fail to cause contractions
D. The endocardium and intracardiac hemorrhage could erode

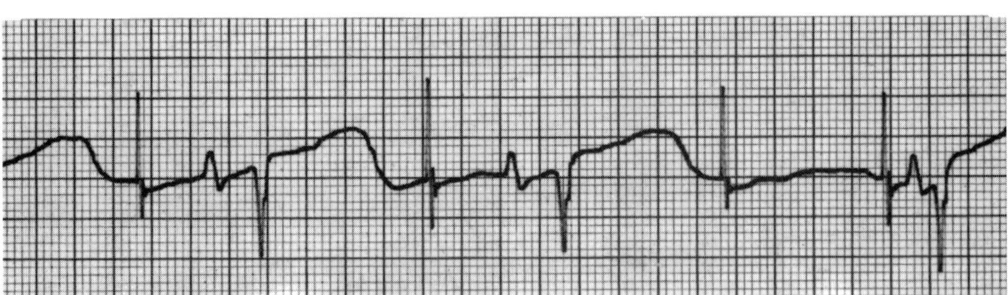

(From Thelan, Davie, Urden, and Lough, 1994.)

104. This rhythm strip demonstrates which problem with Lindsay's pacemaker function?
A. Failure to sense
B. Failure to capture
C. Failure to discharge
D. Failure to pace

105. An 8-year-old child is admitted to the pediatric intensive care unit (PICU) with a history of a fever, skin rash, proteinuria, cervical lymphadenitis, and erythema as well as pain of the hands and feet. His laboratory findings included elevations in this C-reactive protein and erythrocyte sedimentation rate. For which complication should the critical care nurse be alert?
A. Myocarditis
B. Endocarditis
C. Hepatitis
D. Glomerulonephritis

106. Which condition is a common manifestation of cardiac involvement in Kawasaki's disease?
A. Right ventricular hypertrophy
B. Hypertrophic cardiomyopathy
C Aortic stenosis
D. Coronary artery aneurysms

107. When caring for a 10-year-old patient with a pulmonary artery catheter, the critical care nurse notices that the diastolic pressure suddenly drops from 10 mm Hg to 2 mm Hg. Which of the following is the most likely cause?
A. Migration of the catheter tip
B. Balloon rupture in the pulmonary artery
C. Clot formation at the catheter tip
D. Blood in the transducer

108. Following repair of a ventricular septal defect, the patient is returned to the critical care unit intubated, on an FiO_2 of 0.4, intermittent mandatory ventilation (IMV) rate of 10, and positive end expiratory pressure (PEEP) of 2 cm H_2O. The nurse observes an SvO_2 reading of 88% when the pulmonary artery catheter is connected to the monitor for continuous readings. The most appropriate intervention at this point is to:
A. Flush the line by hand, and notify the physician to advance the catheter tip
B. Inflate the balloon for a more accurate reading, and record the reading at end expiration
C. Decrease the FiO_2 to 21%
D. Notify the physician of a possible patch leak

109. A 10-year-old child is admitted to the critical care unit with premature ventricular complexes, nonspecific ST-segment changes, and a decrease in QRS and T-wave voltage. Clinically, the child has decreased peripheral pulses, urinary output of 0.8 mL/kg/hr, and a gallop rhythm. An echocardiogram has ruled out structural heart disease, but identified the presence of pericardial effusion and decreased ventricular motion. The parents state that the child has had flulike symptoms for approximately the last 5 days. The most likely cause of these findings is:
A. Hypertrophic cardiomyopathy
B. Myocarditis
C. Endocarditis
D. Kawasaki's disease

110. A child admitted to the pediatric unit with endocarditis is found to have a vegetative growth on the mitral valve. This child is at risk for all of the following *except*:
A. Pulmonary embolization
B. Renal dysfunction
C. Stroke
D. Arthralgia

111. Which of the following is a priority in assessing the patient with pericarditis?
A. Orthopnea and dyspnea
B. Kussmaul's sign
C. Hepatojugular reflux
D. Decreased peripheral pulses

112. A 18-month-old girl is brought to the emergency room 1 week after being discharged following a Fontan procedure. She has cyanosis, mottled extremities, decreased urine output, listlessness, dyspnea, and a blood pressure of 42/36 mm Hg. The critical care nurse can expect to *immediately* assist with:
A. Insertion of a pulmonary artery catheter
B. Pericardiocentesis
C. Pleural tap
D. Insertion of central venous line

113. A patient having which condition is at higher risk for developing infective endocarditis?
A. Cystic fibrosis
B. Hydrocephalus
C. Patent ductus arteriosus
D. Bronchopulmonary dysplasia

114. A child with Kawasaki's disease is complaining of chest pain unrelieved by positioning or other independent nursing interventions. Which intervention is a priority for the critical care nurse?
A. Administering prescribed analgesics after further pain assessment
B. Obtaining a 12-lead electrocardiogram (ECG) and assessing for ST-segment changes
C. Administering gamma globulin to decrease inflammation
D. Preparing the child for pericardiocentesis

115. A child with hypertrophic occlusive cardiomyopathy (HOCM), also called idiopathic hypertrophic subaortic stenosis (IHSS), has mitral regurgitation, an ejection fraction of 41%, diminished peripheral pulses, and a grade IV/VI systolic ejection murmur heard best along the left sternal border. Which therapy would be indicated?
A. Digoxin to improve ventricular contractility
B. Furosemide to treat congestive heart failure
C. Propranolol to reduce ventricular outflow obstruction
D. Tolazoline to increase cardiac output

116. What would be the safest and most effective oral digitalizing dose for an 11-year-old child with congestive heart failure?
A. 8 to 12 mcg/kg
B. 15 to 25 mcg/kg
C. 18 to 30 mcg/kg
D. 25 to 35 mcg/kg

117. Before administering digoxin, the critical care nurse would assess the ECG for:
I. Prolongation of the QRS complex
II. Depressed ST-segment
III. Elevated ST-segment
IV. Prolongation of the PR interval
A. I and II
B. I and III
C. III and IV
D. II and IV

118. Which finding is most common in infants and children with digoxin toxicity?
A. Bradycardia
B. Nausea and vomiting
C. Diarrhea
D. Blurred vision

119. Which intervention would be appropriate *immediately* after an infant or child goes into ventricular fibrillation?
A. Defibrillation at 4 joules/kg
B. Defibrillation at 2 joules/kg
C. Synchronized cardioversion at 1 joule/kg
D. Synchronized cardioversion at 2 joules/kg

120. A 17-year-old boy is admitted to the intensive care unit following a motor vehicle accident. He received blunt trauma to his chest from the steering wheel. Which findings would indicate cardiac trauma?
I. Elevated CPK-MM
II. Elevated CPK-MB
III. Elevated LDH_5
IV. Elevated LDH_1
A. I and IV
B. II and IV
C. II and III
D. III and IV

121. All of the following would alert the critical care nurse to the possibility of cardiac trauma *except*:
A. ST elevations or depressions
B. Tachycardia
C. T-wave inversion
D. T-wave elevations

122. A 6-year-old patient returns from the operating room after having undergone a Fontan procedure for a single ventricle. He has a wedge pressure of 18 mm Hg, right ventricular pressure of 38/12 mm Hg, cardiac index of 2.8 liters/min/m^2, and heart rate of 185 beats/min. Which drug will most likely improve his cardiovascular function?

A. Dopamine
B. Nitroprusside
C. Epinephrine
D. Amrinone

123. For which condition should the nurse slow or stop an amrinone infusion and notify the physician?

A. Increased pulmonary capillary wedge pressure
B. Decreased cardiac output
C. Cardiac dysrhythmia
D. Increased right ventricular filling pressure

124. The patient you are caring for is diagnosed with digoxin toxicity and supraventricular tachydysrhythmias. All of the following would be part of his treatment plan *except*:

A. Synchronized cardioversion for unstable SVT
B. Enhancement of digoxin excretion
C. Administration of phenytoin to reduce automaticity
D. Prevention of drug absorption

125. All of the following medications could be used to treat hypertensive crises *except*:

A. Nitroprusside
B. Nitroglycerin
C. Dobutamine
D. Hydralazine

NEONATAL-SPECIFIC QUESTIONS

126. Which finding is most common in infants with digoxin toxicity?

A. Nausea and vomiting
B. Diarrhea
C. Seizures
D. Lethargy

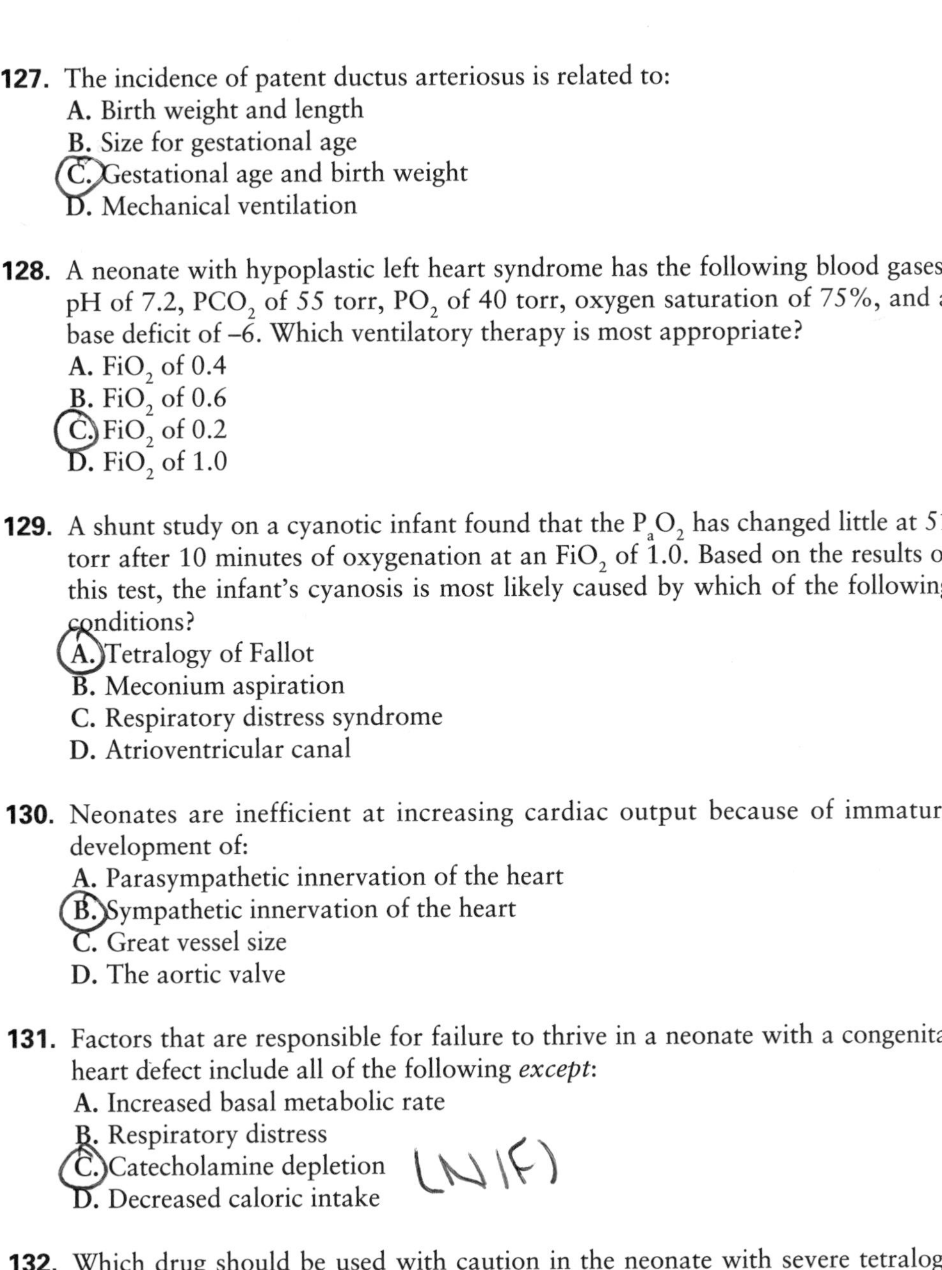

127. The incidence of patent ductus arteriosus is related to:
A. Birth weight and length
B. Size for gestational age
C. Gestational age and birth weight
D. Mechanical ventilation

128. A neonate with hypoplastic left heart syndrome has the following blood gases: pH of 7.2, PCO_2 of 55 torr, PO_2 of 40 torr, oxygen saturation of 75%, and a base deficit of –6. Which ventilatory therapy is most appropriate?
A. FiO_2 of 0.4
B. FiO_2 of 0.6
C. FiO_2 of 0.2
D. FiO_2 of 1.0

129. A shunt study on a cyanotic infant found that the P_aO_2 has changed little at 51 torr after 10 minutes of oxygenation at an FiO_2 of 1.0. Based on the results of this test, the infant's cyanosis is most likely caused by which of the following conditions?
A. Tetralogy of Fallot
B. Meconium aspiration
C. Respiratory distress syndrome
D. Atrioventricular canal

130. Neonates are inefficient at increasing cardiac output because of immature development of:
A. Parasympathetic innervation of the heart
B. Sympathetic innervation of the heart
C. Great vessel size
D. The aortic valve

131. Factors that are responsible for failure to thrive in a neonate with a congenital heart defect include all of the following *except*:
A. Increased basal metabolic rate
B. Respiratory distress
C. Catecholamine depletion
D. Decreased caloric intake

132. Which drug should be used with caution in the neonate with severe tetralogy of Fallot?
A. Propranolol
B. Digoxin
C. Furosemide
D. Prostaglandin E_1

133. A neonate estimated to be at about 30 weeks' gestation is in the neonatal intensive care unit. She has a respiratory rate of 78 breaths/min; a heart rate of 170 beats/min; and the presence of calf, palmar, and plantar pulses. The critical care nurse recognizes these clinical findings as consistent with:

A. Premature closure of the ductus arteriosus
B. A large ventricular septal defect
C. Total anomalous venous return
D. Patent ductus arteriosus

Answers

1. **Correct answer—C.**
   Cardiac output is the amount of blood ejected from the heart over a given amount of time, expressed in liters/minute ($CO = SV \times HR$). Heart rate reflects time; stroke volume reflects the amount of blood pumped. Diastolic, systolic, and end-diastolic pressures are not part of calculating cardiac output.

2. **Correct answer—C.**
   The primary cause of cardiac arrest in infants and children is respiratory, not cardiac, failure. Trauma, congestive heart failure, and cardiac dysrhythmias account for far fewer arrests and deaths than do respiratory problems. Most cardiac arrests actually follow respiratory arrests in infants and children.

3. **Correct answer—D.**
   Stimulation of the sympathetic nervous system increases stroke volume and heart rate to increase cardiac output. The sympathetic nervous system prepares the body for "fight or flight" and therefore is responsible for any activities that increase the output and circulation of blood. Decreasing stroke volume and blood pressure as well as slowing atrioventricular conduction would all serve to decrease output and perfusion.

4. **Correct answer—D.**
   Coarctation of the aorta usually arises around the level of the aorta where the ductus arteriosus enters. Because the narrowing of the aorta results in reduced flow beyond the narrowing, all lower-extremity pulses are weak or absent. Upper-extremity pulses, such as those of the brachial and carotid arteries, are usually still strong because they are supplied by blood above the level of the coarctation.

5. **Correct answer—D.**
   Before surgery can be performed, an infant with coarctation of the aorta is likely to be treated with diuretics and digoxin to aggressively treat congestive heart failure. Dopamine, dobutamine, and sodium bicarbonate would neither help improve the circulation beyond the narrowing nor relieve symptoms of congestive heart failure.

6. **Correct answer—A.**
   Seizures would not be expected unless the infant has a preexisting history of seizure disorders. Sedation is generally given for cardiac catheterization, so observing for respiratory distress related to sedation would be appropriate. Because catheterizations generally are done by cannulating arteries and veins, hematomas or clotting of vessels are also potential complications.

7. **Correct answer—A.**
Cold, pale, and mottled extremities indicate poor cardiac output. Because output is poor, peripheral circulation is decreased as a result of the "clamping down" effect of vasoconstriction; this results in pale coloring which indicates poor perfusion. Cyanosis in all areas indicates either a respiratory problem or a congenital heart defect causing mixed blood flow. Urinary output would be decreased with poor cardiac output from inadequate renal perfusion.

8. **Correct answer—A.**
An expected outcome indicating effective management of a patient with coarctation prior to surgical correction would include adequate hourly urinary output related to adequate or increased peripheral (specifically renal) perfusion. An active precordium is generally a sign of cardiomegaly or ventricular hypertrophy and may be seen with coarctation. Pleural effusions are typically postoperative complications of cardiac surgery. These patients can be acidotic related to poor peripheral perfusion, so a rise in pH would be a positive outcome.

9. **Correct answer—D.**
The best places to assess an infant for fluid overload are over the sacrum, around the eyes, and above the clavicles. Only those who are standing, with their feet dependent, exhibit pedal edema.

10. **Correct answer—B.**
Right-to-left cardiac shunts cause blood to pass directly to the systemic circulation without first passing through the lungs to be oxygenated. These patients are chronically hypoxic, gradually leading to changes such as clubbing of the fingers and toes. Pulmonary edema and hepatomegaly are signs of congestive heart failure. Mottled, gray coloring is characteristic of poor systemic cardiac output.

11. **Correct answer—D.**
In right-to-left cardiac shunts, the diagnostic category Impaired Gas Exchange is a result of decreased pulmonary blood flow. Although less ventilation compared to pulmonary perfusion can cause cyanosis, it is not the mechanism responsible in *cardiac shunting*. Increased pulmonary blood flow occurs in left-to-right shunts. Decreased pulmonary vascular pressure would not impair gas exchange.

12. **Correct answer—A.**
Pulmonary vascular resistance is increased as a result of increased carbon dioxide levels, acidosis, and decreased oxygen levels—all of which mimic fetal circulatory conditions. Hypocapnia, alkalosis, and hyperoxia cause pulmonary vasodilation, which reduces pulmonary vascular resistance.

13. Correct answer—A.
A fixed, split S_2 heart sound is not normal in infants, children, or adults. Physiologic splitting, however, is a normal sound caused by closure of the tricuspid valve late during inspiration, when more blood is returning to the right side of the heart. Systolic murmurs and S_3 heart sounds may be normal findings in young patients and do not necessarily indicate heart dysfunction.

14. Correct answer—B.
An S_3 heart sound is not associated with aortic stenosis. An S_3 sound may be normal in children; it also may indicate a failing ventricle even before rales can be auscultated. Aortic stenosis is associated with an ejection click and systolic thrill or an ejection murmur at the base of the heart 3rd intercostal space to the left of the sternal border.

15. Correct answer—D.
Heart sounds are caused by the closure of valves, whereas murmurs are caused by noisy blood flow, such as turbulence and shunting.

16. Correct answer—A.
Diuretics and digoxin are used to try to medically manage increased pulmonary blood flow. If this treatment is unsuccessful, either corrective surgery or pulmonary artery banding may be performed. Antihypertensive medications would not be effective.

17. Correct answer—B.
Pulmonary vascular resistance is high in the fetus to keep blood flowing to the body, not to unaerated lungs. The foramen ovale and ductus arteriosus both *close* after birth. The foramen ovale is located between the atria, not the ventricles.

18. Correct answer—C.
Symptoms of supraventricular tachycardia are related to poor cardiac output and result in restlessness, poor feeding as a result of the work involved, and tachypnea as a result of cardiac failure. Pulses would be diminished, not bounding.

19. Correct answer—D.
SVT differs from a normal increase in sinus rhythm because it varies little with changes in activity. SVT must have a regular rate greater than 200 beats/min. No abnormal pathway may be detectible by a conventional 12-lead ECG.

20. Correct answer—C.
Wolf-Parkinson-White syndrome should be ruled out before using digoxin to treat SVT. Seizure disorders, bronchopulmonary dysplasia, and premature ventricular beats are not contraindications to the use of digoxin in SVT.

21. Correct answer—A.
Beta-blockers such as propranolol should not be used to treat SVT accompanied by congestive heart failure because they may inhibit naturally circulating catecholamines which are needed to maintain adequate cardiac output. Beta-blockers decrease the effectiveness of catecholamines. SVT can be treated effectively by beta-blockers, but is contraindicated in the presence of congestive heart failure. Cardioversion is a treatment, but not the only effective treatment for SVT.

22. Correct answer—B.
An appropriate nursing diagnosis for SVT is altered tissue perfusion. As the heart rate increases, diastolic filling time, cardiac output, and subsequently tissue perfusion fall. Fluid volume may actually increase as renal perfusion and glomerular filtration fall. No significant change in the risk of infection is related to SVT. Ineffective airway clearance could accompany very late stages of congestive heart failure as pulmonary edema develops, but impaired gas exchange would be a better diagnosis if pulmonary dysfunction occurs.

23. Correct answer—B.
The cardiac index is determined by dividing the cardiac output by body surface area. Multiplying the heart rate by the stroke volume gives the cardiac output. Adding the cardiac output and systolic pressure, or one-third the diastolic pressure do not give any clinically relevant calculations.

24. Correct answer—C.
Infants are not able to increase their stroke volume to increase cardiac output the way older children or adults can. Infants also do not decrease their afterload or increase their preload as compensatory mechanisms to change cardiac output.

25. Correct answer—D.
In complete heart block, the atria and ventricles beat independently. The atrial rate is more rapid and does not influence the pacing of the ventricles. Neither the sinus nor the atrioventricular nodes serve as pacemakers for the heart.

26. Correct answer—C.
Symptomatic congenital heart block is treated by pacing. Digoxin would be ineffective and slow the heart rate even more. Abnormal impulses are not the mechanism of action making beta-blockers inappropriate. Electrocardioversion is indicated in tachydysrhythmias, not a bradydysrhythmia.

27. Correct answer—A.
Congenital heart block is not associated with bronchopulmonary dysplasia. CHB is, however, often associated with maternal SLE, and both myocarditis and endocardial fibroelastosis in the neonate.

28. Correct answer—C.

The most likely cause of this patient's symptoms is cardiogenic shock. These symptoms demonstrate biventricular failure associated with poor myocardial function in cardiogenic shock. This form of shock is associated with critical aortic stenosis from massive increases in left ventricular afterload leading to increased pulmonary pressures and eventually failure of both ventricles. Early septic shock is actually associated with increased renal perfusion. Both hemorrhagic and hypovolemic shock would not show signs of right ventricular failure.

29. Correct answer—C.

An appropriate nursing diagnosis for this patient would be decreased cardiac output related to myocardial dysfunction. Because of the increased afterload on the ventricle, the myocardium hypertrophies and its function is impaired. Ineffective thermoregulation associated with poor perfusion of temperature regulation centers does not occur. Pulmonary vascular volume and pressure are increased, not obstructed or decreased.

30. Correct answer—B.

Vasodilators decrease the afterload, or work that the heart must pump against, but are not effective in a fixed anatomical obstruction like aortic stenosis. Increasing systemic vascular resistance would increase afterload and therefore the heart's work. Dopamine increases the force and rate of myocardial contractions which improves cardiac output in aortic stenosis. Improving renal perfusion does not itself improve cardiac output.

31. Correct answer—C.

Nitroprusside and captopril beta-blocking agents such as propranolol would be contraindicated because they would block the effects of catecholamines, an important compensatory mechanism to increase cardiac output. Digoxin increases the force of contraction, and therefore the output of the heart. Digoxin might be ordered to help the heart pump more effectively past the stenosis until surgery can fix the lesion.

32. Correct answer—A.

Positive outcomes of therapeutic interventions for cardiogenic shock would include adequate urinary output (1 to 3 mL/kg/hr), improvement in arterial oxygen saturation, disappearance of a new S_3 heart sound, and warm, dry skin. All these indicate adequate tissue perfusion and absence of pulmonary congestion. Urinary output of 0.5 cc/kg/hr would not indicate adequate renal perfusion.

33. Correct answer—B.

Normal right-sided pressures are: pulmonary artery pressure 50 to 30/5 to 10 mm Hg; right ventricular pressure 15 to 30/2 to 5 mm Hg; right atrial pressure

1 to 5 mm Hg; and pulmonary capillary wedge pressure 5 to 12 mm Hg. Right-sided heart pressures are used to determine pulmonary hypertension. Left-sided pressures reflect systemic hypertension. A pulmonary capillary wedge pressure reflects left-sided, not right-sided, pressures.

34. Correct answer—B.
Pulmonary artery pressure readings should be recorded at the end of expiration because respirations affect the readings. End expiration is a standard point so that readings over time can be compared.

35. Correct answer—D.
Causes of pulmonary artery waveform dampening include severe hypovolemia, hemorrhage, faulty or wet transducer, kinked or wedged catheter, or a clot in the system. If the tip slips into the ventricle, the waveform will become much greater in size, not dampened.

36. Correct answer—D.
For patients with right-to-left shunts, a pulmonary artery balloon-tipped catheter should be inflated with carbon dioxide, not air, to minimize complications associated with air embolism from balloon rupture. Never inflate a balloon with fluid.

37. Correct answer—A.
The atrioventricular node plays an important part in the cardiac conduction system by delaying, not speeding, the impulse so the ventricles can fill. The sinus node serves as the pacemaker. While the AV node can help delay or block atrial impulses to the ventricles in SVT, it does not prevent SVT.

38. Correct answer—C.
Causes of dysrhythmias in infants and children include hypoxia, sepsis, cyanotic lesions, intubation, intracardiac catheters, hypotension, electrolyte imbalances, congenital conduction defects, cardiac surgical trauma, inflammation of the heart, as well as many medications. Acyanotic lesions are not typically associated with dysrhythmias.

39. Correct answer—A.
When assessing cyanosis, color in peripheral areas such as feet and hands is not as reliable as central areas such as the ears, head, neck, and mucous membranes. Peripheral areas are subject to color changes related to environmental temperature, pain, fear, or vasoconstriction. Central areas such as the ears are less affected by these factors.

40. Correct answer—B.
Uncorrected cyanosis results in polycythemia, brittle hair, dry skin, and clubbed fingers and toes. Rather than becoming obese, most patients with

cyanosis are underweight as a result of increased metabolic demands and decreased caloric intake.

41. Correct answer—B.
Cyanotic lesions associated with decreased pulmonary blood flow need palliation to increase blood flow to the lungs. Pulmonary artery bands are used only for lesions which increase, not decrease, pulmonary flow. Aortoplasty involves treatment of a left-sided heart valve, not associated with tetralogy of Fallot which primarily affects the right heart. Intubation and oxygenation are not likely to significantly improve oxygenation in a lesion which obstructs the flow of blood to the lungs as it tries to get oxygenated. Intubation and oxygenation would only be short-term treatments.

42. Correct answer—D.
A hypercyanotic, or tet, spell occurs when the pulmonary vascular resistance rises and the systemic vascular resistance falls. Because blood will shunt to the lower pressure system, unoxygenated blood flows back out to the body without passing through the lungs for reoxygenation. As carbon dioxide levels rise and oxygen levels fall, the pulmonary vasculature further constricts, exacerbating the shunting.

43. Correct answer—D.
Nitroprusside decreases systemic vascular resistance directly, which would increase right-to-left shunting and further exacerbate the hypercyanosis. Hypercyanotic spells can be effectively treated with a knee-chest or squatting position, because this position increases systemic vascular resistance, therefore decreasing the shunting from the high-pressure pulmonary system. Morphine may be effective because it stops hyperpnea and calms the infant. Sodium bicarbonate can help reduce acidosis and therefore reduce pulmonary hypertension to decrease right-to-left shunting.

44. Correct answer—B.
Stenosis is a problem with valve opening. The aortic valve should open during systole. Therefore, aortic stenosis is a systolic murmur. The aortic valve is best auscultated at the base of the heart, the 3rd right intercostal space.

45. Correct answer—A.
A patent ductus arteriosus produces a continuous machinerylike murmur heard best at the base. Small PDAs may be asymptomatic, but large PDAs result in significant left-to-right shunting which can cause symptoms of congestive heart failure.

46. Correct answer—A.
Cardiogenic shock results from poor pumping of the heart. Afterload and preload are increased as a result of poor pumping action, but these are results, not causes, of cardiogenic shock. While catecholamines are essential

for compensation during shock, inadequate body supplies do not cause cardiogenic shock.

47. Correct answer—C.
Chronotropic agents are used to increase heart rate, while inotropic agents are used to increase the force of contraction. Adrenergic and vasoactive drugs can increase blood pressure, while vasodilators decrease afterload.

48. Correct answer—B.
An infant or child will show signs of hypovolemic shock when fluid loss approaches 7% to 10% of body weight. Infants and children have a larger percentage of extracellular fluid than older children and adolescents who can only lose 5% to 7% of their body weight in fluid.

49. Correct answer—A.
Positive patient outcomes in treating hypovolemic shock would *not* include sunken fontanels which indicate continued hypovolemia. A CVP of 8 and a wedge pressure of 12 indicate adequate circulating volume. Warm, dry skin indicates adequate peripheral circulation reflecting adequate circulating volume.

50. Correct answer—C.
For the child in hypovolemic shock from gastrointestinal fluid losses, the preferred intravenous fluid to maximally increase the intravascular volume is an isotonic crystalloid such as 0.9% normal saline. Dextrose 5% in water and 0.45% normal saline physiologically are hypotonic solutions which move rapidly into the cells, doing little to improve intravascular volume. 7% normal saline is a hypertonic solution which may cause hypernatremia and has not been proven to be more effective than conventional methods of fluid resuscitation.

51. Correct answer—C.
The combination of fluid therapy which is usually most effective in treating hypovolemic shock is crystalloids and colloids. Crystalloids alone do not stay in the vascular space very long. More than 90% may have moved to extravascular spaces in as little as 30 minutes. Even 75% of colloidal solutions leave the vascular space in a few hours. Using crystalloids to restore total body fluid deficits in combination with colloidal solutions which will help draw the fluid into the vascular space is the most effective therapy. Blood replacement is only indicated if blood has been lost.

52. Correct answer—B.
All forms of shock have in common an insufficient tissue perfusion. Decreased cardiac output and renal perfusion may characterize hypovolemic, hemorrhagic, and cardiogenic shock, but increased cardiac output and renal perfusion may be seen in septic shock. Massive vasodilation may also be seen in septic shock, but vasoconstriction is seen in hemorrhagic, hypovolemic, and cardiogenic shock.

53. Correct answer—D.
Hypocalcemia is most likely to develop following multiple transfusions because the preservatives in blood bind ionized calcium leading to decreased levels and clinical symptoms. Hypernatremia and hypokalemia would be unrelated to transfusions; however, hyperkalemia can be associated with stored blood from hemolysis. Phosphate levels tend to move reciprocally with calcium levels, so hyperphosphatemia would be expected with hypocalcemia.

54. Correct answer—C.
Parasympathetic stimulation to the cardiovascular system would produce bradycardia and vasodilation. Unlike the sympathetic nervous system which produces adrenergic responses ("fight or flight"), the parasympathetic system slows heart rate and decreases arterial pressure. Tachycardia, increased systemic vascular resistance, and vasoconstriction would characterize sympathetic stimulation.

55. Correct answer—D.
Tricuspid insufficiency would affect right-sided, pulmonary, and systemic venous pressures. Body surface area, fear, age, blood volume, sodium retention, and heart rate are some of the factors which directly affect arterial pressure.

56. Correct answer—A.
Mean arterial pressure is affected by cardiac output and systemic vascular resistance. Right-sided pressures such as the systemic venous pressure, pulmonary vascular resistance, and pulmonary venous pressures do not directly affect mean arterial pressure, a left-sided pressure.

57. Correct answer—D.
Fetal exposure to alcohol and drugs can have teratogenic effects on fetal cardiac development. However, most congenital cardiac defects are multifactorial in cause. This means no single cause can be determined, but a genetic predisposition and an environmental trigger together probably caused the cardiac maldevelopment. Family history of coronary heart disease or cholesterol ingestion during pregnancy are unrelated to *anatomical or structural* heart disease. Maternal allergies are also not a known risk factor.

58. Correct answer—B.
Inspiration increases venous return (right-sided heart function) and preload by decreasing intrathoracic pressure and drawing venous blood into the heart. Inspiration has no direct effect on ejection fraction or afterload (left-sided heart factor).

59. Correct answer—B.
Vasodilating agents decrease afterload by reducing the pressure that the left side of the heart has to pump against. Aortic valvular stenosis and vasoconstricting agents increase afterload by increasing the force the left ventricle must generate to pump against an increased pressure or obstruction. Polycythemia increases afterload because increased viscosity makes more force necessary to move the blood.

60. Correct answer—B.

Pulsus paradoxus is characterized by a fall of greater than 10 mm Hg arterial pressure during inspiration. Only a decrease of less than 10 mm Hg pressure is normal during inspiration. Alternating strong and weak pulses characterize pulsus alterans. Weak pulses in the presence of normal or increased intravascular volume can indicate coarctation of the aorta, cardiac tamponade, ventricular dysfunction, and hypotension. Weak lower extremity pulses with high blood pressure would be suggestive of coarctation of the aorta.

61. Correct answer—A.

The bell of the stethoscope is used to auscultate low-pitched sounds such as ventricular filling pressure murmurs like S_3 and S_4. The diaphragm of the stethoscope is used to hear high-pitched murmurs, stenotic valvular murmurs, and ejection clicks.

62. Correct answer—B.

Press lightly on the bell to best hear low-pitched sounds. Pressing firmly will not more effectively avoid environmental noise but will actually cause the bell to function as a diaphragm. Holding the bell barely off the chest wall will only pick up grade VI/VI murmurs. No particular technique of holding the stethoscope within your grasp is more effective.

63. Correct answer—C.

Doppler echocardiography allows visualization of blood flow and velocities. Chest x-rays may show increased pulmonary vascularity from increased blood flow associated with a PDA, but this would be a later finding. An electrocardiogram would be able to identify ventricular hypertrophy which might accompany a PDA, but would also be a late finding. Magnetic resonance imaging visualizes structures, but not blood flow.

64. Correct answer—C.

This is a rhythm strip demonstrating complete heart block. Note the regularity of P-waves and QRS complexes, but also the failure of P-waves to pace the ventricles. This is also a very bradycardiac rate. Vagal maneuvers and verapamil are indicated in treating supraventricular tachycardias, not bradycardias. Atropine, not isuprel is the first-line drug of choice.

65. Correct answer—B.

Mitral stenosis would produce a diastolic murmur. Stenosis is a problem with valves opening, and the mitral valve opens during diastole. Both mitral and tricuspid stenosis as well as aortic and pulmonic insufficiency could cause diastolic murmurs. Systolic murmurs could include aortic and pulmonic stenosis as well as mitral and tricuspid insufficiency.

66. Correct answer—B.

Left atrial and pulmonary capillary wedge pressures would be increased in mitral stenosis. These pressures reflect the backup of blood because the left atrioventricular valve does not open effectively. Right atrial and central venous pressures would be elevated in tricuspid stenosis. Left ventricular pressure would be elevated if there were a distal obstruction such as aortic stenosis or coarctation. Elevation in systemic pressure would likely be seen only in a systemic obstruction such as coarctation or interrupted aortic arch.

67. Correct answer—C.

Advantages of magnetic resonance imaging of the heart include that it is safe for pregnant women and children, that there is no need for contrast or ionizing radiation, and that it defines anatomy well, including three-dimensional imaging. Because MRI uses magnets, it is not safe for patients with pacemakers.

68. Correct answer—A.

Prostaglandin E_1 therapy would be most helpful in treating pulmonary atresia by keeping the ductus patent. Because pulmonary atresia does not allow blood to leave the right ventricle and therefore causes poor or absent pulmonary blood flow, a ductus arteriosus is necessary to have a pathway for blood to reach the lungs. A PDA acts as a systemic-to-pulmonary shunt providing pulmonary blood flow. Atrioventricular canal, truncus arteriosus, and patent ductus arteriosus are all lesions that already cause too much pulmonary blood flow through left-to-right shunting.

69. Correct answer—D.

All chest tube systems have a collection chamber, water seal, and suction-control chamber regardless of the specific type or manufacturer's product used. Although bubbling can occur in the water seal chamber, there is no collector for bubbles. Venting of the water seal chamber is necessary, but there is no specific bottle for the purpose of ventilating.

70. Correct answer—C.

Hypoglycemia, hypoxia, and electrolyte imbalances all are possible causes of premature ventricular complexes. Fever, crying, and pain usually cause tachycardia, not premature ventricular complexes. Increased parasympathetic tone causes bradycardia, not ventricular ectopy. Increased arterial pressure is also not usually associated with ectopy.

71. Correct answer—D.

Indications for the use of an umbilical artery catheter include frequent blood gas monitoring, meconium aspiration, surfactant deficiency, congenital cardiac defects, diaphragmatic hernia, persistent pulmonary hypertension, and severe illness.

72. Correct answer—B.

An umbilical vein catheter can be used to monitor central venous pressure. Arterial blood pressure is measured by arterial catheters, or possible umbilical artery catheters. Left atrial pressure is monitored by direct LA lines placed intraoperatively following open heart surgery. Left filling pressures are monitored by the pulmonary artery wedge pressure in the absence of valvular disease.

73. Correct answer—A.
In fetal circulation, the umbilical vein carries oxygenated blood to the right atrium where it mixes with venous blood returning from the fetus. The right atrium, therefore, receives oxygenated blood from the placenta via the vena cava as well as unoxygenated blood from the fetal venous system in order to contain mixed blood. The umbilical arteries carry mixed blood back to the placenta from the left side of the heart (aorta).

74. Correct answer—A.
An umbilical artery line would measure systemic arterial pressures. Central venous pressures could be monitored by an umbilical venous catheter and pulmonary pressures by a pulmonary artery catheter. Renal pressures are not monitored.

75. Correct answer—A.
A patient on prostaglandin E_1 therapy is at risk for apnea, hypotension, and fever. Prostaglandin E_1 is used to treat alterations in tissue perfusion, but is not a cause of this. Ineffective airway clearance is related to an inability to clear secretions, not a problem related to Prostaglandin E_1 therapy.

76. Correct answer—C.
For a full-term infant with hyperbilirubinemia of 15 mg/dL, phototherapy should be instituted. While her levels would decrease with hemodilution, this does not remove total body levels of bilirubin and risks fluid overload. Exchange transfusions are not indicted until a full-term infant's bilirubin level rises above 20 mg/dL.

77. Correct answer—B.
Phototherapy lights should be turned off during sampling to avoid exposure of the blood sample to the lights, which could alter results. Discontinuing the lights for 1 hour before sampling would be contraindicated because it would interfere with therapy. Bilirubin levels are unaffected by the location of the sampling or its relationship to feeding.

78. Correct answer—A.
To avoid the most common problems during an exchange transfusion, the blood pressure and cardiac rhythm need to be closely monitored. Because blood volume is being taken off and replaced, fluctuations in blood pressure can occur. Banked blood can be high in potassium and contains preservatives which can lead to hypocalcemia, causing cardiac dysrhythmias as potential complications. A fall in urinary output would not be routinely anticipated unless cardiac output and renal perfusion fell greatly. Improvements in neurological status will not occur quickly enough to be seen during the exchange, nor would a deterioration in status be expected.

79. Correct answer—A.
An appropriate nursing diagnosis related to the complications would be the potential for decreased cardiac output related to changes in intravascular

volume and electrolytes. Alterations in elimination and hypothermia would not commonly be encountered complications for which the nurse should be actively anticipating. Decreased surfactant production is unrelated to an exchange transfusion, but rather to respiratory distress syndrome.

80. Correct answer—C.
Following exchange transfusion therapy the most appropriate patient outcome would be absence of opisthotonic posturing. This posturing, along with a poor Moro reflex, is seen in hyperbilirubinemia, reflecting the deleterious effect high bilirubin levels have on the newborn. Babinski and extrusion reflexes are normally present in the neonatal period, developing in the fetus at about 28 weeks gestation.

81. Correct answer—B.
Patients in respiratory distress related to increased pulmonary blood flow and elevated pulmonary pressures should be positioned with their head elevated to increase their vital capacity. This position helps the lungs have more room to expand because abdominal contents including an enlarged liver will impinge less on the lungs' space. This position has minimal effects on peripheral perfusion, which in turn does not affect respiratory distress. The work of breathing is not decreased by this position, nor is cardiac output significantly affected.

82. Correct answer—C.
This strip represents supraventricular tachycardia. No P-waves are readily identifiable, and conclusive evidence of a junctional rhythm is not discernible. The narrow QRS complex is inconsistent with ventricular tachycardia.

83. Correct answer—C.
Assessment findings of tachypnea, tachycardia, and respiratory distress all represent congestive heart failure. Differential cyanosis is a difference in coloring between the upper extremities (acyanotic) and lower extremities (cyanotic), commonly seen in coarctation of the aorta. Persistent pulmonary hypertension, diaphragmatic hernia, and transient tachypnea of the newborn would be associated with generalized cyanosis.

84. Correct answer—B.
Therapeutic digoxin levels vary among institutions, but generally fall in the range of 1.1 to 2.2 ng/mL. Levels greater than 3.5 ng/mL are toxic, and levels lower than 1.1 ng/mL are generally not effective.

85. Correct answer—C.
For the patient with a ductal-dependent lesion on prostaglandin E_1, the critical care nurse would assess for a continuous murmur at the base—not apex—of the heart. This murmur is consistent with a *patent* ductus arteriosus which would provide critical blood flow in a ductal-dependent lesion such as coarctation of the aorta, hypoplastic left heart syndrome, pulmonary atresia, critical pulmonary stenosis, and tricuspid atresia. Presence of peripheral pulses are

important, but not as critical as maintaining pulmonary blood flow. Presence of a fixed, split S_2 indicates increased right ventricular volume or resistance to ejection, mitral regurgitation, and prolonged pulmonary closure.

86. Correct answer—B.
Prostaglandin E_1 may be used to improve blood flow and oxygenation in lesions where the ductus is needed to assure blood flow to either the pulmonary or the systemic circulation. Systemic circulation is dependent upon flow through the ductus in hypoplastic left heart syndrome, whereas pulmonary circulation is dependent upon the ductus in pulmonary atresia. Atrioventricular canal usually results in increased pulmonary blood flow and adequate systemic flow without the need for ductal flow. Aortic insufficiency does not obstruct systemic or pulmonary blood flow.

87. Correct answer—A.
Normal total calcium levels for children are 8.8 to 10.8 mg/dL and for newborns 9.0 to 10.6 mg/dL. These clinical findings represent hypocalcemia and increased peripheral vascular resistance secondary to decreased cardiac output. Calcium chloride is the drug of choice to improve cardiac output in the presence of hypocalcemia. Calcium gluconate provides less ionized calcium, which is the active form the body uses. Dobutamine and dopamine do not address the primary problem of decreased cardiac output.

88. Correct answer—D.
The most important *immediate* nursing action would be to assess the patency of the Prostaglandin E_1 infusion. If the tube were displaced or its patency compromised, bilateral breath sounds would not be audible. Increasing the FiO_2 would not be indicated for an unknown precipitous drop in pulse oximetry readings.

89. Correct answer—B.
For the shock patient who is hypotensive, amrinone and dobutamine may further exacerbate the low pressure. Isuprel also produces peripheral dilation and may exacerbate hypotension as well. While all these drugs can increase tachycardia, epinephrine will have the most positive effect on hypotension by increasing systemic vascular resistance.

PEDIATRIC-SPECIFIC ANSWERS

90. Correct answer—B.
Symptoms of a patch leak would be similar to symptoms of a VSD: systolic murmur, congestive heart failure, and tachypnea. Mottling indicates poor cardiac output.

91. Correct answer—B.
Only an echocardiogram would allow direct imaging of blood shunting through the leak. Changes in the electrocardiogram or chest x-ray would be

seen much later. CT scans would not be helpful for most patch leaks because they cannot dynamically record blood flow.

92. Correct answer—A.
A ventricular septal defect over time will cause hypertrophy of one or both ventricles as a result of the increased workload. If a large VSD is left unrepaired, pulmonary hypertension may occur and be irreversible. A VSD results in increased pulmonary blood flow and would not be related to systemic hypertension or AV malformations.

93. Correct answer—A.
Due to the poor cardiac output and perfusion associated with congestive heart failure, both urinary and cardiac outputs drop, the heart enlarges to accommodate increased volume, and the liver enlarges because of systemic venous engorgement.

94. Correct answer—C.
An adrenergic response to congestive heart failure is manifested by tachycardia, tachypnea, cool skin, diaphoresis, and oliguria. These are a result of the body's attempt to increase cardiac output, conserve fluid, and shunt blood to essential organs. Therefore urinary output decreases and blood shunted away from the skin to vital organs leaves it moist and cool. Poor feeding is a manifestation of fatigue, not autonomic system response.

95. Correct answer—D.
The goals of treatment in congestive heart failure include decrease in systemic venous congestion leading to reduced liver size, adequate systemic perfusion resulting in adequate urinary output, and a *decrease* in pulmonary pressures, which will help resolve pulmonary edema and crackles.

96. Correct answer—D.
The most likely cause of these symptoms is congestive heart failure. Hypovolemic shock would not increase liver size or produce respiratory symptoms. Acute renal failure is unlikely in the presence of a low blood urea nitrogen (BUN) and no elevation in the creatinine. Pneumonia is unlikely to cause hepatomegaly.

97. Correct answer—B.
The first intervention the nurse should perform for this patient is to assess airway, breathing, and circulation. This patient is showing problems with all these vital functions with symptoms of respiratory distress and inadequate cardiac output. Arterial blood gases may need to be drawn, oxygen therapy may be indicated, and cardiac monitoring should be instituted. However, these should not be done before her airway, breathing, and circulation are assessed and protected as needed.

98. Correct answer—C.
Echocardiography would be most helpful in confirming her diagnosis, because it can measure ejection fraction as well as evaluate ventricular size and function.

MRI is helpful in determining anatomy, but would not be helpful in assessment of dynamic function. An electrocardiogram would show ventricular hypertrophy, but it also offers little information regarding function. Stress testing is not used to diagnose congestive heart failure.

99. Correct answer—A.

A desired outcome in treating this patient includes that the liver is palpable <2 to 3 cm below the costal margin, not more descended from hepatic engorgement. Hypotension is not associated with her congestive heart failure, so an increase in systemic arterial pressure is not sought. Congestive heart failure is not an infectious process, and no rise in serum creatinine occurs unless severe renal dysfunction occurs.

100. Correct answer—C.

A temperature elevation >38.5°C, leukocytosis >12,000/cm^3, elevation in the ESR >50 mm/hr, pericardial friction rub, effusions in the pericardial sac or the pleural space, and respiratory distress are all consistent with postpericardiotomy syndrome. Speculated to be an autoimmune or inflammatory response following open-heart surgery, postpericardiotomy syndrome is treated with general supportive care and antiinflammatory medications such as aspirin, ibuprofen, or steroids. Viral pneumonia, respiratory syncytial virus, and isolated pericarditis would not be likely to cause pleural effusions.

101. Correct answer—B.

In temporary transvenous endocardial pacing, the catheter is properly placed in the right atrium or right ventricle. However, when complete heart block is present, only the ventricle will provide an appropriate heart rate. The left side of the heart cannot easily be reached from a transvenous approach. Neither the SA nor AV nodes are stimulated for pacing, but rather atrial or ventricular tissue directly.

102. Correct answer—D.

Seizures would not be an expected complication related to pacemaker insertion. Complications associated with transvenous lead placement include hemorrhage from cardiac or vessel trauma, air embolism, and poor pacemaker function. Hiccups are a potential complication if the pacing catheter actually stimulates the diaphragm.

103. Correct answer—A.

When a pacemaker is set on the demand mode, but is failing to sense, this means the pacemaker is unaware of the heart's own intrinsic beats. If the pacemaker is unaware of the heart's own beats, it will stimulate an impulse according to the rate that is set. Without coordinating pacemaker generated beats with the heart's own intrinsic beats, there is a risk that a paced beat will fall on the T-wave and produce serious ventricular dysrhythmias. The pacemaker that does not sense the heart's own beats will generate its own beats according to the set rate and not fail to generate any beats at all. When a pacemaker signals, but fails to generate as beats occur, this is from fibrosis of the catheter, battery failure, fracture of pacing wires, or poor catheter placement. Although catheters can puncture the heart and cause bleeding, this is not a problem associated with failure to sense.

104. Correct answer—B.
This rhythm strip demonstrates failure to capture. When a pacemaker fails to capture, a pacing spike is seen but no cardiac activity follows. Failure to sense is when the pacing spikes are seen despite an adequate intrinsic cardiac rate. Failure to discharge or pace means an absence of pacer spikes.

105. Correct answer—A.
The clinical symptoms of fever, skin rash, proteinuria, cervical lymphadenitis, reddening of lips and buccal mucosa, conjunctivitis, and erythema as well as pain of the hands and feet are indicative of Kawasaki's disease. Laboratory findings include elevations in his C-reactive protein and erythrocyte sedimentation rate in addition to thrombocytosis. Myocarditis is a common complication of this disease. Endocarditis is an infection of the lining of the heart and is commonly associated with congenital cardiac or valvular defects. Hepatitis and glomerulonephritis would not produce these specific physical assessment findings.

106. Correct answer—D.
A common manifestation of myocarditis in Kawasaki's disease is the development of coronary artery aneurysms. Right ventricular hypertrophy is associated with such congenital cardiac defects as tetralogy of Fallot and pulmonary stenosis. Hypertrophic cardiomyopathy affects the heart in general, while it is primarily the coronary arteries that are affected by Kawasaki's disease. Aortic stenosis is often seen with endocarditis.

107. Correct answer—A.
A sudden drop in diastolic pressure from 10 mm Hg to 2 mm Hg in a pulmonary artery catheter is most likely caused by slipping of the catheter tip back to the right ventricle. Balloon rupture in pulmonary artery catheter would prevent the critical care nurse from obtaining a wedge pressure but would not cause a change in diastolic pressure. Clot formation at the catheter tip and blood in the transducer would produce a dampened waveform.

108. Correct answer—D.
A SvO_2 reading of 88% following repair of a ventricular septal defect indicates left-to-right shunting and a probable patch leak or residual VSD. Never flush a pulmonary catheter line by hand—always use the transducer. Inflating the balloon and recording the reading at end expiration is appropriate when obtaining a wedge pressure, not a mixed venous saturation. Decreasing the FiO_2 to

21% could seriously jeopardize oxygenation and acid-base balance and should not be attempted based on mixed venous gases in the presence of a possible left-to-right shunt.

109. Correct answer—B.

Myocarditis often presents following a flulike illness. Common symptoms include dysrhythmias, pericardial effusion, nonspecific ST-segment changes, and a decrease in QRS and T-wave voltage. Often signs and symptoms of shock accompany myocarditis, depending upon the amount of cardiac dysfunction. Hypertrophic cardiomyopathy would be identifiable by echocardiogram as structural heart disease and not accompanied by symptoms of bacterial or viral illness. Endocarditis would not be likely to show electrocardiogram (ECG) changes, but vegetative growths are often easily visualized by echocardiography. Kawasaki's disease usually shows flattening of T-waves and has more specific clinical manifestations of the illness such as erythema and pain in hands and feet.

110. Correct answer—A.

A left-sided vegetative growth can produce systemic emboli which may cause renal artery occlusion, stroke, and arthralgia depending upon where the emboli travel. Pulmonary embolization would occur with a right heart vegetative growth.

111. Correct answer—A.

A finding of orthopnea and dyspnea would be a priority in assessing any patient. Critical assessment and interventions always begin with airway, then breathing, and finally circulation.

112. Correct answer—B.

These symptoms, particularly the narrow pulse pressure, all represent cardiac tamponade. Her history of recent open-heart surgery indicates her risk factor for developing pericarditis with effusion. Although these other interventions may be indicated, immediate relief of the constriction caused by the tamponade must be accomplished.

113. Correct answer—C.

A child with structural heart disease is at highest risk for developing infective endocarditis. Particularly high risk is associated with a VSD, pulmonic stenosis, tetralogy of Fallot, coarctation of the aorta, and transposition of the great vessels.

114. Correct answer—B.

Chest pain associated with Kawasaki's disease could indicate myocardial infarction. Dilated coronary arteries are at risk for thrombosing leading to coronary occlusion and tissue ischemia or necrosis. ST-segment changes can indicate ischemia or infarction. Analgesics for chest pain would not be indicated until the cause has been determined as it could mask a critical symptom. Gamma globulin needs to be administered early in the disease, not in response to development of chest pain. Chest pain associated with pericarditis is usually relieved by sitting up and forward.

115. Correct answer—C.
Propranolol may be effective in reducing ventricular outflow obstruction or myocardial oxygen demands in the child with HOCM (IHSS). Digoxin is contraindicated because it may actually worsen outflow tract obstruction. Diuretics are to be avoided because they may significantly reduce left ventricular preload thereby reducing cardiac output. Tolazoline is a beta-adrenergic blocking agent, which could further reduce cardiac output.

116. Correct answer—A.
For children over 10 years of age, the digitalizing dose is 8 to 12 mcg/kg. Higher digitalizing doses are required in younger patients. Preterm infants, however, require lower doses than full-term infants as a result of their less efficient renal function. Because infants have more red blood cells than older children, there are more binding sites for digoxin requiring higher doses.

117. Correct answer—D.
In digoxin toxicity, the ECG may show depressed ST-segments and prolongation of the PR interval.

118. Correct answer—A.
While all of these are signs and symptoms of digoxin toxicity, bradycardia and other dysrhythmias are the most common in children.

119. Correct answer—B.
The *first* appropriate intervention for the child in ventricular fibrillation is defibrillation at 2 joules/kg. If this is ineffective, defibrillation may be repeated at 4 joules/kg. Synchronized cardioversion is only indicated in supraventricular tachycardias or ventricular tachycardia with a pulse.

120. Correct answer—B.
Elevated CPK-MB and LDH_1 are indicative of myocardial tissue damage. CPK-MM may be elevated in association with any trauma. LDH_5 indicates liver and muscle damage.

121. Correct answer—D.
Cardiac trauma can be manifested by ST elevations or depressions and T-wave inversions which indicate ischemia or infarction as well as tachycardia which is a compensation for cardiac muscle dysfunction. T-wave elevations or tented T-waves may indicate hyperkalemia.

122. Correct answer—D.
Amrinone would be expected to improve cardiac function best in this child because it would increase cardiac output and stroke volume, reduce filling and wedge pressures, and reduce afterload. Both dopamine and epinephrine would not be as helpful because they would cause an increase in systemic vascular resistance and afterload thus increasing left ventricular workload, and exacerbate tachycardia. Nitroprusside would reduce afterload and left

ventricular work, but it can increase heart rate and further decrease cardiac output.

123. Correct answer—C.
An amrinone infusion should be slowed or stopped and the physician notified if dysrhythmias develop. It is used to treat elevations in pulmonary capillary wedge pressure, decreased cardiac output, and increased ventricular filling pressures.

124. Correct answer—A.
Treatment of digoxin toxicity and supraventricular tachydysrhythmias would include enhancement of digoxin excretion, phenytoin to reduce automaticity, and prevention of drug absorption. Synchronized cardioversion in the presence of digoxin toxicity could cause a deterioration of the rhythm to a more lethal rhythm-like ventricular fibrillation.

125. Correct answer—C.
Nitroprusside, nitroglycerin, reserpine, diazoxide, hydralazine, and propranolol are all commonly used to treat hypertensive crises in children. These medications all have a direct dilatory effect on venous and/or arterial vessels. Although dobutamine decreases systemic vascular resistance, it would not be used to treat hypertension.

NEONATAL-SPECIFIC ANSWERS

126. Correct answer—D.
The most common signs and symptoms of digoxin toxicity in infants are lethargy and drowsiness. Nausea, vomiting, diarrhea, and dysrhythmias may also occur. Seizures would not be expected in digoxin toxicity.

127. Correct answer—C.
The incidence of patent ductus arteriosus is related to gestational age and birth weight. Incidence is highest in premature infants weighing less than 1 kilogram.

128. Correct answer—C.
For a newborn infant with hypoplastic left heart syndrome, a drastic rise in PO_2 will increase acidosis. Because oxygen is a potent pulmonary vasodilator, a rise in PO_2 will dilate pulmonary vessels and further increase pulmonary flow at the expense of systemic flow. Because systemic flow will be decreased, systemic acidosis will increase. These infants are best maintained on room air, ventilated, and on prostaglandin E_1.

129. Correct answer—A.
In a shunt study, the arterial oxygen levels are compared between room air and after 5 to 10 minutes on 100% O_2. For a cyanotic infant with a right-to-left cardiac shunting defect, the P_aO_2 will change little even with oxygenation at an

FiO_2 of 1.0. If oxygen levels improve with 100% O_2, then the cause of cyanosis is most likely pulmonary. An atrioventricular canal defect is generally a left-to-right shunt and would not be associated with cyanosis.

130. Correct answer—B.

The newborn is not greatly able to increase cardiac output because of immaturity of the development of sympathetic innervation of the heart. Sympathetic innervation of the heart is responsible in part for increased heart rate and stroke volume. Parasympathetic innervation plays no role in increasing cardiac output. Both great vessel size and the aortic valve are appropriately mature in a normal newborn to function effectively in delivering blood flow and maintaining systolic or diastolic pressures.

131. Correct answer—C.

Factors that are responsible for failure to thrive in a neonate with a congenital cardiac defect include an increase in the basal metabolic rate related to increased ventricular work, respiratory distress related to congestive heart failure, and decreased caloric intake related to fatigue during feeding. Catecholamine depletion is not a factor.

132. Correct answer—B.

Digoxin would be used with caution in the neonate with severe tetralogy of Fallot because it could increase right outflow tract obstruction by increasing the force of myocardial contraction. Propranolol is often used to treat hyperdynamic obstructive lesions to decrease the impediment to flow. Furosemide would be appropriate to treat congestive heart failure, and prostaglandins would help maintain ductal flow and increase systemic oxygenation.

133. Correct answer—D.

These clinical findings, especially the presence of pulses (such as the calf pulses, which usually are not present), indicate a patent ductus arteriosus. A rapid upstroke and wide pulse pressure related to the PDA cause hyperdynamic and easily palpable peripheral pulses. A large VSD or total anomalous pulmonary venous return would result in increased pulmonary flow, but not accentuated peripheral pulses. Premature closure of the ductus arteriosus occurs in utero.

CHAPTER 2

Pulmonary Care Problems

Passkeys

GENERAL PRINCIPLES OF PULMONOLOGY

Pediatric and neonatal lungs are different from adult lungs in the following ways:

- Lungs require longer gestation time to form than other body systems. They are not capable of gas exchange until about 22 to 24 weeks gestation. See normal lung anatomy in Fig. 2-1.
- The actual number of alveoli increase after birth and continue until adulthood.
- The chest wall in older children and adults is relatively rigid; however, in infants it is very flexible. Intercostal muscles stabilize the chest wall. Contraction of the diaphragm with respiratory dysfunction actually leads to retractions of intercostal spaces and sternum, which further impairs inflation of the lungs. (See Fig. 2-2.)
- Pediatric arrests usually occur from primary respiratory or shock problems, not cardiac arrest.
- Acute disease of the respiratory tract is the most common cause of illness in infancy and childhood.

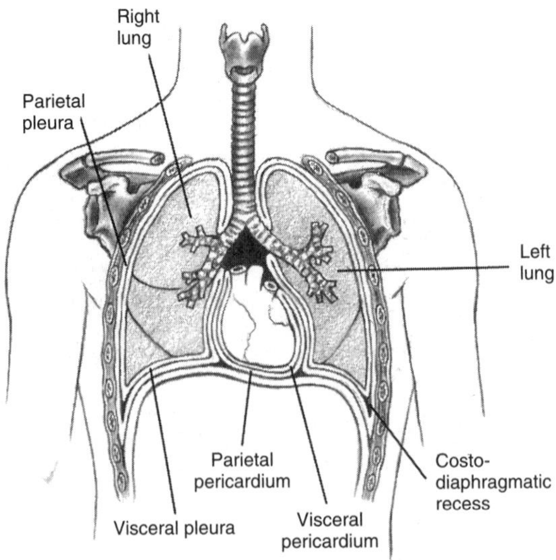

Fig. 2-1 Chest cavity and related structures, anterior view. (From Thompson JM and others: Mosby's clinical nursing, ed 3, St Louis, 1993, Mosby.)

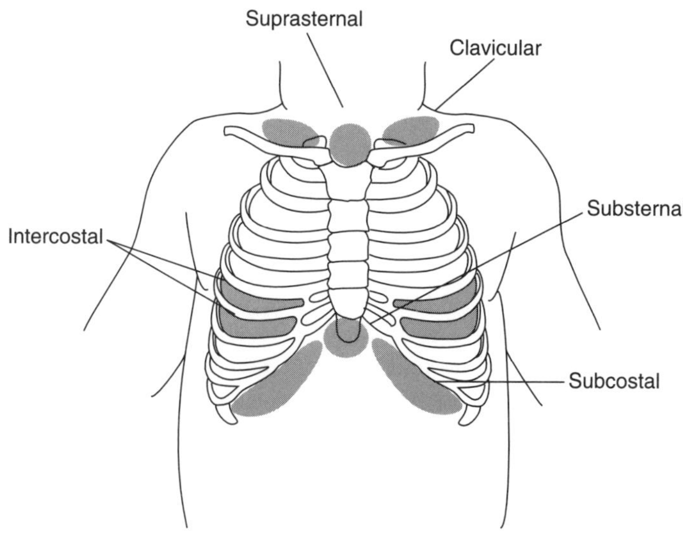

Fig. 2-2 Location of retractions. (From Wong DL: Whaley and Wong's nursing care of infants and children, ed 5, St Louis, 1995, Mosby.)

- Fetal pulmonary vascular resistance (PVR) is high. Within 24 hours after birth, PVR normally falls to ½ systemic vascular resistance (SVR). It reaches adult levels within weeks after birth.

- Neonates breathe through their noses rather than their mouths. Insertion of nasogastric tube can compromise ventilatory efforts.

- Alveolar hypoxia promotes pulmonary vasoconstriction, which in turn leads to more hypoxemia. Use of oxygen therapy is important to prevent pulmonary vascular reactivity leading to pulmonary hypertension and persistent fetal circulation. Oxygen demand and therefore cardiac output is highest at birth, rapidly decreasing in the first 8 weeks (to ½ at birth) and then tapering more gradually.

- Respiratory alkalosis in infants and children is unusual. Most often it results from hyperventilation (crying) or mechanical ventilation. Organic problems leading to respiratory alkalosis may be CNS injury, aspirin ingestion, Reye's syndrome, and hepatic encephalopathy.

- Respiratory acidosis may result from sedation, obstruction, or muscle weakness.

- Muscles in the lower airways are underdeveloped in infants, which causes a greater susceptibility to collapse.

- A respiratory rate within age appropriate limits in a stressed, ill, or injured infant or child is *not* normal. This can be a sign of impending arrest.

Ventilation-Perfusion Association

- Ventilation-Perfusion (V/Q) ratio describes the relationship between pulmonary perfusion (blood flow through the lungs that comes in contact with alveoli) and pulmonary ventilation (aerated alveoli).
- The normal V/Q ratio is 0.8, which reflects slightly more blood flow than aerated alveoli.
- A decrease in the V/Q ratio indicates decreased ventilation in relation to perfusion. This decreased V/Q is seen with atelectasis, respiratory distress syndrome (RDS), pneumothorax, aspiration pneumonia, asthma, epiglottis, pleural effusion, and other conditions that increase physiologic dead space.
- An increase in the V/Q ratio indicates a decrease in perfusion in relation to ventilation. This increase in V/Q may be seen with severe pulmonary stenosis, tricuspid atresia, severe right ventricular outflow tract obstruction, pulmonary emboli, and cardiogenic shock.

Maturational Development of the Lungs

- Alveolar sacs are not formed until 22 to 24 weeks gestation. Only then do the critical elements required for gas exchange develop.
- Before 22 to 24 weeks gestation the fetal lungs are unable to support life as a result of inadequate development.
- By 34 to 36 weeks gestation the fetal lungs are developed enough to avoid the development of idiopathic respiratory distress syndrome (hyaline membrane disease).

Principles of Oxygen and Respiratory Therapy

- The goal of oxygen therapy is to increase oxygen delivery. Nursing interventions need to include strategies to reduce oxygen demand such as preventing elevations in temperature, decreasing stress, treating pain, avoiding shivering, and conserving energy.
- Compliance is an important concept in lung distensibility and inflation. It is decreased in respiratory distress syndrome, pulmonary edema, pneumonia, pneumothorax, hemothorax, atelectasis, and pulmonary fibrosis.
- Lung compliance is directly related to age—the younger the age, the lower the compliance.
- Lung compliance is determined by surfactant and elasticity of lung tissue.

- Oxygen in a mild to moderate *intracardiac* shunt (right-to-left—O_2 arterial oxygen saturations of 85% to 90%) is usually not helpful. However, oxygen in a severe shunt (60% to 75% arterial oxygen saturations) may be helpful.

- Oxygen therapy is effective in a patient with an *intrapulmonary* shunt.

- Normal physiologic shunting results from the fact that the upper lobes of the lungs are better aerated and the lower lobes are better perfused. The matchup between lung aeration and lung perfusion is not perfect (normal V/Q ratio is $\frac{4}{5}$ or 0.8).

- Physiologic shunting results in hypoxemia, but not hypercapnia because CO_2 diffuses much more easily than O_2.

- Physiologic shunting can be from atelectasis, edema, pneumonia, pneumothorax, and other conditions that decrease aerated alveoli.

- Alveolar respiration is influenced by both chemical and neural factors. Chemical factors are the CO_2 centers in the brainstem and O_2 sensors in the carotid bodies. Neural factors include parasympathetic and sympathetic innervation and respiratory centers in the brain.

- Normal A-a (arterial-alveolar) O_2 gradient is <50. This calculation is used to estimate hypoxemia and intrapulmonary shunting.

- Positive end expiratory pressure (PEEP) and continuous positive airway pressure (CPAP) help keep alveoli open and move fluids out of the critical alveoli-arterial interface.

Airways

- Overextension or flexion of the neck can cause airway obstruction. An infant's or small child's airway can easily be occluded by hyperextension or flexion of the neck.

- Airways in young children and infants are much smaller than in adults. The presence of mucus or edema causes much greater obstruction in younger patients.

- Airway resistance is increased in asthma, cystic fibrosis, bronchitis, bronchiolitis, bronchopulmonary dysplasia, tracheal stenosis, and increased airway resistance.

- The small airways are predominantly innervated by the parasympathetic (cholinergic) system. The sympathetic system plays a lesser role. Adrenergic substances cause bronchodilation and a decrease in the production of mucus; cholinergic substances cause bronchoconstriction and an increase in the production of secretions.

Ventilation

- Tidal volume = the volume of air inspired and expired during normal breathing.
- Minute ventilation = tidal volume × breaths/min.
- Vital capacity = maximal expiratory volume following maximal inspiration.
- Total lung capacity = amount of air in lungs with maximal inspiration.
- Functional residual capacity = gas in lungs following normal expiration.
- Inspiratory reserve volume = the volume of air that can be inspired after a normal inspiration.
- Expiratory reserve volume = the volume of air that can be expired after a normal expiration.
- Residual volume = the amount of air remaining in the lungs after maximal exhalation.

Dead space:

- Portions of the lungs where no gas exchange is occurring.
- Anatomic dead space in cubic centimeters = weight in pounds.
- Physiologic dead space is where gas exchange should be taking place, but is not.

Intubation

- Intubation should be accomplished early when treating respiratory distress in infants and children.
- Do not use atropine routinely before intubation to avoid vagal-induced bradycardias. Some bradycardias during intubation occur from hypoxemia, and atropine masks this.
- The tip of an endotracheal tube should be no lower than 1 to 2 cm above the carina and no higher than the 1st rib.
- Cuffed endotracheal tubes are not generally used in infants or small children. The cricoid area of the larynx forms a natural seal around the tube in these age groups.

- Size of the endotracheal tube can be estimated by using the infant's or child's little finger as an approximation or by taking the child's age (in years) and dividing by 4 and adding 4:

$$[(age/4) + 4].$$

- Multiply the endotracheal tube size by 2 to pick the correct size suction catheter.

Oxyhemoglobin Dissociation

Fig. 2-3 shows the relationship between oxygen affinity and changes in blood pH.

- A shift to the right in the oxyhemoglobin dissociation curve means that hemoglobin will more readily give up the oxygen it holds. This process is seen in hyperthermia, acidosis, and hypercapnia.

- A shift to the left in the oxyhemoglobin dissociation curve means that hemoglobin will hold onto oxygen more tightly. This process is seen in hypothermia, alkalosis, and hypocapnia.

- Fetal hemoglobin naturally is "shifted to the left" compared with adult hemoglobin. Fetal hemoglobin disappears by 4 to 6 weeks of age.

Respiratory Failure

- Signs of respiratory failure are summarized in the box on p. 99.

- In most acute cases of respiratory failure, the pCO_2 is normal or even decreased. Hypoxemia, but not hypercapnia, is typically seen on the blood gases.

- Hypoxemia = pO_2 <80 Hypercapnia = pCO_2 >45

- Hypercarbia, not hypoxemia, is a hallmark of airway obstruction.

- Most respiratory problems are characterized by hypoxemia, not hypercarbia.

- Cyanosis is a very late sign of hypoxemia. Anemic individuals may never appear cyanotic because cyanosis is a function of deoxygenated hemoglobin. In anemia, there simply may not be enough hemoglobin to clinically show cyanosis. Visible cyanosis is not apparent until the arterial O_2 saturation is 75% to 80%. Inspect the oral membranes and tongue as the most reliable sites.

- Hypercapnia causes cerebral vasodilation, which increases cerebral blood flow and intracranial pressure (ICP). Hypocapnia of pCO_2 generally in the low 30s is desirable in head injury patients.

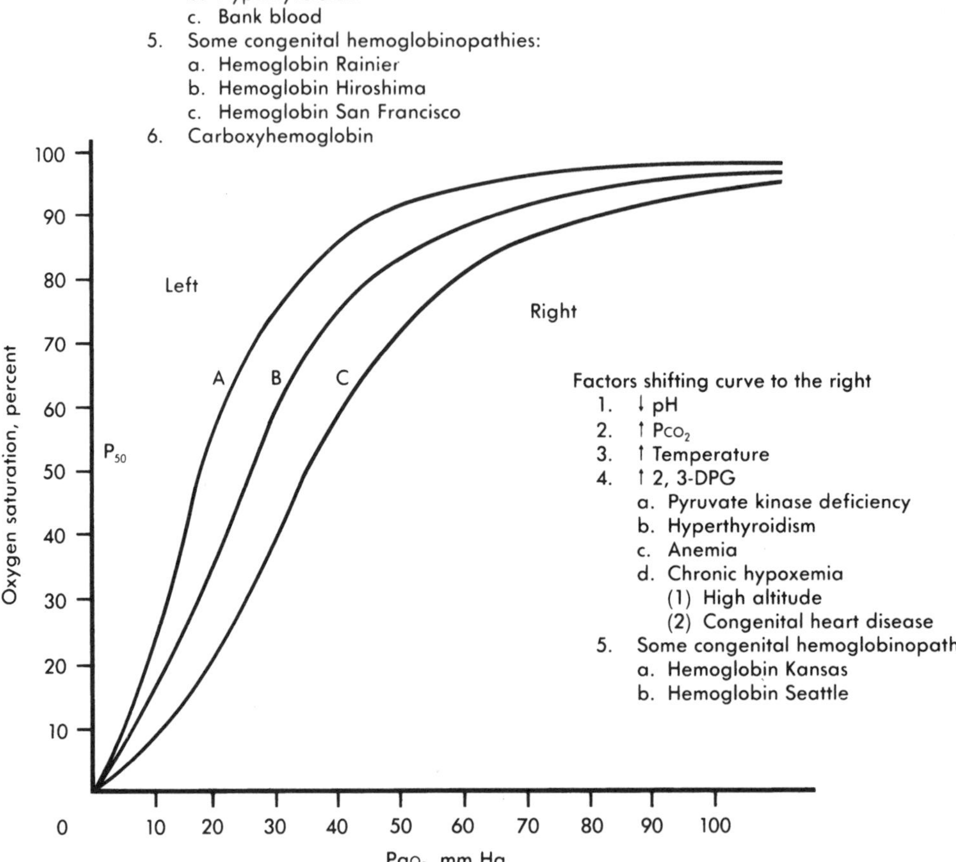

Fig. 2-3 Curve B is the standard oxyhemoglobin dissociation curve. Curve A shows the curve shifted to the left because of hemoglobin's increased affinity for oxygen. Curve C shows the curve shifted to the right because of hemoglobin's decreased affinity for oxygen. Factors responsible for shifting the curve are listed adjacent to curves A and C. (From Thelan LA, Davie JK, Urden LD, and Lough ME: Critical care nursing: diagnosis and management, ed 2, St Louis, 1994, Mosby.)

Signs of Respiratory Failure

Cardinal Signs

Restlessness

Increase in respiratory effort

Tachypnea

Tachycardia

Diaphoresis

Early but Less Obvious Signs

Mood changes, such as euphoria or depression

Headache

Altered depth and pattern of respirations

Hypertension

Exertional dyspnea

Anorexia

Increased cardiac output and renal output

Central nervous system symptoms (decreased efficiency, impaired judgment, anxiety, confusion, restlessness, irritability, depressed level of consciousness)

Flaring nares

Chest wall retractions

Expiratory grunt

Wheezing and/or prolonged expiration

Absent or decreased breath sounds

Signs of More Severe Hypoxia

Hypotension or hypertension

Dimness of vision

Somnolence

Stupor

Coma

Dyspnea

Depressed respirations/agonal respirations

Bradycardia

Cyanosis, peripheral or central

Apnea

From Wong DL: Whaley and Wong's nursing care of infants and children, ed 5, St Louis, 1995, Mosby.

- With lung disease and poor lung compliance, diaphragmatic excursion can cause sternal and intercostal retractions without inflating the lungs.

Mechanical Ventilation

Indications for mechanical ventilation include the following:
- Refractory hypoxemia
- Hypercapnia
- Inadequate ventilation as evidenced by inappropriate ventilatory rate or depth
- Respiratory acidosis
- Severe dyspnea causing excessive work of breathing

- Positive pressure ventilation is the principle behind most ventilators. The superior and anterior lung fields are better inflated in the typical critical care patient (supine or semifowlers position).

- Positive pressure ventilation causes an increase in intrathoracic pressure which may decrease systemic and pulmonary venous return leading to a decrease in cardiac output. Ensure that the patient is adequately hydrated to assist in cardiac output. This is especially true when PEEP is used.

- Most ventilators are pressure, volume, time, or flow driven. Only inhalation is truly controlled by mechanical ventilation. Exhalation is passive. This is an important concept when treating respiratory diseases associated with air trapping, such as asthma.

- Ventilatory modes include control, assist/control, intermittent mandatory volume, synchronized intermittent mandatory volume, pressure-support ventilation, and high frequency ventilation (both jet and oscillatory).

- Tidal volume is typically 6 to 15 cc/kg body weight. Assess that the volume is adequate by watching good chest wall movement.

- Increased peak inspiratory pressures can indicate respiratory distress syndrome, decreasing lung compliance, pneumothorax, secretions in airways or tubing, or kinks in tubing.

- Fluid therapy is conservative during mechanical ventilation to prevent excess lung fluid; however, this must be balanced when using PEEP to prevent a decrease in cardiac output from decreased right-sided filling.

- Nutritional support related to ventilatory therapy includes relatively low carbohydrates (to avoid increasing CO_2), judicious use of intralipids (to avoid increasing serum triglyceride levels which can compromise gas exchange and increase hypoxemia), and high fat sources for calories.

- Extracorporeal membrane oxygenation (ECMO) is a form of both cardiac and ventilatory support. Liquid ventilation and nitric oxide are newer ventilatory therapies that are still technically experimental and offered only at select clinical sites.

Positive End Expiratory Pressure (PEEP)

- Positive end expiratory pressure (PEEP) is used for ventilated patients and continuous positive airway pressure (CPAP) is used for patients with spontaneous respirations.
- Positive effects and indications for PEEP include the following: increases functional residual capacity (FRC), prevents or reopens atelectatic areas, enhances alveolar ventilation, improves ventilation perfusion match, decreases intrapulmonary shunting, and moves pulmonary water (edema) out where it does not interfere with gas exchange.
- PEEP increases intrathoracic pressure and can decrease pulmonary and systemic venous return, leading to a decrease in cardiac output.
- Avoid high levels of PEEP—they increase the chance of air leaks and can increase intracranial pressure by impairing cerebral venous return. The lowest effective level of PEEP is the best amount.
- When using PEEP make sure the patient has an adequate circulating volume to compensate for potential decreased cardiac output related to decreased venous return from higher intrathoracic pressure.
- PEEP should always be maintained during suctioning! It can take 20 to 30 minutes to regain the therapeutic effect of PEEP if it is lost even for a few seconds. A closed suctioning system may help prevent critical loss of PEEP. Preoxygenation and hyperventilation should be done before suctioning unless a plug is suspected.
- Be on guard for inadvertent, or intrinsic, PEEP. This occurs when there is a flow obstruction and inadequate exhalation time, both of which result in air trapping. This is especially seen in bronchiolitis or chronic lung disease. Signs include rising CO_2 and poor chest wall movement.

Assessment of the Mechanically Ventilated Infant or Child

Check the following carefully:

- Appropriate heart rate and blood pressure
- Overall color and indicators of perfusion
- Chest wall movement
- Bilateral and equal breath sounds with equal pitch
- Level of consciousness
- End-tidal CO_2

- When in doubt, hand ventilate until the function of the ventilator can be verified.

- Obstruction of the tube, migration of the tube, or development of a pneumothorax accounts for many cases of acute deterioration.

- Breath sounds are easily transmitted in infants and small children—note change in pitch from one side to the other as a clue to pneumothorax, atelectasis, and consolidation.

Weaning

Criteria for weaning include the following:

- Normal blood gases
- Spontaneous tidal volume >5 mL/kg
- Vital capacity >10 mL/kg
- PEEP <4 to 6 cm H_2O
- Resolution of acute respiratory condition that caused failure
- Adequate cardiovascular function
- Adequate neurological function

- Steroid therapy may be beneficial before and after extubation to reduce or prevent airway obstruction from edema.

- Avoid oral intake and chest physiotherapy for 2 to 4 hours before and after extubation to reduce the potential for aspiration.

- Racemic epinephrine, nebulized saline, and helium-oxygen mixtures are effective in treating upper airway edema, especially following extubation.

Oxygen Toxicity

- Free oxygen radicals are formed in the presence of high levels of oxygen therapy. Ideally the FiO_2 is kept less than 0.4.

- Free radicals can combine with nonradicals to form new free radicals. This process can continue with the use of high oxygen levels and result in lung damage.

- Lung damage associated with oxygen toxicity includes alveolar damage, increased capillary leak, interstitial edema, infiltration with inflammatory cells, increased numbers of type II pneumocytes, and eventually pulmonary interstitial fibrosis.

Apnea of Prematurity

- Immaturity of the nervous system may account for apnea observed in the premature infant. One mechanism may be an inability of the immature nervous system to produce a stimulation that can result in a ventilatory muscle response. General decreased levels of catecholamines also may be responsible. Respiratory muscle fatigue related to the more difficult work of breathing also may account for apnea.

- Disorders of almost all body systems have been associated with apnea—secondary apnea.
- Increased or changed ambient temperature and vagal stimulation by gagging or suctioning may precipitate apnea.
- To decrease the risk of apnea, the premature infant should be protected from temperature variances. Increased core temperature may result from phototherapy lights or incubators, which are maintained in the high normal temperature range. Decreased core temperature may be related to unwarmed oxygen therapy.
- Gentle stimulation by touch should be used to stimulate an infant during an apneic episode. Vigorous shaking or loud banging should be avoided.
- When tactile stimulation has not been successful, bag-mask ventilation is indicated during an apneic episode. However, vigorous bagging can actually exacerbate apnea. Water bed flotation mattresses may help reduce, but not eliminate, apneic episodes.
- CPAP at low pressures (3 to 5 cm H_2O) may be used to treat apnea.
- Aminophylline, theophylline, and caffeine may be used to treat primary apnea of prematurity. They do not work by affecting pulmonary function but rather by providing central nervous system stimulation.

Persistent Pulmonary Hypertension (PPHN: Persistent Fetal Circulation)

- Persistent pulmonary hypertension (PPHN) is a failure in transition to postnatal circulation. Right-to-left shunting of blood occurs through the patent foramen ovale (PFO) and patent ductus arteriosus (PDA) as a result of persistently high pulmonary vascular pressures.
- Right-to-left shunting is manifested by cyanosis, hypoxia, and acidosis.
- Increased pCO_2, decreased pO_2, and acidosis all facilitate pulmonary vasoconstriction and pulmonary hypertension. A cycle of increasing hypoxemia and acidosis resulting from pulmonary vasoconstriction leads to further pulmonary vasoconstriction.
- PPHN develops primarily in the term or postterm infant. Smooth muscle function in the pulmonary vessels is not sufficient to cause pulmonary hypertension in the preterm infant.
- PPHN is associated with (1) meconium aspiration, (2) transient tachypnea of the newborn, (3) sepsis, (4) diaphragmatic hernia, (5) hypoglycemia, (6) maternal

ingestion of ibuprofen, dilantin, lithium, and aspirin, (7) asphyxia, (8) anemia, (9) hypothermia, (10) pneumonia, and (11) alveolar hypoventilation.

- Intubation and mechanical ventilation aimed at increasing pO_2, decreasing pCO_2, and producing respiratory alkalosis may help decrease pulmonary vascular resistance. This type of respiratory management generally requires sedation and/or paralysis.

- Tolazoline, nitroprusside, nitroglycerine, adenosine, and prostaglandin E_1 may be effective in reducing pulmonary vascular resistance. These should be administered in a scalp vein to drain into the superior vena cava.

- Systemic vasoconstrictors also may be used to treat PPHN to reduce right-to-left shunting by raising the systemic vascular resistance. These may include dopamine and epinephrine.

- It is important to minimize stimulation, agitation and crying, which can increase pulmonary vascular resistance and, in turn, increase hypoxemia.

Diaphragmatic Hernia

- Most infants with a congenital diaphragmatic hernia (CDH) are born at term and full birth weight. They present soon after delivery in severe respiratory distress.

- Most diaphragmatic hernias affect primarily the left side. The protrusion of abdominal contents into the chest displaces the heart to the right side of the chest.

- The lungs of an infant with CDH are hypoplastic as a result of impingement of the abdominal organs on the lungs from very early in fetal life.

- Ineffective ventilation is related to hypoplasia and compression of lung tissue.

- Crying and respiratory distress actually worsen the clinical course of CDH by increasing the amount of air in the intestines and increasing negative pressure within the chest, which causes increased impingement of the bowel into the thorax.

- Treatment of CDH includes immediate ventilatory support with low pressures to prevent pneumothorax and decompression of the stomach. Extracorporeal membrane oxygenation may be required.

- Surgical correction may be accomplished immediately or following a period of stabilization.

- Presence of a CDH is often associated with persistent pulmonary hypertension of the newborn.

- Try to prevent the infant with CDH from crying, which can exacerbate the amount or volume of abdominal contents in the chest cavity.

- Upright positioning may help promote downward displacement of abdominal contents and facilitate diaphragmatic excursion.

- Positioning on the right side increases aeration of the left lung and perfusion of the right lung. Conversely, positioning on the left side increases aeration of the right lung and perfusion of the left lung.

- Postoperatively, position on the affected side (usually left) to promote expansion of the unaffected lung.

- Chest tubes may need to be placed preoperatively as a result of the high occurrence of pneumothoraces. A nasogastric tube may need to be placed to decompress the stomach.

- During surgical repair, a chest tube is placed on the affected side without suction to allow gradual reexpansion and drainage of accumulated fluid or blood. The tube is placed to water seal only to prevent mediastinal shift from rapid changes in intrathoracic contents and pressures.

- Dopamine infusions may be required postoperatively to improve cardiac output. Tolazoline infusions may be required to reduce pulmonary vasoconstriction in the infant with persistent pulmonary hypertension. Nitroglycerine, adenosine, nitroprusside, and prostaglandin E_1 also may be used to reduce pulmonary vasoconstriction.

- Despite hypoplasia, the lung of an infant with CDH will often develop and grow normally.

Tracheoesophageal Fistula (TEF)

- A tracheoesophageal fistula (TEF) occurs where there is abnormal communication between the trachea and the esophagus.

- Because the infant has a complete or partial obstruction of the esophagus, there is often a history of polyhydramnios, profuse oral secretions, and severe coughing and distress with feeding.

- Generally, passage of a nasogastric or oral gastric tube is impossible as a result of either a blind ending to the esophagus or abnormal coursing to communicate with the trachea.

- A tube should be passed into the esophagus near the point of obstruction and connected to low suction to prevent accumulation of oral secretions that would increase the risk of aspiration. Position upright to help decrease this risk. Make sure nothing is administered via the tube.

- Antibiotic therapy is used to prevent pneumonia from aspiration.
- Coughing and cyanosis may develop during feeding related to entrance of fluid into the trachea and laryngospasms.
- Pacifiers are not used preoperatively or early in the postoperative period because they stimulate oral secretions.

PEDIATRIC-SPECIFIC PRINCIPLES

RESPIRATORY DISTRESS SYNDROME (RDS)

- Pediatric respiratory distress syndrome (RDS) is not a primary disease. It is a consequence of lung injury from trauma, sepsis, metabolic disturbances, infections, and other lung or systemic maladies.
- The pathophysiology includes pulmonary capillary leak, pulmonary edema, the production of free oxygen radicals, inflammation, infiltration with leukocytes, intrapulmonary shunting, impaired surfactant production, and fibrin infiltration leading to severe respiratory compromise and/or dysfunction.
- Signs and symptoms include hyperventilation, dyspnea, decreased pO_2 and pCO_2, and alkalosis early on. Later the pCO_2 may rise and be accompanied by acidosis.
- RDS is treated with intubation, PEEP, decreasing oxygen demands (treat fever, thermal neutral environment, paralysis, sedation), somewhat negative fluid balance (50 to 60 mL/kg/day of fluid), diuretic therapy, and other supportive measures.
- Trends in treating RDS include use of surfactant, nonsteroidal antiinflammatory drugs, liquid ventilation, high frequency ventilation, and monoclonal antibodies.

CROUP (LARYNGOTRACHEALBRONCHITIS—LTB)/EPIGLOTTIS

- Avoid procedures and parental separation that will cause anxiety and crying. These further stress the child, increase oxygen demands, and may increase airway obstruction. See Fig. 2-4.
- Epiglottis is a medical emergency! The cough is weaker and the voice quieter than in LTB. Drooling, higher fever, and more severe dyspnea help differentiate epiglottis. NO EXAMINATION OF THE AIRWAY SHOULD OCCUR WITHOUT HIGHLY SKILLED PROFESSIONALS AT THE BEDSIDE READY TO INTUBATE! INTUBATION IS PERFORMED ONCE THE DIAGNOSIS IS CONFIRMED BY X-RAY.

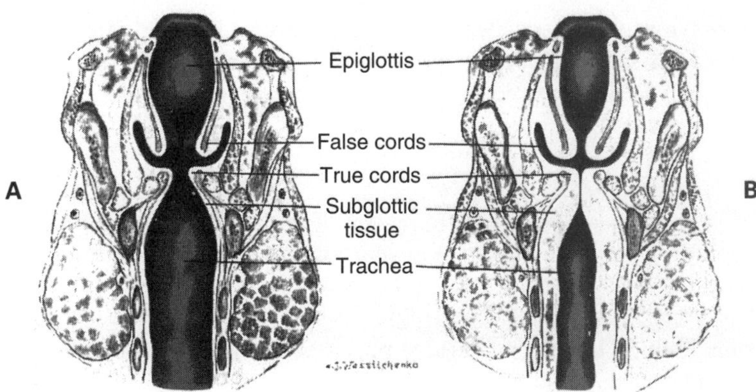

Fig. 2-4 **A,** Normal larynx. **B,** Obstruction and narrowing resulting from edema of croup. (From Wong DL: Whaley and Wong's nursing care of infants and children, ed 5, St Louis, 1995, Mosby.)

- Position comfortably, usually in parent's arms, sitting upright, even leaning forward.

BRONCHIOLITIS

- Bronchiolitis, a lower respiratory tract infection, is usually seen in small infants and characterized by increased mucous production leading to obstructed bronchioles. Commonly it is caused by respiratory syncytial virus (RSV).
- Symptoms develop following a brief period of coldlike symptoms. Dyspnea characterized by tachypnea, wheezing, rales, and retractions is seen. The liver may even be palpable because the lungs are hyperinflated as a result of air trapping.
- Treatment is largely supportive, including oxygen therapy, intubation as indicated, albuterol or terbutaline, aminophylline, and good hydration.
- When treating infants and children with RSV, Ribovirin® (antiviral agent) may be used in intubated or nonintubated patients. Caution: it may crystallize in the tubing of ventilators.

CHEST TRAUMA

- Rib and sternal fractures are less common as a result of their increased flexibility in children. The lack of rib or sternal fractures does *not* rule out lung contusions.
- Look for pericardial tamponade, pneumothorax, hemothorax, tension pneumothorax, rupture of larynx, lacerations of lungs, bronchioles, and vessels, and ruptured diaphragm.
- Lung contusions can cause bleeding and fluid shifts into interstitial and intraalveolar spaces.

- Signs and symptoms associated with chest trauma include paradoxical respirations, tracheal shift, dyspnea, pain, abnormal breath sounds, absent breath sounds, pulsus paradoxus, poor perfusion, and new murmur.

ASTHMA

- Air trapping occurs as a result of severe airway constriction. Increased mucous production is associated with acute attacks.

- Symptoms include cough, wheezing, prolonged expiration, mucous production, dyspnea, tachycardia, and tachypnea.

- All asthma attacks are associated with hypoxemia. Mild attacks have decreased pCO_2 and increased pH as a result of tachypnea. Moderate attacks may have normal pCO_2 and pH as a result of decreased ability to get rid of CO_2 even with tachypnea. Only severe attacks are associated with increased pCO_2 and decreased pH.

- Beta-agonist drugs and corticosteroids are standard treatments. Inhalation or intravenous administration may be used. Aminophylline may be helpful.

- Chest physiotherapy is not used during an acute attack because it places further stress on the child. Chest PT is used after the attack has acutely resolved.

AIRWAY OBSTRUCTION

- Risks for airway obstruction include (1) intubation, (2) ingestion or inhalation of foreign bodies or irritating fumes, (3) croup, (4) epiglottis, (5) anaphylaxis, (6) impaired neurological status, (7) tonsilar disease, (8) sedation, (9) anesthesia, (10) trauma to head, neck, or chest, and (11) excessive mucous production.

- Airway obstruction can occur with exhalation (asthma) or inhalation (choking).

- Signs of airway obstruction are mottling (less often cyanosis) and lethargy or irritability.

- Permit the child with upper airway obstruction to assume a position of comfort.

- Alternatively, position the child in a sitting position, leaning forward.

- Symptoms of airway obstruction following extubation may be as a result of subglottic stenosis. This peaks at 8 to 24 hours after extubation. If severe symptoms are seen in as little as 2 hours elective reintubation should occur quickly.

- All infants and children with respiratory distress should be positioned upright. A car seat or infant seat is helpful for babies.
- Upper airway obstruction caused by epiglottis is a medical emergency.
- Do not encourage, but rather *avoid* coughing in the child with epiglottis.
- A significant cause of airway obstruction in the infant or preschool child is laryngospasm or bronchospasm.

ASPIRATION PNEUMONIA

- Signs and symptoms of aspiration pneumonia are related to the nature of the aspirant.
- Hydrocarbon aspiration (gasoline, nail polish, solvents, propellants) usually causes a chemical pneumonitis as manifested by severe dyspnea, violent coughing, wheezing, pulmonary edema, and cyanosis. Bronchospasms, atelectasis, air trapping, and necrosis of tissue may occur. Induction of vomiting after ingestion is *not* indicated.
- Aspiration of oral secretions and insert substances does not cause a chemical pneumonitis. Hypoxemia and impaired gas exchange do occur. Symptoms include coughing, cyanosis, dyspnea, and pulmonary edema.
- Aspiration of upper airway secretions can cause infection and is usually manifested by cough, dyspnea, fever, and abnormal sputum production. Treatment involves antibiotic therapy.
- Treatment for aspiration pneumonia generally is similar to treatment for respiratory distress syndrome.

FOREIGN BODY ASPIRATION

- Signs and symptoms of foreign body aspiration in the larynx or trachea include severe dyspnea, stridor, cough, retractions, and inability to make sounds in complete obstruction.
- Signs and symptoms of foreign body aspiration in the bronchi include cough, wheezing, dyspnea, cyanosis, air trapping, and decreased breath sounds.
- Chest x-rays will show differentiated aeration of lungs. If the object is metallic or radiopaque it may be visualized.

- Following removal of a foreign body, observe for airway obstruction as a result of developing edema.

NEONATAL-SPECIFIC PRINCIPLES

- Premature infants may respond differently to hypoxemia. The initial response may be rapid, deep respirations; however, these are followed by bradypnea or even apnea.

- Surfactant serves to reduce surface tension and promote alveolar patency. It also helps increase lung compliance and keep the alveoli free of fluid, and it plays a role in pulmonary perfusion at the capillary level.

- Factors that may result in decreased surfactant function include mechanical ventilation, acidosis, hypercarbia, shock, hypoxia, maternal diabetes, and multiple births.

- Surfactant metabolism is actually increased in the following: some maternal diabetes, premature rupture of membranes, placental dysfunction, abruptio placenta, and maternal hypertension.

IDIOPATHIC RESPIRATORY DISTRESS SYNDROME (IRDS)

- The most common factor in the development of idiopathic respiratory distress syndrome (IRDS) is prematurity. Other factors include male gender, persistent pulmonary hypertension of the newborn, degree of prematurity, multiparity, and maternal health problems.

TRANSIENT TACHYPNEA OF THE NEWBORN (TTN)

- In transient tachypnea of the newborn (TTN), large amounts of fluid remain in the lungs obstructing airways and preventing the bronchioles from opening normally, which results in air trapping.

- Lungs are normally fluid filled before birth. During normal vaginal delivery much of this fluid is squeezed out by chest compressions or, alternatively, absorbed.

- Infants at risk for TTN include those born by cesarean section or with a maternal history of a precipitous delivery.

- Onset is usually within a few hours after birth and is manifested by respiratory distress—tachypnea, dyspnea, grunting, nasal flaring, retractions, and cyanosis.

- Oxygen therapy to correct hypoxemia and acidosis is critical. Adequate and effective therapy will help prevent pulmonary vasoconstriction and persistence of pulmonary circulation.

- Absorption of lung fluid will occur with supportive therapy via the lymphatic system.

CHOANAL ATRESIA

- Bilateral choanal atresia is an acute problem that usually manifests in the delivery room because infants are obligate nose breathers.
- Dyspnea, which increases with closure of the infant's mouth, is indicative of choanal atresia.
- Intubation or use of an oropharyngeal airway is indicated until surgical correction can take place.

PULMONARY INTERSTITIAL EMPHYSEMA (PIE)

- Pulmonary interstitial emphysema (PIE) results from ruptured alveoli allowing gas to accumulate in the interstitial tissue.
- Pulmonary interstitial emphysema impairs both ventilation and perfusion.
- All of the following may predispose an infant to pulmonary interstitial emphysema: (1) spontaneous alveolar rupture, (2) positive pressure ventilation, (3) idiopathic respiratory distress syndrome, (4) aspiration, (5) diaphragmatic hernia, (6) hypoplasia of the lungs, (7) meconium aspiration, (8) positive end expiratory pressure, (9) continuous positive airway pressure, and (10) manual ventilation with a bag.
- Treatment includes supportive therapy in mild cases to intubation of the affected lung in severe cases. The use of high frequency ventilation is important therapy for PIE.

MECONIUM ASPIRATION

- Asphyxia in utero causes gastrointestinal peristalsis in the fetus releasing meconium into the amniotic fluid.
- Aspiration of meconium occurs most frequently in utero when repeated episodes of hypoxia lead to gasping respirations of the fetus.
- The lung disease associated with meconium aspiration is atelectasis with ball-valve air trapping and hyperinflation of the lungs. Increased lung volumes are seen on chest x-ray.
- Chemical pneumonitis often accompanies meconium aspiration. This may be as a result of the bile salt content of meconium.
- Meconium aspiration is often associated with persistent pulmonary hypertension of the newborn, probably as a result of acidosis and hypoxia.

- Meconium aspiration is most often seen in full-term or postterm infants. It is rarely seen earlier than 36 weeks gestation.
- Signs and symptoms of meconium aspiration are the clinical presentation of respiratory distress. These include tachypnea, nasal flaring, retractions, barrel-shaped chest, prolonged expiration, rales, rhonchi, and mixed metabolic and respiratory acidosis.
- Complications associated with meconium aspiration include air leaks from air trapping, persistent pulmonary hypertension, pneumonia, bronchopulmonary dysplasia, hypoglycemia, acidosis, hypocalcemia, and polycythemia.
- Ventilator management often includes low PEEP as well as increased respiratory rate to decrease acidosis and prevent PPHN. Air leaks are a frequent complication.

BRONCHOPULMONARY DYSPLASIA (BPD)

- The following boxes summarize risk factors for the development of bronchopulmonary dysplasia (BPD) and describe the classification system for BPD.
- Treatment goals for BPD focus on reducing factors that produce injury. Therapy is supportive and includes preventing fluid overload and closing PDAs.
- Bronchodilator therapy has not definitively been proven effective in treating BPD, probably as a result of neonates' immature smooth muscle layer in bronchioles leaving them unable to respond to pharmacological therapy. Bronchodilator therapy has not been proven effective until 12 to 30 months of age.
- Aerosol treatments such as albuterol, cromolyn, and terbutaline may be effective.
- Theophylline may be effective in ventilator-dependent infants with BPD because of its ability to improve lung compliance and reduce resistance to expiration.

Risk Factors for the Development of Bronchopulmonary Dysplasia

Oxygen toxicity	Nutritional deficiencies
Positive pressure ventilation	Low birth weight
Left-to-right shunting	Family history of asthma
Early fluid volume overload	Prematurity

Classification System for Bronchopulmonary Dysplasia

Stage I

Early interstitial changes

Air bronchogram

Resembles respiratory distress syndrome

First 3 days of life

Stage II

Diffuse haziness on chest x-ray

Cardiac markings are obscured on x-ray

Regeneration and proliferation of bronchial epithelium

Alveolar epithelium shows necrosis and early fibrosis

First 3 to 10 days of life

Stage III

Beginning of chronic disease

Bronchial and bronchiolar metaplasia

Signs of emphysema

Interstitial edema

Pulmonary hypertension

Cyst formations within opaque lungs and cardiac borders

First 10 to 20 days of life

Stage IV

Obliterative bronchiolitis

Interstitial fibrosis

Hyperexpansion on chest x-ray

Increase in size and number of cysts

After 28 days of life

- Methylxanthine may aid in weaning.
- Diuretic therapy and fluid restriction are important to reduce pulmonary edema and right-sided heart failure often seen with BPD.
- Caloric needs are high as a result of increased metabolism and work of breathing.
- Effectiveness of steroids therapy is controversial, but may help increase compliance.
- Tracheostomy may be required after 6 to 8 weeks of not being able to wean from the ventilator. It allows oral feeding and reduces the risks of tracheomalacia and bronchomalacia.

Questions

GENERAL PULMONARY CARE QUESTIONS

1. Surfactant performs all of the following functions *except*:
   A. Increase surface tension to prevent alveolar collapse
   B. Decreases surface tension to increase lung compliance
   C. Decreases opening pressure
   D. Increases fluid clearance from the alveoli

2. Which of the following would increase the ventilation/perfusion ratio?
   A. Pulmonary emboli
   B. Atelectasis
   C. Pulmonary edema
   D. Meconium aspiration

3. The goal of oxygen therapy is to:
   A. Increase inspired oxygen
   B. Decrease carbon dioxide levels
   C. Increase oxygen delivery
   D. Decrease oxygen consumption

4. Pulse oximetry is effective in measuring:
   A. Arterial oxygen content
   B. Hemoglobin oxygen saturation
   C. Amount of oxygen dissolved in plasma
   D. Arterial oxygen tension

5. The critical care nurse observes continuous, noisy bubbling in the water seal chamber of the chest tube drainage system. The most appropriate action would be:
   A. Check the suction tubing for any kinks or clots obstructing drainage
   B. Milk the chest tube gently to remove clots
   C. Raise the tubing between the patient and the collection system to empty stagnant drainage
   D. Clamp tube at insertion site briefly to observe for cessation of bubbling

6. A patient with the following blood gases is admitted to the critical care unit. Which of the following changes in ventilatory therapy would be most likely to improve the blood gases?
pH: 7.31
pO_2: 88 torr
pCO_2: 53 torr
HCO_3: 19 mEq/L
A. Increase the FiO_2 by 10%
B. Increase the respiratory rate
C. Decrease the peak inspiratory pressure
D. Increase the inspiratory/expiratory ratio

7. The critical care nurse observes fluid fluctuations in the water seal chamber during respirations. The most appropriate action in the care of this patient with a chest tube and drainage system would be:
A. Milk the chest tube gently to remove clots which may have formed
B. Note that the drainage system is functioning properly
C. Immediately observe the patient for respiratory distress
D. Disconnect the system and hand ventilate the patient until the system can be replaced

(Not)

8. Two hours after returning from surgery, the critical care nurse observes a decreased level of responsiveness in her patient. He is breathing spontaneously on room air. Blood gases are obtained and are as follows:
pH: 7.22
pO_2: 90 torr
pCO_2: 63 torr
HCO_3^-: 23 mEq/L
Base excess: +2
Which of the following actions would be most appropriate based on these findings?
A. Administration of 100% oxygen by facial mask to improve hypoxia
B. Administration of narcotic analgesics to decrease pain and improve deep breathing
C. Administration of sodium bicarbonate to correct acidosis
D. Administration of naloxone to reverse effects of anesthesia

9. An intubated and ventilated patient suddenly shows a decrease in the pulse oximetry reading from 95% saturation to 81%. The patient is exhibiting nasal flaring, intercostal retractions, tachypnea, and use of accessory respiratory muscles despite the ventilator showing an adequate tidal volume and absence of peak pressure alarms. Which of the following actions should the critical care nurse do *first*?
A. Disconnect from the ventilator and manually bag the patient
B. Immediately suction the endotracheal tube
C. Increase the FiO_2 to 100%
D. Auscultate breath sounds

10. Which of the following ventilators is *most* effective for an infant or small child?
A. Pressure cycled
B. Volume cycled
C. Time cycled
D. Negative pressure

Case Study

Michael was a 3460 gram full-term infant with a history of meconium stained amniotic fluid noted 2 hours prior to delivery. He was suctioned at birth and found to have meconium below the cords. Apgar scores were 7 at one minute and 8 at five minutes. He was tachypneic with nasal flaring and expiratory grunting. His pulse oximetry reading on his right finger was 98% saturation while the pulse oximetry on his right toe was only 65%. His blood gases by umbilical artery catheter on 80% hood were as follows:

pH: 7.32
pO_2: 72 mm Hg
pCO_2: 40 mm Hg

Questions 11 to 13 refer to this case study.

---

11. Which of the following is the most likely explanation for the differences in pulse oximetry readings between his upper and lower extremities?
A. Coarctation of the aorta
B. Persistent pulmonary hypertension
C. Poor reading on the lower extremity pulse oximeter
D. Poor peripheral circulation related to acidosis

12. After the infant was intubated, what pH level in analyzing the blood gases would the nurse view as the best outcome of ventilatory therapy?
A. 7.35 (too low)
B. 7.47
C. 7.50
D. 7.67 (too alkalotic)

13. Based on the desired outcome of the pH level in question 12, for what complications would the critical care nurse be alert?
A. Hyponatremia
B. Hypocalcemia
C. Hyperkalemia
D. Hypermagnesemia

14. Which of the following would the critical care nurse recognize as the *earliest* sign of impending respiratory problems?
A. Tachypnea
B. Grunting
C. Nasal flaring
D. Intercostal retractions

15. An infant was admitted to the critical care unit for meconium aspiration and was intubated on 80% oxygen for the last 3 days. Upon examination, the nurse finds decreased breath sounds over the lung fields, lethargy, restlessness, dyspnea, and an increasing A-a gradient. No increase in secretions, fever, or wheezing are noted. These findings are most consistent with the development of:
A. Pneumonia
B. Foreign body aspiration
C. Oxygen toxicity
D. Airway obstruction

16. All of the following would be helpful in promoting airway clearance *except*:
A. Restricting fluids to minimize formation of secretions
B. Suctioning airway
C. Providing humidification
D. Cupping and postural drainage

17. While caring for an intubated and mechanically ventilated patient, the critical care nurse notices sudden, profound cyanosis with bradycardia. She observes asymmetrical chest excursion and decreased amplitude of the QRS complex, and auscultates shifted breath sounds. What *immediate* action should the critical care nurse take?
A. Elevate the head of the bed and increase the FiO_2 to 1.0
B. Suction the endotracheal tube to remove any obstruction
C. Call for a stat x-ray to check tube placement
D. Prepare to administer epinephrine

18. All of the following are related to the development of bronchopulmonary dysplasia *except:*
A. Patent ductus arteriosus
B. High inspired oxygen levels
C. Positive pressure ventilation
D. Negative pressure ventilation

19. Which of the following types of medications is NOT used to treat bronchopulmonary dysplasia?
A. Diuretics
B. Beta-blockers
C. Vasodilators
D. Cortiocosteroids

Case Study

A neonate is admitted to the critical care unit appearing pale with retractions, tachypnea, grunting, nasal flaring, and use of accessory muscles. The chest x-ray is described as ground-glass in appearance. Breath sounds by auscultation are decreased. Blood gases are as follows:

pH: 7.30
pO_2: 53 torr
pCO_2: 49 torr
HCO_3: 18 mEq/L

Questions 20 to 23 refer to this case study.

20. This infant is showing signs and symptoms of:
A. Aspiration pneumonia
B. Persistent pulmonary hypertension
C. Respiratory distress syndrome
D. Bronchopulmonary dysplasia

21. Treatment goals for this infant would include:
I. Reduce hypoxemia to decrease metabolic acidosis
II. Decrease ambient temperature to decrease metabolic demands
III. Increase pCO_2 to correct bicarbonate deficit
IV. Increase pH to correct acidosis
A. I, II, and IV
B. I and IV
C. I and II
D. III and IV

22. An important factor in the development of respiratory disease in this patient is the pathophysiology of:
A. Decreased surfactant production
B. Decreased 2,3-DPG production
C. Increased surfactant metabolism
D. Increased 2,3-DPG production

23. Which of the following would contribute to the work of breathing in this infant?
I. Placement of a nasogastric tube
II. Decreased compliance of the lungs
III. Decreased chest wall compliance
IV. Administration of oxygen
A. I and IV
B. II and III
C. I and II
D. III and IV

24. Positive end expiratory pressure (PEEP) improves the respiratory status by:
A. Opening collapsed bronchioles
B. Moving edema from the site of gas exchange
C. Assuring airway patency
D. Improving the ventilatory effort

25. Which of the following findings would indicate proper endotracheal tube placement immediately after intubation?
A. Presence of breath sounds over the upper left quadrant
B. Bronchial breath sounds over the trachea
C. Good excursion of the right chest during ventilation
D. Bilateral chest expansion with manual ventilation

26. Grunting is often observed with respiratory distress. This breathing technique:
A. Increases vital capacity to decrease hypoxemia
B. Increases end expiratory pressure to promote gas exchange
C. Decreases large airway obstruction to decrease air trapping
D. Decreases the work of breathing to decrease oxygen demands

27. Infants and children in respiratory distress need to be positioned upright or allowed to assume a position of comfort to:
A. Increase lung volume
B. Decrease work of breathing
C. Prevent aspiration
D. Decrease oxygen consumption

28. Atropine should not be used routinely during intubation to prevent vagal bradydysrhythmias because it may:
A. Cause laryngospasms and airway obstruction
B. Increase hypoxia by decreasing respiratory drive and chest wall excursion
C. Mask bradydysrhythmias from hypoxia associated with intubation
D. Increase the risk of aspiration as a result of increased production of secretions

29. Vesicular breath sounds are normally auscultated over which areas of the lungs?
A. Trachea and distal lungs
B. Bronchioles and small airways
C. Peripheral lung fields
D. Large and small airways

30. Postoperative care of a patient who has undergone repair of a tracheoesophageal fistula would include:
A. Deep suctioning to avoid leakage of gastric secretions into the trachea
B. Use of a pacifier to maintain oral stimulation in absence of oral feedings
C. Suctioning only to the end of the endotracheal tube
D. Use of a gastrostomy tube for feeding

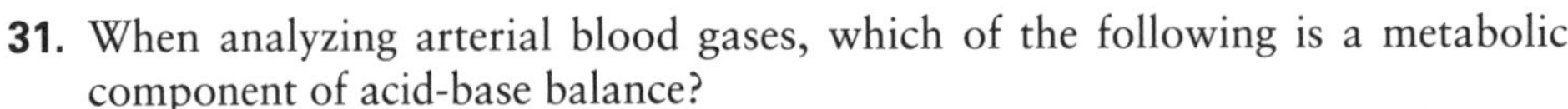

31. When analyzing arterial blood gases, which of the following is a metabolic component of acid-base balance?

A. pH
B. pCO_2
C. pO_2
D. HCO_3^-

32. Which of the following calculations of fluid therapy is optimal for normovolemic neonate with respiratory distress syndrome who is intubated and mechanically ventilated?

A. 50% of maintenance fluid requirements
B. 75% of maintenance fluid requirements
C. 100% of maintenance fluid requirements
D. 125% of maintenance fluid requirements

33. Nasal continuous positive airway pressure therapy is effective because it:

A. Increases the tidal volume
B. Decreases residual volume
C. Decreases anatomic dead space
D. Increases functional residual capacity

34. Which of the following may be used to treat persistent pulmonary hypertension?

A. Tolazoline
B. Dopamine
C. Isoproterenol
D. Dobutamine

35. A patient's arterial blood gases are the following:

pH: 7.30
pO_2: 55 mm Hg
pCO_2: 55 mm Hg
HCO_3: 29 mEq/L
% sat: 86%

These results show:

A. Uncompensated metabolic alkalosis
B. Compensated metabolic acidosis
C. Compensated respiratory alkalosis
D. Uncompensated respiratory acidosis

36. An afebrile, acyanotic patient returned 12 hours ago from surgical repair of an omphalocele. During suctioning, the critical care nurse observes for the first time thick, clear to white secretions. Which nursing action would be most effective in promoting airway clearance?

A. Assess adequacy of humidification
B. Send sputum for culture and sensitivity
C. Use saline lavage to thin secretions
D. Use sterile suction technique only

37. In caring for the patient with a newly inserted tracheostomy, which of the following is critical to ensure maintenance of the airway?
A. Snugly secure the ties around the tracheostomy tube so that only a small gauze fits between the tube and the skin
B. Keep a tracheostomy tube one size smaller at the bedside
C. Secure the tracheostomy tube with a bow to prevent knotting of the ties
D. Secure the tie at the side of the neck to provide easy access in emergencies

38. Which of the following is the most critical complication immediately following a tracheostomy?
A. Tenacious secretions
B. Infection
C. Speech delays
D. Decannulation

39. Which of the following is required in order to use facial CPAP on a patient with respiratory insufficiency?
A. Adequate respiratory excursion
B. Endotracheal or nasotracheal tube
C. Oral-nasal airway
D. Atelectatic lung fields

40. Which of the following represents effective postoperative management of chest tubes in the infant who has undergone repair of a congenital diaphragmatic hernia?
A. Chest tube on affected side to water seal
B. Chest tube on unaffected side to water seal
C. Chest tube on affected side to low suction
D. Chest tube on unaffected side to low suction

41. An infant with a history of polyhydramnios is noted soon after birth to have copious oral secretions. The critical care nurse recognizes which of the following conditions as the most likely cause of these symptoms:
A. Down syndrome
B. Cleft lip
C. Tracheoesophageal fistula
D. Fulminant pulmonary edema

42. What condition do the following blood gas results indicate?
pH: 7.33
pO_2: 62 mm Hg
pCO_2: 30 mm Hg
HCO_3: 14 mEq/L
SaO_2: 89%
A. Respiratory acidosis
B. Respiratory alkalosis
C. Metabolic acidosis
D. Metabolic alkalosis

43. A patient's peak inspiratory pressures have increased steadily over the last 24 hours. This can indicate a/an:
A. Increase in lung compliance
B. Decrease in lung compliance
C. Improvement in lung disease
D. Decrease in oxygen requirements

44. After endotracheal intubation, the critical care nurse notes decreased pulse oximetry readings, absent breath sounds, and no excursion in the left chest, and high peak pressure alarms on the ventilator. The critical care nurse suspects the patient has a:
A. Left pulmonary embolus
B. Pneumothorax
C. Pneumomediastinum
D. Right bronchial intubation

45. Which of the following parameters increases with bronchopulmonary dysplasia?
A. Functional residual capacity
B. Vital capacity
C. Tidal volume
D. Lung compliance

46. During suctioning for patients on mechanical ventilation with PEEP, the critical care nurse takes what additional measure to maintain PEEP?
A. Oxygenates with 100% O_2 prior to suctioning
B. Avoids suctioning to prevent interruption of PEEP
C. Uses a closed suctioning system
D. Routinely suctions every 2 hours to prevent atelectasis

47. Apnea of prematurity is primarily caused by:
A. Underdevelopment of primary and accessory respiratory muscles
B. Ineffective central nervous system response to increased pCO_2
C. Decreased surfactant metabolism resulting in respiratory insufficiency
D. Failure to clear fluid from lungs in the immediate neonatal period

48. Which of the following is an optimal level of PEEP? A level that:
A. Maintains the PaO_2 >85 mm Hg
B. Decreases lung compliance
C. Achieves the highest pO_2
D. Reduces intrapulmonary shunting

49. Which of the following conditions increases lung compliance?
A. Asthma
B. Pneumothorax
C. Atelectasis
D. Pulmonary edema

50. A neonate is found at birth to be severely tachypneic (rate of 115) with severe sternal retractions, nasal flaring, central cyanosis, and largely absent breath sounds. A chest x-ray demonstrates bowel located in the chest, an underdeveloped left lung, and the appearance of dextrocardia. The critical care nurse recognizes these symptoms as most consistent with:

A. Pneumothorax
B. Diaphragmatic hernia
C. Respiratory distress syndrome
D. Meconium aspiration

51. During early management of the infant with congenital diaphragmatic hernia affecting primarily the left lung, where should the nurse obtain information about arterial oxygenation/saturation?

I. A pulse oximetry probe on the right hand
II. A pulse oximetry probe on the left foot
III. An arterial blood gas from the umbilical artery catheter
IV. An arterial blood gas from the right radial artery

A. I and II
B. I and IV
C. II and III
D. II and IV

52. Postoperative ventilatory management of a 3200 gram neonate with congenital diaphragmatic hernia includes mechanical ventilation with:

A. Peak inspiratory pressure of 30 cm H_2O
B. Tidal volume of 80 cc
C. Positive end expiratory pressure of 10 cm H_2O
D. Tidal volume of 30 cc

53. What is the purpose of underwater drainage for chest tube drainage systems?

A. To prevent air from leaving the lungs
B. To prevent air from entering the pleural space
C. To maintain sterility
D. To prevent a hemothorax

54. Increasing the inspiratory/expiratory ratio through mechanical ventilation has which of the following therapeutic benefits?

A. Improves refractory hypercarbia
B. Decreases bronchospasm
C. Recruits atelectatic lung areas
D. Decreases oxygen toxicity

55. Administering 100% oxygen at rapid ventilatory rates to the infant suspected of having persistent pulmonary hypertension is helpful in:

A. Improving PaO_2 as a result of recruitment of lung areas
B. Improving PaO_2 by dilating pulmonary vessels
C. Confirming the diagnosis because the PaO_2 is not improved
D. Improving refractory hypercarbia

56. Which of the following *most* influences oxygen exchange during mechanical ventilation?
A. Changes in tidal volume
B. Changes in respiratory rate
C. Changes in mean airway pressure
D. Changes in oxygen consumption

PEDIATRIC-SPECIFIC QUESTIONS

Case Study

A 7-year-old boy is brought to the hospital with respiratory distress and is diagnosed with croup. Questions 57 to 60 refer to this case study.

---

57. Which of the following clinical findings do *not* characterize croup?
A. Rales and crackles
B. Dyspnea and stridor
C. Hoarseness or husky voice
D. Cough and "barking"

58. The ventilation-perfusion (V/Q) mismatch observed in this child would be related to:
A. Decreased perfusion as a result of capillary leak
B. Decreased ventilation as a result of airway obstruction
C. Decreased ventilation as a result of air trapping
D. Decreased perfusion related to decreased cardiac output

59. Which of the following clinical findings would the critical care nurse recognize as an emergency?
A. Sternal retractions
B. Subcostal retractions
C. Drooling
D. Abdominal breathing

60. For the child with suspended epiglottis, which of the following potential orders would the critical care nurse best defer until an x-ray is obtained?
A. Listening to breath sounds
B. Starting humidified oxygen
C. Obtaining a urine sample
D. Drawing arterial blood gases

61. A 12-year-old child with cystic fibrosis is admitted to the pediatric intensive care unit with severe hemoptysis, BP 88/40, a sinus rate of 118, respiratory rate of 22, a capillary refill time of 4 seconds, 2+ femoral pulses, and equivocal bilateral dorsalis pedis pulses. A central line is placed and volume expanders are infused at 20 mL/kg. The BP following 30 minutes of fluid resuscitation is 86/38, heart rate of 122, and respiratory rate of 22. The nurse can anticipate which of the following to be initiated immediately:
A. Placement of indwelling arterial and pulmonary catheters
B. Initiation of arminone at 5 mcg/kg/min
C. Administration of whole blood at 30 mL/kg
D. Initiation of a dopamine drip at 5 mcg/kg/min

62. In a patient with pulmonary hemorrhage, which of the following will assist in restoring functional residual capacity and minimize FiO_2 requirements?
A. Increasing tidal volume
B. Using positive end expiratory pressure
C. Increasing respiratory rate
D. Decreasing inspiratory/expiratory ratio

63. A 9-year-old patient is brought to the critical care unit in status asthmaticus. He has a productive cough that raises thick, white, tenacious secretions. Wheezing is audible without a stethoscope. Dyspnea is apparent from nasal flaring, tachypnea, and use of accessory respiratory muscles. While admitting the patient, the nurse observes decreased wheezing and increased lethargy. Which of the following immediate actions would be most appropriate?
A. Continue to observe the patient as his condition improves
B. Prepare for immediate intubation
C. Prepare for chest tube insertion
D. Begin an epinephrine infusion

64. A 14-year-old boy is diagnosed with acute respiratory failure secondary to pulmonary trauma from a pedestrian accident. He is intubated and placed on a mechanical ventilator. In order to minimize multisystem organ failure, which of the following treatments would be most effective?
A. Maintain a hematocrit greater than 40% to increase oxygen delivery
B. Maintain PaO_2 greater than 90% to minimize hypoxemia
C. Maintain low normal cardiac index to decrease cardiac work
D. Increase the FiO_2 to 1.0 to maximize oxygen delivery

65. Which of the following respiratory abnormalities would be expected in a patient with status asthmaticus?

I. Increased inspiratory/expiratory ratio
II. Decreased inspiratory/expiratory ratio
III. Increased functional residual capacity
IV. Decreased functional residual capacity

A. II and III
B. I and IV
C. I and III
D. II and IV

66. Which of the following is critical during aerosol therapy to meet the ventilatory demands of an acute asthma attack?

A. Maintain an FiO_2 >0.4
B. Ensure adequate oxygen flow
C. Perform chest physiotherapy to clear secretions
D. Monitor terbutaline levels

67. The goal of treatment in status asthmaticus includes all of the following *except*:

A. Increase oxygen delivery
B. Improve ventilation
C. Increase residual volume
D. Decrease airway obstruction

68. A 14-year-old girl is brought to the hospital following a motor vehicle-bicycle accident. She is complaining of chest pain exacerbated by inspiration and has shallow respirations. Upon close observation, the critical care nurse notices paradoxical respirations. These are most likely as a result of:

A. Pneumothorax
B. Hemothorax
C. Flail chest
D. Fractured rib

69. In administering aerosol bronchodilators, the critical care nurse observes for all of the following side effects *except*:

A. Bradycardia
B. Restlessness
C. Nausea
D. Dysrhythmias

70. Which of the following foreign body aspirants will be readily visible on a chest x-ray, facilitating diagnosis?

A. Popcorn
B. Hot dog
C. Paper clip
D. Pencil eraser

71. Normal serum levels of aminophylline are:
A. 5 to 10 mcg/mL
B. 10 to 20 mcg/mL
C. 20 to 30 mcg/mL
D. 25 to 35 mcg/mL

72. The hypoxia associated with asthma is a result of:
A. Ventilation/perfusion mismatch
B. Hypoventilation
C. Left-to-right shunting
D. Increased oxygen demands

73. Beta-agonists are used to treat asthma. These are most often administered:
A. Orally
B. Intravenously
C. Intramuscularly
D. By aerosol

74. Which of the following medications used to treat asthma is *not* given by aerosol?
A. Epinephrine
B. Isoproterenol
C. Atropine
D. Aminophylline

75. A 3-year-old girl is brought to the emergency department after her mother said she swallowed a coin. Her respiratory rate is 50 breaths per minute, her blood pressure is 96/60, and her pulse rate is 130 beats per minute. She appears anxious, is clinging to her mother, and has difficulty cooperating with the examination. An intermittent nonproductive cough and sternal retractions as well as use of accessory muscles to breathe are noted during the examination. As the critical care nurse is examining her, she becomes quiet and her respiratory rate slows to 16. The nurse recognizes this as:
A. Possible resolution of the obstruction
B. Adaptation to the hospital setting
C. Impending respiratory arrest
D. Development of pneumothorax

76. The critical care nurse recognizes as possible complications following foreign body airway obstruction all of the following *except*:
A. Infection
B. Obstruction
C. Hoarseness
D. Cyanosis

77. When caring for a child who has an end-tidal CO_2 monitoring ($P_{ET}CO_2$) device in place, the critical care nurse notices the reading rapidly falling to near 0 levels. This is most likely as a result of:
A. A mucous plug in the endotracheal tube
B. Migration of the endotracheal tube into the right bronchus
C. Falling PaO_2 levels
D. Hypoventilation

78. An 8-month-old infant was admitted to the intensive care unit with clear nasal discharge, a respiratory rate of 56, cough, temperature of 100.4°F (38°C), poor feeding, and dyspnea. Examination of the pulmonary system revealed subcostal retractions, nasal flaring, and use of accessory muscles to breathe. Crackles, wheezes, and decreased breath sounds were auscultated on admission. The chest x-ray showed hyperinflated lungs and atelectatic areas. The critical care nurse suspects the patient has:
A. Bacterial pneumonia
B. Bronchiolitis
C. Aspiration pneumonia
D. Bronchopulmonary dysplasia

79. When examining a child who may have epiglottis, the critical care nurse would avoid all of the following *except*:
A. Administration of humidified oxygen before blood gas analysis
B. Examining the throat for the possibility of overlooked foreign body obstruction
C. Drawing blood gases to evaluate respiratory failure
D. Asking the parents to leave because the child is clinging to them too much to be examined

---

Case Study

A 14-year-old boy is admitted to the pediatric intensive care unit following a pedestrian accident. He has known chest trauma as evidenced by bruising over the sternum and tenderness over the 3rd, 4th, and 5th ribs, left midclavicular line.

Questions 80 to 83 refer to this case study.

---

80. In assessing for a pneumothorax, the critical care nurse would look for:
A. Distant breath sounds, change in pitch, and tracheal deviation to the right
B. Hyperresonant breath sounds, crackles, and midline trachea
C. Distant breath sounds, change in pitch, and tracheal deviation to the left
D. Hyperresonant breath sounds, stridor, and midline trachea

81. When the critical care nurse performs a full respiratory assessment, the patient is found to have complaints of chest pain, coarse breath sounds, and a slightly increased respiratory rate accompanied by nasal flaring. There is no use of accessory muscles. The nurse suspects this patient most likely has:
A. Hemothorax
B. Rib fracture
C. Chylothorax
D. Lung contusion

82. Twelve hours after admission to the unit, the patient begins to be somewhat combative and very restless. An emergent examination reveals a gradually decreasing blood pressure over the last 90 minutes to 88/78, jugular vein distension, and cold, pale extremities with weak and thready peripheral pulses. The critical care nurse prepares to immediately assist with:
A. Tapping the pleural space
B. Pericardiocentesis
C. Insertion of a chest tube
D. Rapid infusion of colloids

83. A child with aspiration pneumonia from hydrocarbons would be expected to present with:
A. Severe dyspnea, wheezing, cardiac dysrhythmias, somnolence
B. Fever, irritability, tachycardia, cough
C. Seizures, frothy sputum, cough, fever
D. Acute agitation, nasal flaring, sternal retractions, fever

84. An 11-month-old child with bronchopulmonary dysplasia is most likely to be at risk for developing:
A. Aspiration pneumonia
B. Pneumothorax
C. Bronchiolitis
D. Pulmonary hemorrhage

85. Values obtained by monitoring end-tidal CO_2 ($P_{ET}CO_2$) in patients without lung disease reflect all of the following *except*:
A. Alveolar pCO_2
B. $PaCO_2$
C. Serum CO_2
D. Exhaled CO_2

86. A mixed venous blood gas sample is drawn from a pulmonary artery catheter. The critical care nurse interprets the results of the mixed venous pO_2 of 38 mm Hg as indicating:
A. Hypoxia and probable shock
B. Adequate peripheral perfusion
C. Hypoventilation and hypoxia
D. Respiratory acidosis

87. A 9-year-old boy with respiratory distress syndrome has a fiberoptic pulmonary artery catheter in place to measure continuous mixed venous oxygen saturation (SvO_2). A value of 55% would most likely indicate:
- A. Decreased oxygen delivery
- B. Decreased oxygen demand
- C. Optimal oxygen balance
- D. Decreased hemoglobin levels

88. All of the following are characteristic of respiratory distress syndrome in children except:
- A. Air trapping
- B. Atelectasis
- C. Decreased compliance
- D. Infection

89. Hypoxemia associated with respiratory distress syndrome in children results from:
- A. Right-to-left shunting through a patent foramen ovale
- B. Intrapulmonary shunting past inadequately aerated alveoli
- C. Inadequate perfusion of the lungs as a result of pulmonary capillary leakage
- D. Hypoventilation from poor ventilatory effort

90. A 17-month-old child was intubated and mechanically ventilated for 16 days with severe bronchiolitis. Two hours following extubation the child developed sternal retractions, nasal flaring, and used accessory muscles for breathing. What is this child most at risk for to explain these respiratory findings?
- A. Exacerbation of bronchiolitis
- B. Development of pneumonia
- C. Subglottic edema
- D. Rebound bronchoconstriction

NEONATAL-SPECIFIC QUESTIONS

91. An infant with persistent pulmonary hypertension and a patent ductus arteriosus is at risk for developing:
- A. Ascites
- B. Pleural effusion
- C. Pulmonary hemorrhage
- D. Hepatomegaly

92. Which of the following is not associated with the development of idiopathic respiratory distress syndrome (IRDS)?
- A. Lecithin/sphingomyelin (L/S) ratio of 3:1
- B. Prematurity
- C. Persistent fetal circulation
- D. Low birth weight

93. The pathology of transient tachypnea of the newborn (TTN) involves:
- A. Progressive fulminant pulmonary edema
- B. Development of hyaline membrane disease
- C. Formation of an air leak
- D. Persistent presence of lung fluid

94. Which of the following infants is at greatest risk for developing TTN?
- A. Spontaneous vaginal delivery: 36 weeks gestation
- B. Cesarean section delivery: 41 weeks gestation
- C. Induced vaginal delivery: 43 weeks gestation
- D. Vaginal delivery with epidural anesthesia: 38 weeks gestation

95. In order to mobilize secretions in the posterior upper right lobe, the critical care nurse would position an infant on:
- A. Right side elevated 45 degrees and prone
- B. Left side elevated 45 degrees and prone
- C. Right side elevated 45 degrees and supine
- D. Left side elevated 45 degrees and supine

96. Which of the following is proper suctioning procedure of the neonate who does not have an artificial airway?
- A. Perform chest physiotherapy, suction the nasopharyngeal airway, then suction the mouth
- B. Suction the mouth, suction the nasopharyngeal airway, then perform chest physiotherapy
- C. Suction the mouth, perform chest physiotherapy, then suction the nasopharyngeal airway
- D. Perform chest physiotherapy, suction the mouth, then suction the nasopharyngeal airway

97. Prolonged inspiration in relation to expiration provides more efficient ventilation and better arterial oxygenation. A complication associated with prolonged inspiration is:
- A. Atelectasis
- B. Air leak
- C. Decreased V/Q ratio
- D. Bronchial collapse

98. High frequency ventilation is helpful in reducing barotrauma by:
- A. Using large tidal volumes delivered at low pressures
- B. Using large tidal volumes delivered at reduced peak inspiratory pressures
- C. Using small tidal volumes delivered at the mean airway pressure
- D. Using normal tidal volumes delivered at low pressures

99. A premature infant was just intubated for apnea of 30 seconds, unresponsive to tactile stimulation and manual ventilation. When auscultating breath sounds, the critical care nurse hears good breath sounds in the right chest, but absent breath sounds on the left. Which of the following is the best immediate action?

A. Continue to advance the tube until breath sounds are heard bilaterally
B. Remove the tube and manually ventilate until the infant can be reintubated
C. Call for a stat x-ray and continue to manually ventilate the infant
D. Pull the tube back slowly until breath sounds are heard bilaterally

100. During weaning from mechanical ventilation, which of the following parameters is usually lowered *first*?

A. FiO_2
B. Respiratory rate
C. Inspiratory time
D. Tidal volume

101. A premature infant on long-term ventilatory therapy requiring high positive pressure support to achieve an adequate tidal volume develops an air leak accompanied by severe respiratory distress. Which of the following interventions would the critical care nurse anticipate first in treating this infant?

A. Immediate reduction of pressure support
B. Atropine to treat bradycardia
C. Lower the head of the bed
D. Needle aspiration of air

102. Bronchopulmonary dysplasia is *least* likely to be associated with which of the following?

A. High FiO_2 administration
B. Hypovolemia
C. Infection
D. Prematurity

103. Theophylline is used in the neonate to:

A. Treat asthma
B. Improve lung compliance
C. Stimulate surfactant formation
D. Increase tidal volume

104. An infant of 30 weeks gestation exhibits periods of apnea lasting 5 to 10 seconds and periods of breathing of 10 to 15 seconds. What is the most likely cause of this pattern?

A. Periodic breathing
B. Apnea of prematurity
C. Transient tachypnea
D. Apneustic breathing

105. An infant is admitted to the neonatal intensive care unit and the critical care nurse observes acrocyanosis. The best action for the nurse to take next would be to:
A. Administer ¼ liter flow of oxygen by nasal cannula
B. Place the infant in 30% oxygen via hood
C. Suction mouth and nose
D. Observe for central cyanosis

106. Which of the following increases the risk and occurrence of apnea in the premature infant?
I. Use of phototherapy resulting in increased temperature
II. Continuous positive airway pressure
III. Intraventricular hemorrhage
IV. Feeding
A. II, III, IV
B. I, III, IV
C. I, II, III
D. I, II, III, IV

107. For which of the following is an infant of 32 weeks' gestation at the *least* risk?
A. Persistent pulmonary hypertension
B. Patent ductus arteriosus
C. Apnea of prematurity
D. Hypoglycemia

108. An infant with persistent pulmonary hypertension requires sedation to achieve optimal ventilation. Which of the following would be most appropriate?
A. Phenobarbital at 7 mg/kg
B. Phenobarbital at 0.7 mg/kg
C. Fentanyl at 0.4 mcg/kg
D. Fentanyl at 4 mcg/kg

109. Which of the following tests would *not* help identify a metabolic cause of apnea in a premature infant?
A. Arterial blood gases
B. Ionized calcium level
C. Serum magnesium level
D. Complete blood count

110. Increasing the respiratory rate in an intubated infant with persistent pulmonary hypertension has which of the following effects:
A. Decreases pCO_2, causes vasodilation of the pulmonary vessels, and decreases right-to-left shunting
B. Increases pO_2, causes vasodilation of the pulmonary vessels, and decreases right-to-left shunting
C. Increases pCO_2, causes vasodilation of the systemic vessels, and decreases left-to-right shunting
D. Increases pO_2, causes vasodilation of the systemic vessels, and decreases left-to-right shunting

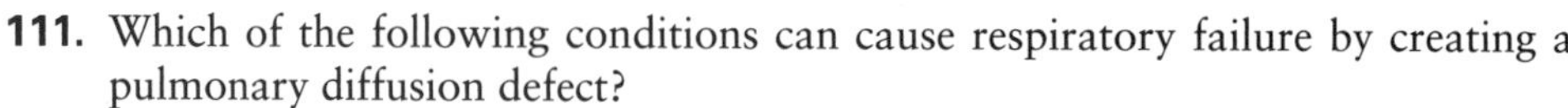

111. Which of the following conditions can cause respiratory failure by creating a pulmonary diffusion defect?
- A. Tracheal stenosis
- B. Apnea of prematurity
- C. Pulmonary edema
- D. Airway obstruction

112. An infant in respiratory distress will assume which of the following positions when possible?
- A. Fetal position
- B. Sniffing position
- C. Knee-chest position
- D. Neck flexion position

113. A premature infant is receiving 30% oxygen via hood. In order to monitor the effectiveness of therapy and prevent complications related to oxygen therapy, which of the following is required?
- A. Arterial blood gases once a shift
- B. Continuous SvO_2 monitoring
- C. Ongoing assessment for cyanosis
- D. Continuous pulse oximetry monitoring

114. Infants at risk for developing pulmonary hemorrhage include all of the following *except:*
- A. Asphyxia
- B. Sepsis
- C. Low birth weight
- D. Oxygen toxicity

115. A 3-day-old infant is diagnosed with acute respiratory failure secondary to apnea of prematurity. In order to minimize multisystem organ failure, which of the following treatments would be most effective?
- A. Maintain a hematocrit greater than 40% to increase oxygen delivery
- B. Maintain PaO_2 greater than 90% to minimize hypoxemia
- C. Maintain low normal cardiac index to decrease cardiac work
- D. Increase stimulation to avoid apneic episodes

116. An infant with aspiration pneumonia from oral secretions would be expected to increase his oxygen consumption as a result of which of the following clinical conditions?
- A. Fever
- B. Seizures
- C. Shivering
- D. Decreased pO_2

Case Study

A full term newborn is admitted to the neonatal intensive care unit in septic shock. The infant appears pale, femoral and brachial pulses are weak, the heart rate is 200, respiratory rate is 70 with nasal flaring and retractions. The infant is electively intubated based on clinical evaluation of the work of breathing as well as blood gases. Questions 117 and 118 refer to this case study.

---

117. At suctioning, the nurse notes large amounts of bright red blood in the catheter. Which of the following is most likely the cause of bleeding?

A. Trauma from intubation
B. Pulmonary hemorrhage
C. Pulmonary hemosiderosis
D. Trauma related to suctioning

118. Initial treatment of this infant would include fluid resuscitation to achieve a CVP of:

A. 10 cm H_2O
B. 5 cm H_2O
C. 15 cm H_2O
D. 2 cm H_2O

Case Study

At birth an infant is noted to have severe respiratory distress, pronounced heart sounds in the right chest, and a scaphoid abdomen. Questions 119 to 121 refer to this case study.

---

119. At birth the infant is judged to need immediate ventilatory assistance. Which of the following would be contraindicated?

A. Ventilation with a bag and mask
B. Intubation and mechanical ventilation at high rates
C. Intubation and mechanical ventilation at low pressures
D. Mechanical ventilation with paralysis

120. All of the following are priorities for the critical care nurse to monitor in this infant *except*:

A. Preductal saturations
B. Postductal saturations
C. Arterial blood gases
D. Capillary blood gases

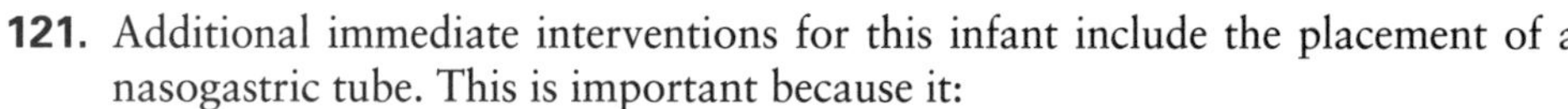

121. Additional immediate interventions for this infant include the placement of a nasogastric tube. This is important because it:
- A. Provides a route for feeding
- B. Prevents aspiration
- C. Decreases compression of lungs
- D. Decreases shunting

122. Most preterm infants demonstrate which mechanism of apnea?
- A. Central apnea
- B. Obstructive apnea
- C. Neural apnea
- D. Mixed apnea

123. All of the following are risk factors related to apnea of preterm infants *except*:
- A. Feeding
- B. Nasogastric intubation
- C. Infection
- D. Periodic breathing

124. A 32-week gestation infant is in a 30% oxygen hood and has been noted to have periods of apnea. When the critical care nurse responds to the apnea alarm, the infant is found to have a heart rate of 72 and slight circumoral cyanosis. The first intervention the nurse should do is:
- A. Gently stimulate the infant by touch
- B. Make a loud noise by clapping or banging
- C. Ventilate the infant with a mask and bag
- D. Prepare for intubation

125. During feedings, a 33-week gestation infant is noted to have periods of apnea. Which of the following is *not* a probable cause?
- A. Poor coordination of sucking and swallowing
- B. Swallowing of air during feeding
- C. Gastroesophageal reflux
- D. Flexion of the neck during feedings

126. Which of the following positions aids in improving ventilation-perfusion matching?
- A. Prone
- B. Supine
- C. Left lateral
- D. Knee-chest

127. A preterm infant is being treated with a methylxanthine for apnea. Which of the following is not a toxic or side effect of this drug?
A. Hypotension and tachycardia
B. Paradoxical apnea
C. Exacerbation poor nutritional status
D. Seizures

128. Theophylline would be used with caution in an infant with which of the following conditions?
A. Hypovolemia
B. Apnea of prematurity
C. Central apnea
D. Congenital heart block

129. Continuous positive airway pressure (CPAP) is a respiratory therapy often used to treat apnea in newborns. For which of the following types of apnea is CPAP *not* effective?
A. Obstructive apnea
B. Mixed apnea
C. Apnea of prematurity
D. Central apnea

130. Which of the following provides the best information about the adequacy of tidal volume for a mechanically ventilated infant?
A. Calculated tidal volume of 10 cc/kg
B. Peak inspiratory pressure of 18 cm H_2O
C. Adequate chest wall movement
D. PaO_2 of greater than 90 mm Hg

131. A 4-hour-old infant is admitted to the neonatal intensive care unit (NICU) with a respiratory rate of 110, nasal flaring, grunting, retractions, and central cyanosis. The nurse notices apneic periods of 12 to 16 seconds. Which of the following would the nurse anticipate doing immediately?
I. Prepare for intubation
II. Draw blood cultures
III. Begin a tolazoline infusion
IV. Begin a dopamine infusion
A. I, II
B. I, II, III
C. III, IV
D. II, IV

132. For neonates who require intubation, high pressures, and high FiO_2, oxygenation should be monitored by:
A. Arterial blood gases at least every 2 to 4 hours and continuous pulse oximetry
B. Arterial blood gases at least every hour and continuous transcutaneous oxygen monitoring
C. Preductal and postductal arterial blood gas sampling every 6 hours and transcutaneous oxygen monitoring
D. Umbilical arterial and venous blood gas sampling every 8 hours and continuous pulse oximetry

133. Use of an umbilical artery catheter has been associated with all of the following *except*:
A. Necrotizing enterocolitis
B. Embolic incidents
C. Hypertension
D. Intracranial hemorrhages

134. Which of the following does *not* increase oxygen consumption in the neonate?
A. Hypothermia
B. Sepsis
C. Fever
D. Chemical paralysis

135. Which of the following natural compensatory mechanisms in infants mimics the therapeutic use of continuous distending pressure?
A. Nasal flaring
B. Grunting
C. Use of accessory muscles
D. Tachypnea

136. Which of the following signs would the nurse look for as an adverse response to the use of positive end expiratory pressure in an infant undergoing mechanical ventilation?
A. Decrease in chest wall movement
B. Decreased peripheral pulses
C. Decreased breath sounds over the left lung field
D. Increased right-to-left shunting

137. When analyzing blood gases, which of the following findings would the nurse recognize as a problem associated with the use of positive end expiratory pressure?
A. Increase in pCO_2
B. Decrease in pO_2
C. Increase in pH
D. Decrease in arterial saturation

138. A term neonate has been diagnosed with persistent pulmonary hypertension. Treatment includes intubation and mechanical ventilation with high ventilatory rates. Despite mechanical ventilation, oxygenation remains inadequate and right-to-left shunting is significant. Which of the following would the nurse anticipate being used next to improve oxygenation and decrease shunting?

A. Further increase ventilatory rate
B. Sedation and paralysis
C. Increase the FiO_2 and tidal volume
D. Decrease the respiratory rate

139. Which of the following may be helpful in preventing atelectasis after extubation following prolonged mechanical ventilatory support?

A. Nasal CPAP
B. Racemic epinephrine
C. Aminophylline
D. Caffeine

140. During chest physiotherapy for the preterm infant with respiratory distress syndrome, what should the nurse be continuously monitoring?

A. Breath sounds
B. Respiratory rate
C. Electrocardiogram
D. Pulse oximetry

141. A 28-week gestation infant was intubated and mechanically ventilated for 2 weeks for respiratory distress syndrome. Despite aggressive respiratory management, the neonate's need for an FiO_2 of 0.6 and pressures of 36/6 were constant and progress in weaning was poor. What diagnostic test would be indicated to rule out another commonly associated pathology?

A. Echocardiogram
B. Electrocardiogram
C. Renal ultrasound
D. Liver enzyme tests

142. Which of the following would be used to help medically close a patent ductus arteriosus?

A. Prostaglandin E_1 at .05 to 0.1 mcg/kg/min
B. Prostaglandin E_1 at .05 to 0.1 mcg/kg/dose
C. Indomethacin 0.1 to 0.3 mg/kg/dose
D. Indomethacin 0.1 to 0.3 mg/kg/min

(Not close it)

143. Patterns of pathological aeration associated with meconium aspiration include:
   I. Areas of atelectasis
   II. Areas of air trapping
   III. Air leaks
   IV. Decrease in functional residual capacity
   A. I only
   B. II only
   C. I, II, III
   D. I, II, III, IV

144. A neonate with congenital bilateral choanal atresia should also have which of the following diagnostic tests?
   A. Liver function tests
   B. Echocardiogram
   C. Renal ultrasound
   D. Barium swallow

145. Which of the following therapies is most effective in reducing the development of chronic lung disease and bronchopulmonary dysplasia in neonates?
   A. FiO_2 >0.5 to reduce hypoxemia
   B. PEEP levels of 8 to 10 cm H_2O to prevent airway collapse
   C. Maintenance fluid therapy of 105 mL/kg/day to prevent tenacious secretions and airway obstruction
   D. Indomethacin therapy to close a patent ductus arteriosus

146. Nutritional support is critical in infants with bronchopulmonary dysplasia for all of the following reasons *except:*
   A. An increase in oxygen consumption
   B. To prevent fractures
   C. To prevent infection
   D. To increase metabolic demand

Answers

1. Correct answer—A.
Surfactant decreases surface tension to increase lung compliance, decreases opening pressure of the alveoli, and helps promote clearance of fluid from the alveoli. Surfactant does not decrease surface tension which would promote collapsing of the alveoli.

2. Correct answer—A.
Pulmonary emboli would increase the ventilation/perfusion ratio by decreasing the amount of circulation available to aerated alveoli in relation to the number of aerated alveoli. If the normal V/Q ratio is $\frac{4}{5}$ or 0.8, decreasing the denominator (the amount of perfusion) actually increases the ratio. If normal perfusion falls from 5 to 3, then the ratio itself becomes $\frac{4}{3}$ which is greater than $\frac{4}{5}$. All of the other conditions decrease ventilation rather than perfusion, which results in a decrease in the V/Q ratio.

3. Correct answer—C.
The goal of oxygen therapy is to increase oxygen delivery to the tissues and cells. Increasing inspired oxygen only addresses oxygen levels within the airways, and does not guarantee that increased oxygen is reaching the tissues. Continuous positive airway pressure and positive end expiratory pressure are two examples of therapies that may need to be used in conjunction with oxygen therapy because increased oxygen alone would not be effective in increasing oxygen delivery. Carbon dioxide levels are decreased by either increasing respiratory rate, decreasing air trapping, or increasing expired volume. Oxygen therapy is not effective in reducing CO_2 levels. Oxygen consumption is reduced by decreasing cellular demand.

4. Correct answer—B.
Pulse oximetry measures hemoglobin oxygen saturation. The arterial oxygen tension (PaO_2) is measured by blood gas analysis or by using an oxygen dissociation curve with a known arterial oxygen saturation.

5. Correct answer—D.
Continuous bubbling in the water seal chamber indicates a leak in the system between the water seal and the patient. If leaking stops with brief clamping at the insertion site, continue to move the clamp closer at regular, small intervals and clamp briefly to see if bubbling stops. If bubbling stops at all points along the path of the collection tubing, the patient most likely has an intrapleural air leak. Unclamp the tube immediately to prevent a pneumothorax and notify the physician who may need to change the tube. Kinks in the suction tubing would create an absence of bubbling in the suction control chamber. Milking the chest tube gently to remove clots would be indicated if a clot in the chest tube was suspected. An absence of either fluctuation or mild bubbling in the water

seal chamber can indicate clotting of the chest tube. Raising the tubing between the patient and the collection system to empty stagnant drainage would be indicated if an unexpected decrease in chest drainage were observed.

6. **Correct answer—B.**
   These blood gases indicate respiratory acidosis related to hypercarbia. Increasing the respiratory rate would increase the exhalation and elimination of CO_2. Increasing the FiO_2 would improve the PaO_2, but not change the patient's pH or CO_2 levels which are the greater problem. Decreasing the peak inspiratory pressure would further increase the $PaCO_2$, and increasing the I/E ratio would not significantly affect the $PaCO_2$. Carbon dioxide is primarily eliminated by adequate respiratory rate and tidal volume.

7. **Correct answer—B.**
   Fluid fluctuations in the water seal chamber during respirations are normal and indicate the system is functioning properly. Milking the chest tube gently would be indicated if there was no fluctuation in the water seal chamber. Disconnecting the system and manually ventilating the patient would be contraindicated. There would be no need to suspect the patient is in respiratory distress.

8. **Correct answer—D.**
   These blood gases most likely represent hypoventilation associated with the effects of anesthesia. Administration of oxygen would not improve hypercarbia and respiratory acidosis. Administration of narcotic analgesics this early in the postoperative period associated with a decreased level of consciousness would only exacerbate hypoventilation. Administration of sodium bicarbonate can actually worsen respiratory acidosis. Naloxone reverses the effects of anesthesia and would be expected to reverse hypoventilation associated with central respiratory depression.

9. **Correct answer—D.**
   Assessing the ventilation of the patient by auscultating breath sounds immediately would be the most important intervention in determining the cause and the corrective action. A sudden deterioration of an intubated and ventilated patient can be caused by a number of factors such as ventilator failure, tube obstruction, and tube displacement. The most appropriate action would be to auscultate breath sounds bilaterally to determine if both lungs are being ventilated. In the event of tube obstruction or displacement, increasing the FiO_2 or manually ventilating the patient would be ineffective. Immediate suctioning of the endotracheal tube would only be helpful in the case of obstruction. If tube displacement or ventilator failure were the causes of respiratory distress, this intervention would not be effective.

10. **Correct answer—A.**
    Pressure cycled ventilators are most effective for an infant or small child because of the small tidal volumes. Volume cycled ventilators work best when

larger tidal volumes are required. Time cycled ventilators are not sensitive enough to the pressures or volumes delivered and therefore are not as safe in infants and children. Negative pressure ventilators are not commonly used in critical care. They are large and limit access to the critically ill infant's or child's body.

11. Correct answer—B.

The most likely explanation for the differences in pulse oximetry readings between his upper and lower extremities is persistence of fetal circulation (PFC). Because the patent ductus arteriosus (PDA) remains open in PFC, venous blood is shunted from the right ventricle directly into the aorta through the PDA beyond the subclavian arteries. This makes saturations in the lower extremities much lower because blood delivered here is mixed arterial-venous blood. Coarctation of the aorta or inaccurate pulse oximetry readings can account for differing saturations, but the history of meconium aspiration is consistent with persistent pulmonary hypertension. Poor peripheral circulation from massive peripheral arterial constriction would not cause a difference between upper and lower extremity readings.

12. Correct answer—C.

A pH of 7.50, which is slightly alkalotic, would be the best outcome of ventilatory therapy for this infant. A slightly alkalotic arterial pH promotes pulmonary arterial dilation in the newborn period rather than persistence of pulmonary hypertension or vasoconstriction. A pH of 7.35 or 7.47 would be too low to achieve this effect. A pH of 7.67 is too alkalotic and would cause other multisystem problems.

13. Correct answer—B.

Alkalosis is associated with hypocalcemia because an increase in the pH causes increased calcium protein binding, leaving less ionized calcium available. Hypocalcemia is associated with hypomagnesemia. Alkalosis also is associated with hypokalemia because as hydrogen ions leave the cells to raise serum pH, potassium ions enter the cells to replace the positive charges lost. Hyponatremia is not closely related to alkalosis.

14. Correct answer—A.

Tachypnea, or an increase in respiratory rate, is the first compensatory mechanism. Later compensatory actions include nasal flaring, retractions, and grunting.

15. Correct answer—C.

These symptoms and the infant's history are most consistent with oxygen toxicity. Pneumonia most likely would be accompanied by fever and increased secretions, and crackles would be noted. Acute foreign body aspiration or airway obstruction would be accompanied by coughing, stridor, and wheezing or, in total obstruction, absent breath sounds.

16. Correct answer—A.
Restricting fluids would only thicken any secretions formed and make removal by coughing or suctioning more difficult. Suctioning, humidification to loosen and thin secretions, and chest physiotherapy all would promote removal of pulmonary secretions.

17. Correct answer—A.
Increasing the FiO_2 and elevating the head of the bed promotes more effective ventilation. These findings, especially asymmetrical chest excursion and shifted breath sounds, are consistent with a pneumothorax or air leak. Suctioning would not be effective and only increase hypoxemia. Calling for a stat x-ray even with tube displacement does not address the immediate distress the patient is exhibiting. Epinephrine would be indicated if there were no pulse, not with bradycardia.

18. Correct answer—D.
Negative pressure ventilation is not associated with the development of bronchopulmonary dysplasia. Patent ductus arteriosus, high levels of oxygen therapy, positive pressure ventilation, fluid overload in the neonatal period, family history of asthma, and prematurity are all implicated in the development of bronchopulmonary dysplasia.

19. Correct answer—B.
Beta-blockers would not be used because they promote bronchoconstriction. Diuretics, beta-adrenergic agonists (bronchodilators), cortiocosteroids, and vasodilators are all used in the treatment of BPD.

20. Correct answer—C.
Symptoms of respiratory distress, blood gases revealing respiratory and metabolic acidosis, and a classic chest x-ray with a ground-glass appearance is indicative of respiratory distress syndrome (RDS). Aspiration pneumonia would typically manifest with wheezing rather than decreased breath sounds and the chest x-ray would show diffuse infiltrates. Persistent pulmonary hypertension would manifest with cyanosis, no ground-glass appearance to the x-ray, and a PDA shunt murmur without decreased breath sounds. Bronchopulmonary dysplasia typically develops later as a sequelae to RDS. The chest x-ray would show linear infiltrates, and symptoms of right-sided heart failure would be common.

21. Correct answer—B.
The goals of therapy would be to reduce hypoxemia to decrease metabolic acidosis resulting from anaerobic metabolism and increase the pH to correct the acidosis. Decreasing the ambient temperature would stress the infant and increase metabolic demands, oxygen consumption, and therefore metabolic acidosis. Increasing the pCO_2 would further increase the acidosis, not offset a bicarbonate deficit.

22. Correct answer—A.
An important factor in the development of respiratory distress syndrome is the decrease in surfactant metabolism. 2,3-DPG is a critical component in binding and releasing oxygen from hemoglobin, but is not involved in respiratory distress syndrome.

23. Correct answer—C.
Because infants are obligate nose breathers, placement of a nasogastric tube would increase the work of breathing by serving as an obstruction. Decreased compliance of the lungs occurs with RDS and increases the work of breathing by increasing the pressures the infant needs to create by breathing to allow adequate ventilation. Decreased chest wall compliance would actually decrease the work of breathing by having a more stable cavity to allow less diaphragmatic movement to exchange gases. Oxygen administration would improve hypoxia, thereby reducing respiratory distress associated with hypoxemia.

24. Correct answer—B.
Positive end expiratory pressure (PEEP) improves the respiratory status by opening atelectatic *alveoli* and moving edema from the site of gas exchange into areas of the lungs where gas exchange does not occur. Continuous positive airway pressure (CPAP) does not ensure the patency of an airway; intubation or the use of a nasal or oral airway performs this function. Adequate ventilatory effort on the part of the patient must be present or mechanical support is required.

25. Correct answer—D.
Proper endotracheal tube placement immediately after intubation is best determined by noting bilateral chest expansion with manual or mechanical ventilation. Presence of breath sounds over the upper left quadrant indicates air is entering the esophagus. Bronchial breath sounds over the trachea would give no information about whether the trachea, not the right bronchus, has been intubated. Good excursion of the right chest during ventilation indicates adequate ventilation of the right lung, but gives no information about expansion and ventilation of the left lung. Right mainstem bronchus intubation is a common problem as a result of the angle it comes off the mainstem bronchus.

26. Correct answer—B.
Grunting increases end expiratory pressure to promote gas exchange and prevent collapse of small—not large—airways and alveoli. Vital capacity is the maximal amount of air that can be forcibly exhaled after maximal inhalation and would not be measured in a patient in respiratory distress. Grunting does not significantly reduce the work of breathing to decrease oxygen demands.

27. Correct answer—A.
Infants and children in respiratory distress need to be positioned upright or allowed to assume a position of comfort to increase vital capacity and

therefore lung volume. The work of breathing and oxygen consumption are not significantly reduced by positioning, but respiratory efforts are more effective.

28. Correct answer—C.
Atropine should not be used routinely during intubation to prevent vagal bradydysrhythmias because it may mask bradydysrhythmias from hypoxia associated with intubation. Atropine does not cause laryngospasms or decrease respiratory efforts. It does decrease the production of secretions.

29. Correct answer—C.
Vesicular breath sounds are normally auscultated over the peripheral lung fields. Bronchial breath sounds are heard over large airways, and bronchovesicular breath sounds are heard between the large airways and peripheral lung fields.

30. Correct answer—C.
Postoperative care of a patient who has undergone repair of a tracheoesophageal fistula would include suctioning only to the end of the endotracheal tube or a level of 8 cm with oral suctioning to prevent damage to the surgical anastomosis site. Pacifiers are not used because they increase oral secretions. A gastrostomy tube is not always required postoperatively.

31. Correct answer—D.
HCO_3^- is the metabolic component of acid-base balance found in arterial blood gases. The pH measures the acid-base balance in general, while the pCO_2 is a respiratory component. The pO_2 is not directly related to acid-base balance.

32. Correct answer—B.
Maintenance fluid requirements of 75% are optimal for a normovolemic neonate with respiratory distress syndrome who is intubated and mechanically ventilated. A slightly dry state is desirable to reduce the development of pulmonary edema. Less than ⅔ maintenance fluid requirements would not be recommended because of the effect on circulating volume, and mechanical ventilation would further decrease venous return and cardiac output. Amounts greater than 75% are likely to increase the development of pulmonary edema.

33. Correct answer—D.
Nasal continuous positive airway pressure therapy is effective because it increases functional residual capacity and discourages collapse of the alveoli. Tidal volume is related more to respiratory effort or delivered volume by mechanical ventilation. Decreasing residual volume would promote alveolar collapse, and anatomic dead space is a fixed amount of the respiratory system where gas exchange cannot occur.

34. Correct answer—A.
Tolazoline, nitroprusside, nitroglycerin, adenosine, and prostaglandin E_1 may be used to treat persistent pulmonary hypertension. These all promote pulmonary vasodilation.

35. Correct answer—D.
These results show uncompensated respiratory acidosis. The pH is less than 7.35 indicating acidosis that is uncompensated. The pCO_2 and HCO_3^- are elevated supporting a respiratory basis and the start of metabolic compensation.

36. Correct answer—A.
Thick, white secretions within 12 hours of surgery are unlikely to be caused by infection. The use of saline instillations does not thin secretions for suctioning. Sterile technique should always be used in suctioning.

37. Correct answer—B.
In caring for the patient with a newly inserted tracheostomy, it is important to keep a tracheostomy tube one size smaller at the bedside in the event of accidental decannulation. Recannulation in a fresh tracheostomy is best achieved with a smaller tube until the tract made by the surgical placement is well healed days later. The tube should be secured with a knot at the back of the neck to prevent accidental unfastening. The tube should be secured allowing the width of a little finger to prevent excessive pressure which could lead to tissue damage.

38. Correct answer—D.
Immediately following a tracheostomy, the most critical complication is decannulation. Recannulation with a freshly placed tracheostomy is difficult as a result of edema and the lack of a tract formation. Tenacious secretions from bypass of upper airway humidification processes, infection, and speech delays all develop later.

39. Correct answer—A.
Adequate respiratory effort is required in order to use facial CPAP. CPAP only maintains positive airway pressure; it does not provide ventilation. Intubation and airways are not required. CPAP may be used to treat or prevent atelectasis.

40. Correct answer—A.
Following surgery for an infant who has undergone repair of a congenital diaphragmatic hernia, the chest tube should be placed on the affected side and to water seal only for drainage of fluids and blood as well as gentle reexpansion. Suction can cause a mediastinal shift and compromise lung and cardiac function.

41. Correct answer—C.
A history of polyhydramnios and copious oral secretions after birth are consistent with tracheoesophageal fistula. The infant is unable to swallow amniotic fluid or normal oral secretions. Down syndrome and cleft lip can cause feeding problems but are not typically associated with failure to handle oral secretions. Pulmonary edema could produce frothy sputum; however, it also would be associated with severe respiratory distress.

42. Correct answer—C.

These blood gases indicate metabolic acidosis. A pH of <7.35 indicates acidosis. This is supported by a lack of metabolic bases in the HCO_3^- value of 14 mEq/L. There is some respiratory compensation seen by a decrease in pCO_2 to 30 mm Hg. A decreased saturation of 89% and hypoxemia of 62 mm Hg suggest that metabolic acids are accumulating as a result of anaerobic metabolism.

43. Correct answer—B.

A steady increase in peak inspiratory pressures over 24 hours indicates a decrease in lung compliance and a worsening of pulmonary disease. Stiff, noncompliant lungs will require increasing pressures to deliver a required amount of volume. There is no evidence of a decrease in oxygen needs.

44. Correct answer—D.

These symptoms and history are consistent with right bronchial intubation, a frequent complication of intubation that usually manifests early after the procedure. Because the right main bronchus comes off the trachea at a straighter angle, passing the tube too far will result in intubation of only one lung, usually the right.

45. Correct answer—A.

Functional residual capacity (FRC) increases with bronchopulmonary dysplasia as a result of air trapping. The amount of air remaining at the end of expiration (FRC) increases as air is trapped and effectively reduces vital capacity and tidal volume. Lung compliance is decreased in BPD.

46. Correct answer—C.

During suctioning for patients on mechanical ventilation with PEEP, the critical care nurse uses a closed suctioning system to prevent interruption of PEEP. Almost all patients who are mechanically ventilated benefit from preoxygenation at 100% before suctioning. Suctioning should not be done routinely, but also should not be avoided when assessments indicate the need.

47. Correct answer—B.

Apnea of prematurity is primarily caused by ineffective central nervous system response to increased pCO_2. A rise in the pCO_2 fails to stimulate respiration. Respiratory muscles are able to respond to central nervous system stimulus when present. Surfactant is a factor in the development of RDS. Failure to clear fluid from the lungs results in transient tachypnea of the newborn.

48. Correct answer—D.

An optimal level of PEEP is a level that reduces intrapulmonary shunting. The ideal PEEP is the lowest level that increases oxygen delivery, not levels that achieve the highest PaO_2 or hemoglobin saturation. Ideally, PEEP will achieve a pO_2 >70 to 80 mm Hg and an SaO_2 >92% without decreasing cardiac output. PEEP should increase, not decrease, lung compliance.

49. Correct answer—A.
Asthma actually increases lung compliance whereas pneumothorax, atelectasis, and pulmonary edema decrease compliance.

50. Correct answer—B.
These clinical findings and the chest x-ray are consistent with a diaphragmatic hernia. Severe respiratory distress, absence of breath sounds, shifting of chest contents, and acidosis characterize this anomaly. Presence of bowel in the chest cavity as seen by x-ray is diagnostic. None of the other conditions would cause bowel to shift to the thorax.

51. Correct answer—A.
The infant with congenital diaphragmatic hernia is at risk for developing persistent fetal circulation. In order to effectively monitor oxygenation and detect persistent pulmonary hypertension, the readings should compare preductal and postductal blood flow. Lower extremities are supplied by blood below the ductal level, upper extremities are supplied by preductal flow. The umbilical artery measures postductal blood flow, the radial artery preductal flow.

52. Correct answer—D.
Postoperative ventilatory management of a neonate with congenital diaphragmatic hernia includes mechanical ventilation with low PIP and PEEP pressures as well as conservative tidal volumes. The hypoplastic lungs cannot be expanded too rapidly and are at high risk for barotrauma and air leaks.

53. Correct answer—B.
Underwater drainage helps prevent air from entering the pleural space during inhalation which generates a negative, or pulling pressure, otherwise, air would be pulled into the chest. This prevents a pneumothorax, not a hemothorax.

54. Correct answer—C.
Increasing the inspiratory/expiratory ratio through mechanical ventilation helps recruit atelectatic lung areas by discouraging collapse during full expiration. An increased I/E ratio improves refractory hypoxemia. Increasing respiratory rate and tidal volume would improve refractory hypercarbia. Bronchospasms are not affected by the I/E ratio. Oxygen toxicity can only be prevented by avoiding elevated FiO_2 settings.

55. Correct answer—B.
Administering 100% oxygen at rapid ventilatory rates to the infant suspected of having persistent pulmonary hypertension will result in respiratory alkalosis and pulmonary artery vasodilation. PPHN is not characterized by atelectatic lung areas that need to be recruited. If the PaO_2 is not improved by hyperventilation and hyperoxia, then a diagnosis of a congenital cardiac defect associated with right-to-left shunting is likely. Refractory hypoxemia more than hypercarbia characterizes persistent pulmonary hypertension.

56. Correct answer—C.
Oxygen exchange during mechanical ventilation is most influenced by changes in the mean airway pressure. Mean airway pressure is a function of the peak inspiratory, positive end expiratory pressure, inspiratory time, and expiratory time. Changes in tidal volume and respiratory rate most affect carbon dioxide gas exchange during assisted ventilation. Changes in oxygen consumption do not influence gaseous exchange, but rather influence oxygen demand.

PEDIATRIC-SPECIFIC ANSWERS

57. Correct answer—A.
Rales and crackles characterize distal lung field disease. Croup is an upper airway problem that affects the vocal cords, epiglottis, trachea, subglottic area, or bronchi. Croup is characterized by dyspnea, cough, stridor, and hoarseness.

58. Correct answer—B.
The ventilation-perfusion (V/Q) mismatch observed in this child would be related to decreased ventilation as a result of small airway obstruction. Ventilation would be decreased resulting in a decline in the V/Q ratio. Inhalation and inspiration are a greater problem than air trapping in croup. A decrease in cardiac output would be late related to shock and impending respiratory arrest.

59. Correct answer—C.
Drooling would be a clinical finding indicative of an emergency because the oropharynx is so obstructed that secretions cannot be swallowed. It is usually found in epiglottitis. Epiglottitis is a medical emergency and is associated with a high risk of respiratory arrest, which may be refractory to endotracheal intubation.

60. Correct answer—D.
Drawing arterial blood gases would be deferred until an x-ray was obtained to rule out epiglottis. Any painful or stressful procedures would be avoided until epiglottitis is ruled out to avoid acute worsening or airway occlusion. Breath sounds can be auscultated providing this does not cause the child to be too anxious, and humidified oxygen may improve oxygenation and reduce inflammation. A urine sample would not be a priority for treating a child with this suspected diagnosis.

61. Correct answer—A.
For a child with bleeding, unstable vital signs, and symptoms of poor systemic perfusion unresponsive to fluid therapy at 20 mL/kg, direct pressure monitoring is indicated. Increasing fluid therapy or initiating vasoactive drugs is not indicated until more information is available about systemic arterial pressure and filling pressures of the heart. Dopamine would not be indicated in the presence of continued hypovolemia. The vasodilatory effect of amrinone could exacerbate hypotension.

62. Correct answer—B.

The use of positive end expiratory pressure in a patient with pulmonary hemorrhage helps restore functional residual capacity, recruit atelectatic areas, minimize FiO_2 requirements, and reduce the risks of oxygen toxicity. Because blood acts as a diffusion barrier in the alveoli, gas exchange is impaired. Increasing the tidal volume and respiratory rate will not maintain an increased pressure in the alveoli at end expiration so FRC is not increased and atelectasis is not minimized. Decreasing the inspiratory/expiratory ratio will increase expiratory time and decrease FRC.

63. Correct answer—B.

A decrease in wheezing and lethargy in an asthma patient with previous signs and symptoms of respiratory distress is an ominous finding which heralds respiratory arrest. A chest tube would be indicated only if a pneumothorax was present. An epinephrine intravenously is not indicated without severe hemodynamic compromise.

64. Correct answer—B.

In order to minimize multisystem organ failure in a child with respiratory failure, a goal of therapy is to maintain the arterial saturation greater than 90% to minimize hypoxemia to organs. The hematocrit should be maintained between 30% and 40%, and the cardiac index should be supported to be normal or slightly above normal to increase oxygen delivery. The FiO_2 should be adjusted to maintain an adequate pO_2 and arterial saturation, not automatically set at any predetermined level.

65. Correct answer—A.

In a patient with status asthmaticus, the inspiratory/expiratory ratio is decreased as a result of the difficulty in exhaling trapped air. Air trapping leads to an increased functional residual volume.

66. Correct answer—B.

During an acute asthma attack, respiratory rate and ventilatory efforts are greatly increased. There is no predetermined oxygen level required. Chest physiotherapy is not indicated early in an attack because it increases the risk of exacerbating airway obstruction. Serum terbutaline levels are not measured.

67. Correct answer—C.

Residual volume in the lungs increases with air trapping. It would not be a goal of therapy to further increase air trapping. The goal of treatment in status asthmaticus includes increasing oxygen delivery, improving ventilation, and decreasing airway obstruction.

68. Correct answer—C.

Chest pain exacerbated by inspiration, shallow respirations, tenderness, and paradoxical respirations is most likely related to flail chest or multiple rib fractures. The chest wall becomes unstable with multiple fractures and flail chest resulting in chest expansion during exhalation rather than inhalation. Contraction of the chest wall occurs during inhalation. A single fractured rib, pneumothorax, and hemothorax would not produce paradoxical respirations.

69. Correct answer—A.
In administering aerosol bronchodilators, the critical care nurse observes for tachycardia, restlessness, nausea, vomiting, headache, vertigo, decreased pO_2, and other signs of adrenergic-sympathetic stimulation.

70. Correct answer—C.
Because a paper clip is metal, it is radiopaque and easily visualized on x-ray. Objects such as food and nonmetal objects such as an eraser are not easily imaged by x-ray.

71. Correct answer—B.
The normal serum level of aminophylline is 10 to 20 mcg/mL.

72. Correct answer—A.
The hypoxia associated with asthma is a result of ventilation/perfusion mismatch. Aeration of alveoli is decreased while perfusion is largely unchanged. Blood from the right intracardiac side of the heart fails to come in contact with aerated alveoli, decreasing the V/Q ratio. Patients in acute respiratory distress such as asthma actually have increased, not decreased, ventilatory efforts. Left-to-right shunting would not be associated with hypoxemia. While there are increased oxygen demands, they do not account for hypoxemia in asthma.

73. Correct answer—D.
Beta-agonists are used to treat asthma and are most often administered by aerosol. Because of their sympathomimetic action, they are bronchodilators.

74. Correct answer—D.
Aminophylline is administered orally or intravenously but not by aerosol. Medications to treat asthma, which can be given by aerosol, include epinephrine, racemic epinephrine, isoproterenol, atropine, isoetharine, metaproteronol, terbutaline, and albuterol.

75. Correct answer—C.
Whenever a child who is demonstrating signs and symptoms of acute respiratory distress suddenly decreases his respiratory and cardiac rates, becomes lethargic, or drools, impending arrest must be suspected. The work of breathing can become so difficult and tiring that respiratory arrest develops. A previously anxious child who becomes quiet or a quiet child who becomes agitated may be an indication of hypoxia or impending arrest. Resolution of the obstruction would be unlikely without raising the object, and is unlikely to cause abnormally low respiratory and heart rates. Adaptation to the hospital setting for a 3-year-old in this length of time also is not likely. Development of a pneumothorax would increase respiratory distress.

76. Correct answer—D.
Possible complications following foreign body airway obstruction include infection, further obstruction from edema or broken pieces of the original object, hoarseness, and cough. Cyanosis would indicate further respiratory distress and require immediate attention.

77. Correct answer—A.
A rapid fall to near 0 levels in end-tidal CO_2 monitoring ($P_{ET}CO_2$) is most likely as a result of partial obstruction of the airway or an air leak in the system. A falling PaO_2 is not directly linked to a falling $P_{ET}CO_2$. Hypoventilation and migration of the tube would cause a gradual rise in the $P_{ET}CO_2$.

78. Correct answer—B.
Symptoms such as nasal discharge, tachypnea, nonproductive cough, low grade fever, poor feeding, hypercapnia, respiratory acidosis, retractions, nasal flaring, use of accessory muscles to breath, in addition to adventitious and decreased breath sounds are all indicative of bronchiolitis. Bronchiolitis is a viral infection that predominantly affects the lower airways or small bronchioles and causes air trapping leading to emphysema-like conditions. It typically starts with or is associated with upper respiratory tract infections. Bacterial pneumonia and aspiration pneumonia are unlikely to be associated with upper respiratory tract symptoms such as nasal discharge. Bronchopulmonary dysplasia does not present as an infectious process.

79. Correct answer—A.
When examining a child who may have epiglottitis, the critical care nurse would avoid examining the throat because of the risk of inducing gagging and causing acute airway obstruction. Performing a painful procedure such as drawing blood gases to evaluate respiratory failure would be avoided because it also could precipitate laryngospasm or exacerbate airway obstruction. Parents should be encouraged to remain with the child because fear and anxiety also can precipitate acute obstruction. Administration of humidified oxygen is indicated to treat hypoxemia and may help treat the edematous epiglottis.

80. Correct answer—A.
In assessing for a pneumothorax, the critical care nurse would look for distant breath sounds, change in pitch, and tracheal deviation to the right. Tracheal deviation is away from the affected lung as a result of the increase in lung volume on the affected side from trapped air. Breath sounds are not hyperresonant because the air is trapped in the pleural space. Crackles and wheezes are sounds that originate in the airway, not in trapped spaces where pneumothoraxes occur.

81. Correct answer—D.
Complaints of chest pain, coarse breath sounds, and a slightly increased respiratory rate accompanied by nasal flaring without use of accessory muscles in a chest trauma patient suggests a lung contusion. A hemothorax generally

produces distant sounds or change in pitch and is likely to be associated with more severe respiratory distress. A rib fracture, which is uncomplicated, may cause decreased breath sounds associated with hypoventilation secondary to pain while breathing, not an increased respiratory rate with nasal flaring. A chylothorax is more commonly seen following thoracic surgery but may present similarly to a hemothorax.

82. Correct answer—B.
Pericardial tamponade is the accumulation of fluid or blood in the pericardial sac, which constricts the pumping action of the heart and prevents adequate diastolic filling and reduces cardiac output. Classic signs and symptoms are related to both right- and left-sided heart failure such as combativeness, restlessness, hypotension, jugular vein distension, poor peripheral perfusion, and narrow pulse pressure. Treatment is to directly tap the pericardial space and remove the fluid or air that is constricting the heart.

83. Correct answer—A.
Most commonly, hydrocarbon ingestion produces severe dyspnea, wheezing, cardiac dysrhythmias, and central nervous system depression. Hydrocarbons include gasoline, lighter fluid, motor oil, nail polish removers, refrigerants, propellants, and furniture polish. Seizures can occur with aromatic hydrocarbons, but frothy sputum and fever are not typical. Dyspnea is usually so severe it would not be restricted to nasal flaring and sternal retractions.

84. Correct answer—C.
Children with bronchopulmonary dysplasia are most likely to be at risk for developing bronchiolitis related to the respiratory syncytial virus and its underlying chronic airway disease. They have no increased risk factors for aspiration or pulmonary hemorrhage. Pneumothoraxes would not be common.

85. Correct answer—C.
Values obtained by monitoring of $P_{ET}CO_2$ in patients without lung disease reflect the alveolar pCO_2, $PaCO_2$, and amount of CO_2 in exhaled gases. The serum CO_2 reflects bicarbonate levels and is not a measurement of CO_2 as a respiratory gas.

86. Correct answer—B.
A mixed venous pO2 of 38 mm Hg is within the normal range of 35 to 40 mm Hg. This blood sample is venous, not arterial, so the pO_2 would be expected to be much less. Because this value is within the normal limits, there is no reason based on the mixed venous pO_2 to suspect hypoxia, shock, hypoventilation, or respiratory acidosis.

87. Correct answer—A.
The normal range for SvO_2 is about 60% to 80%. A mixed venous oxygen saturation (SvO_2) of 55% in a patient with respiratory distress syndrome most

likely would indicate decreased oxygen delivery as a result of pulmonary disease. Decreased oxygen balance would result in an increase in the SvO_2. Optimal oxygen demand would require a more normal SvO_2. Decreased hemoglobin levels would not be discernable directly from the SvO_2 because this value is a percentage.

88. Correct answer—A.
Air trapping occurs in asthma and obstructive lung diseases, not respiratory distress syndrome. Characteristics of respiratory distress syndrome in children include atelectasis, decreased lung compliance, infection, decreased surfactant production, and decreased functional residual capacity. Right-to-left intrapulmonary shunting also occurs.

89. Correct answer—B.
Hypoxemia associated with respiratory distress syndrome in children results from intrapulmonary shunting past inadequately aerated alveoli. Right-to-left shunting occurs because unoxygenated blood from the right side of the heart passes through the lungs to the left heart without being adequately oxygenated. A foramen ovale is not normally patent in children. While capillary leak in the lungs is associated with RDS, generally there is not a lack of perfusion. Most patients with RDS are breathing rapidly and deeply to compensate for hypoxia, and therefore do not hypoventilate.

90. Correct answer—C.
A child who has been intubated and mechanically ventilated for a prolonged period is at risk for developing subglottic edema following extubation. Development of an infectious process is likely to be less acute. Rebound bronchoconstriction may occur following the use of beta-agonist nebulizer therapy.

NEONATAL-SPECIFIC ANSWERS

91. Correct answer—C.
An infant with persistent pulmonary hypertension and a patent ductus arteriosus is at risk for developing pulmonary hemorrhage as a result of left-sided failure from increased blood flow to and work of the left ventricle. With left ventricular failure, the left ventricular end diastolic pressure rises and causes a backup to the point of raising the pulmonary capillary pressure which leads to a risk of pulmonary hemorrhage. Hepatomegaly and ascites will result from right-sided, not left-sided, pressure. Pleural effusion results from accumulation of fluid in the intrapleural space.

92. Correct answer—A.
An L/S ratio greater than 2:1 is not associated with the development or IRDS. An increased L/S ratio shows lung fluid has moved well into the amniotic fluid preparing the lungs more effectively to function adequately after birth. Factors

which are associated with the development of IRDS include prematurity, persistent fetal circulation, low birth weight, male sex, multiple gestations, and a variety of maternal health problems.

93. Correct answer—D.
TTN develops when normal fetal lung fluid remains in the lungs following birth causing an obstructive and air trapping lung disease. While fluid is present, it is not the result of leaky capillaries as in pulmonary edema. Hyaline membrane disease (idiopathic respiratory distress syndrome) is not associated with fetal lung fluid.

94. Correct answer—B.
Transient tachypnea of the newborn is seen most typically in term or near term infants who are born by cesarean section or who have a precipitous delivery. Normal vaginal delivery causes compressions of the chest which help eliminate fetal lung fluid. Time during delivery also allows for resorption of fluid. In TTN, fluid remains in the neonate's lungs and obstructs airways.

95. Correct answer—A.
In order to mobilize secretions in the posterior upper right lobe, the critical care nurse would position an infant with the right side elevated 45 degrees and prone. The left side elevated 45 degrees and prone would drain the posterior upper left lobe. The right side elevated 45 degrees and supine would drain the anterior upper right lobe while having the left side elevated 45 degrees and supine would drain the anterior upper left lobe.

96. Correct answer—D.
Chest physiotherapy should be performed first to loosen secretions within the chest which can then be cleared. Suctioning the mouth first is important to prevent aspiration. When the nares are stimulated with a catheter, reflex inspiration occurs which could lead to aspiration of oral contents. Therefore, physiotherapy followed by oral and then nasopharyngeal suctioning is most effective in removing pulmonary secretions and minimizing the risk of aspiration.

97. Correct answer—B.
Prolonged inspiration in relation to expiration is associated with air leaks as a result of pressure, volume, and time. Atelectasis may be treated effectively by increasing the I/E ratio, but is not a risk associated with increasing the I/E ratio. Because ventilation is improved and perfusion is not negatively affected, the V/Q ratio remains stable or improves. Bronchial collapse would not occur in the presence of further inspiratory time which promoted expansion of airways.

98. Correct answer—C.
High frequency ventilation is helpful in reducing barotrauma by using small tidal volumes delivered at the mean airway pressure. Small tidal volumes and low pressures such as the mean airway pressure aid in reducing trauma to the lungs.

99. Correct answer—D.

A common complication associated with intubation is advancement of the tube too far into the right bronchus. The right bronchus comes off the trachea at a straighter angle than the left bronchus, making intubation of the right bronchus likely when the tube is placed too far. Removing the tube is unnecessary at this point when simply withdrawing the tube slowly can be effective. A chest x-ray is helpful in determining correct positioning, but the time taken to get one would result in serious respiratory compromise.

100. Correct answer—A.

Because two of the greatest risks associated with mechanical ventilation are barotrauma and retinopathy associated with long-term oxygen therapy, the FiO_2 and pressure support are reduced as soon as possible.

101. Correct answer—D.

Evacuation of the pneumothorax needs to be accomplished immediately to improve the respiratory status. Reduction of pressure support would only further compromise the ability to ventilate the infant. While bradycardia does accompany severe respiratory distress from air leaks, treatment should be aimed at the cause and removal of trapped air. Lowering the head of the bed will further compromise respiratory-diaphragmatic excursion and exacerbate the distress.

102. Correct answer—B.

Bronchopulmonary dysplasia is associated with high FiO_2 administration, infection, mechanical ventilation, prematurity, family history of asthma, and ligation of a patent ductus arteriosus.

103. Correct answer—B.

Theophylline is used in the neonate to improve lung compliance and decrease the resistance to expiration. Asthma is a disease of pediatrics, not neonates. Surfactant replacement therapy studies are currently being done, but theophylline plays no role in the stimulation of surfactant metabolism.

104. Correct answer—A.

Periods of apnea lasting 5 to 10 seconds followed by periods of breathing of 10 to 15 seconds are most likely due to periodic breathing. This is a normal pattern of breathing in neonates and occurs because the respiratory centers and central nervous system are not fully developed.

105. Correct answer—D.

Acrocyanosis is cyanosis in the peripheral aspects of the body such as fingers, hands, toes, and feet. This is a normal finding in the first 24 hours of life. Central cyanosis is best assessed in the mucous membranes, around the mouth, and in the trunk and is not a normal finding. Oxygen would not be indicated unless central cyanosis was confirmed. Suctioning without indications by auscultation may actually cause hypoxia.

106. Correct answer—D.

The risk and occurrence of apnea in the premature infant are increased by conditions in virtually all body systems. Some common conditions include use of phototherapy (as a result of changes in body temperature), continuous positive airway pressure, intraventricular hemorrhage, sepsis, meningitis, respiratory distress syndrome, hypoglycemia, hypocalcemia, congestive heart failure, polycythemia, anemia, gastroesophageal reflux, central nervous system depressants, rapid increase of ambient temperature which phototherapy or isolettes may cause, suctioning, sleep, stooling, and necrotizing enterocolitis.

107. Correct answer—A.

An infant of 32 weeks gestation is at the least risk for persistent pulmonary hypertension because the vessel muscles in the lungs have not yet developed. Immature muscular development makes vessels unable to vasoconstrict to create persistent pulmonary hypertension. An infant of this gestational age would be at greater risk for a PDA, apnea, and hypoglycemia.

108. Correct answer—A.

Sedation can be achieved with a variety of drugs including phenobarbital (5 to 7 mg/kg), fentanyl (2 to 4 mcg/kg), or pancuronium bromide (30 to 60 mcg/kg). The other doses listed here are not therapeutic.

109. Correct answer—D.

A metabolic cause of apnea in a premature infant may be identified by serum electrolyte levels and arterial blood gases. Serum electrolyte levels that may be responsible for apnea include potassium, sodium, magnesium, chloride, calcium, and phosphate. Serum glucose levels also may help identify a metabolic component of apnea. A complete blood count would help identify an infectious cause.

110. Correct answer—A.

Increasing the respiratory rate in an intubated infant with persistent pulmonary hypertension decreases pCO_2 by increasing the amount being "blown off." A decreased level of pCO_2 causes vasodilation of the pulmonary vessels which lowers the pulmonary pressure in relation to the systemic pressure leading to a decrease in right-to-left shunting. Increasing the respiratory rate decreases pCO_2 without significantly raising the pO_2 on room air. A decreased pCO_2 generally causes vasoconstriction in systemic vessels.

111. Correct answer—C.

A pulmonary diffusion defect can lead to respiratory failure by interfering with gaseous exchange across the alveoli and pulmonary capillaries. Pulmonary edema, pulmonary infection, anemia, and hemorrhage are all conditions which affect the exchange of oxygen and carbon dioxide across the alveoli and pulmonary capillaries. Tracheal stenosis and airway obstruction can lead to respiratory failure by obstructing the entrance and exit of gas to the respiratory system.

Apnea of prematurity is a problem with immaturity of the central respiratory control centers and a failure to signal ventilatory efforts.

112. Correct answer—B.
An infant in respiratory distress will assume the sniffing position whenever possible. The sniffing position is when the infant hyperextends the neck and assumes a position which looks like a person sniffing or smelling. By straightening the airway, resistance is lowered allowing air to more easily enter and leave the airway. The fetal position and neck flexion would promote occlusion and obstruction of the airway more than opening. The fetal position does not facilitate breathing.

113. Correct answer—D.
To monitor the effectiveness of therapy and prevent complications related to oxygen therapy, a continuous method of measuring arterial oxygenation such as pulse oximetry or transcutaneous oxygen monitoring must be used. Arterial blood gases once a shift is not often enough to evaluate the therapeutic effectiveness or guard against oxygen toxicity. Continuous SvO_2 monitoring measures venous oxygenation and gives more information about oxygen consumption than arterial oxygen levels. This is also seldom available in infants. Finally, assessment for cyanosis is very inadequate in early detection of optimal oxygen therapy.

114. Correct answer—D.
Infants at risk for developing pulmonary hemorrhage are those with asphyxia, sepsis, low birth weight, infection, congenital heart defects, arteriovenous fistula, foreign body aspiration, persistent pulmonary hypertension, and a variety of immunological problems. Oxygen toxicity is *not* recognized as increasing the risk of pulmonary hemorrhage.

115. Correct answer—B.
In order to minimize multisystem organ failure in an infant with respiratory failure, a goal of therapy is to maintain the PaO_2 greater than 90% to minimize hypoxemia to organs. The hematocrit should be maintained between 30% and 40%. Higher levels increase blood viscosity and may increase cardiac work and impair microcapillary circulation. The cardiac index should be supported to be normal or slightly above normal to increase oxygen delivery. Stimulation should be avoided because it increases oxygen consumption and therefore worsens the respiratory failure.

116. Correct answer—A.
Aspiration pneumonia from oral secretions is associated with infection which may be accompanied by fever. Hyperthermia increases oxygen consumption. Seizures and shivering also increase oxygen consumption, but are not usually associated with pneumonia. A decrease in pO_2 may result from increased oxygen consumption. A decrease in SvO_2 is more strongly related to an increase in oxygen consumption.

117. Correct answer—B.

Moderate to large amounts of bright red blood with suctioning indicate pulmonary hemorrhage. Risk factors in this patient include sepsis. Other common risk factors in the neonate include asphyxia, hypothermia, and intracranial hemorrhage. Trauma from intubation and suctioning are less likely to result in this quantity of blood, but rather blood-tinged secretions. Pulmonary hemosiderosis is a diffuse type of alveolar hemorrhage that is seen in older children.

118. Correct answer—A.

Initial treatment of this infant would include fluid resuscitation with red packed cells and colloids to achieve a CVP of 10 cm H_2O. CVP readings less than 8 to 10 cm H_2O will not provide adequate filling pressures and indicate continued hypovolemia. Elevated CVP readings risk right heart failure.

119. Correct answer—A.

Ventilation with bag mask is contraindicated for an infant with a congenital diaphragmatic hernia because it will increase the amount of air entering the gut exacerbating the hernia. Intubation with mechanical ventilation at high rates and low pressures with sedation helps prevent trauma to hypoplastic lungs while adequately ventilating the alveoli.

120. Correct answer—D.

Because a congenital diaphragmatic hernia can result in severe right-to-left shunting, it is important that both preductal and postductal saturations are measured to detect and estimate the shunt. Arterial blood gases are critical in an infant with profound hypoxemia and hypercarbia leading to severe acidosis. Capillary blood gases are not sensitive enough or provide direct enough information to be helpful in monitoring an infant with this degree of respiratory disease.

121. Correct answer—C.

Placement of a nasogastric tube for the infant with congenital diaphragmatic hernia helps prevent further compression of and impingement on the lungs by decompressing the bowel. The bowel tends to fill with air with crying and respiratory distress, increasing the volume of the bowel and the herniation. Feeding by gut is contraindicated as a result of the respiratory work associated with feeding, lack of bowel function, and risk of increasing air swallowing. While the risk of aspiration may be decreased with placement of a nasogastric tube, it is not the primary reason for immediate placement. The degree of shunting is not directly affected or decreased by placement of the tube.

122. Correct answer—D.

Many preterm infants demonstrate mixed apnea. This is apnea caused by both the central nervous system and obstructive components. The central nervous system fails to cause respiratory muscles to ventilate. Obstructive apnea occurs when airflow ceases even with chest wall movements. The upper airways of infants are particularly prone to obstruction at the pharyngeal and hypopharyngeal levels. While either central (neural) apnea or obstructive apnea may alone account for apneic episodes, most often they are both factors in apnea.

123. Correct answer—D.
Risk factors related to apnea of preterm infants include feeding, nasogastric intubation, infection, sleep, hypoxemia, metabolic disorders, changes in temperature, gastroesophageal reflux, intracranial pathology, and many medications. Periodic breathing, while characterized by periods of apnea, is normal in preterm infants and does not by itself represent an increased risk factor.

124. Correct answer—C.
A preterm infant noted to have a period of apnea, which is associated with bradycardia and cyanosis, should be immediately ventilated with a mask and bag. Gentle stimulation is not adequate when the infant is already symptomatic, such as bradycardic and cyanotic. Noxious stimuli such as clapping and banging are never indicated. Preparing for intubation does not address the infant's immediate ventilatory needs and may not be required.

125. Correct answer—B.
Apnea during feedings is most often related to poor coordination of sucking and swallowing, gastroesophageal reflux, and hyperflexion of the neck during feedings. Swallowing air into the stomach is not associated with apnea.

126. Correct answer—A.
Ventilation-perfusion matching is improved by prone positioning. Knee-chest positioning can be useful in pulmonary hypertensive crises such as a hypercyanotic, or tet, spell.

127. Correct answer—B.
Toxic and side effects associated with a methylxanthine include hypotension, tachycardia, increased metabolic demand which can worsen nutritional status, fever, tachypnea, and seizures.

128. Correct answer—A.
Because of the potential for hypotension, theophylline would be used with caution in an infant with hypovolemia. It is used to treat various forms of central or neural apnea. If indicated, its use in a child with congenital heart block would not be contraindicated since it can cause tachycardia, not bradycardia.

129. Correct answer—D.
Continuous positive airway pressure (CPAP) is a respiratory therapy often used to treat apnea in newborns that is obstructive or mixed. It is not effective in treating centrally or neural mediated apnea. CPAP works by physically maintaining the patency of large and small airways, but is not effective in stimulating ventilatory movement from the respiratory center in the brain.

130. Correct answer—C.

The best information about the adequacy of the tidal volume administered by mechanical ventilation is provided by observing adequate chest wall movement. While 10 cc/kg may usually be enough calculated tidal volume or a peak pressure of 18 cm H_2O may be normal, in the presence of lung disease these may not be appropriate. An adequate PaO_2 is related more to the FiO_2, perfusion, shunting, and other factors and does not provide direct information about the adequacy of tidal volume.

131. Correct answer—A.

An infant admitted to the NICU with a respiratory rate of 110, nasal flaring, grunting, retractions, and central cyanosis with apneic periods of 12 to 16 seconds is at high risk for respiratory failure. These signs and symptoms may also be associated with sepsis, hypothermia, hypoglycemia, anemia, polycythemia, and many other conditions. Tolazoline is used to treat persistent pulmonary hypertension of the newborn. There is insufficient evidence here to being an infusion. There are also no indications from the case study that would support dopamine infusion at this time.

132. Correct answer—A.

For neonates who require intubation, high pressures, and high FiO_2, oxygenation should be monitored by arterial blood gases at least every 2 to 4 hours (and with changes in treatment) and continuous pulse oximetry. Adequate oxygenation needs to be monitored frequently through arterial sampling and continuously through pulse oximetry or transcutaneous monitoring. Preductal and postductal arterial blood gas sampling would only be indicated in those cases in which shunting through the ductus arteriosus was suspected. Umbilical arterial blood gas sampling may be used, but arterial sampling from any site is usually satisfactory.

133. Correct answer—D.

Use of an umbilical artery catheter has been associated with necrotizing enterocolitis if the mesenteric artery is involved, and embolic incidents and hypertension if the renal artery is involved. Intracranial hemorrhages have not been implicated in the use of umbilical artery catheters.

134. Correct answer—D.

Oxygen consumption is increased in the neonate with hypothermia, sepsis, fever, respiratory disease, and seizures. Chemical paralysis is one therapy used to decrease oxygen consumption by decreasing oxygen demand.

135. Correct answer—B.

Grunting is a natural compensatory mechanism in infants that mimics the therapeutic use of continuous distending pressure. Continuous distending pressure therapy refers to continuous positive airway pressure and positive and expiratory pressure. Grunting is the active exhalation against a partially closed glottis which creates continuous distending pressure in the lungs. Intubation eliminates grunting in infants and may actually lower the pO_2 because continuous distending pressure is lost unless CPAP or PEEP is a part of the respiratory therapy.

136. Correct answer—B.

Decreased peripheral pulses, decreased urine output, increased intracranial pressure, air leaks, and hepatomegaly are some of the adverse responses to the use of positive end expiratory pressure in an infant undergoing mechanical ventilation. PEEP increases the intrathoracic pressure and impedes systemic vascular return and return of venous blood from the brain as well as increases the risk of air leaks. Intracranial pressure may rise and cardiac output may fall, resulting in either intracranial bleeding or poor systemic perfusion.

137. Correct answer—A.

When analyzing blood gases, an increase in CO_2 should be recognized as a problem associated with the use of positive end expiratory pressure. PEEP may decrease tidal volume and therefore elevate the pCO_2. PEEP is used to treat a decrease in pO_2, but is not a cause of decreased pO_2. An increase in pH represents an alkalotic state and would not be associated with a rise in pCO_2. Arterial saturation would be expected to rise with the use of PEEP.

138. Correct answer—B.

Sedation and paralysis are indicated to treat persistent fetal circulation when the pO_2 remains low and right-to-left shunting is great despite intubation and mechanical ventilation. Agitation may be increased by both mechanical ventilation and high rates, which increase oxygen demand, consumption, and shunting. Sedation and paralysis may decrease oxygen demand and oxygen consumption, increasing the pO_2 which has a vasodilatory effect on the pulmonary vasculature.

139. Correct answer—A.

Nasal CPAP may be helpful in preventing atelectasis after extubation following prolonged mechanical ventilatory support. By maintaining continuous distending pressure, atelectasis is discouraged and atelectatic areas may be recruited. Racemic epinephrine is used to treat laryngeal edema following extubation. Aminophylline and caffeine may be used to treat apnea in preterm infants.

140. Correct answer—D.

During chest physiotherapy (PT) for the preterm infant with respiratory distress syndrome pulse oximetry readings need to be continuously monitored. For many of these fragile infants, vigorous stimulation such as that associated with chest PT will cause a significant decline in arterial saturation. Breath sounds would not give any indication of a drop in arterial saturation. While the respiratory rate would likely increase in the absence of sedation or paralysis, it would not be a sensitive indicator of arterial desaturation. The electrocardiogram may show ectopy in the presence of a drop in saturation, but it would not be a sensitive indicator. Pulse oximetry and/or transcutaneous monitoring of oxygen are more sensitive and earlier indicators.

141. Correct answer—A.

A patent ductus arteriosus is often (15% to 30%) found in infants with respiratory distress syndrome. The presence of a PDA has been associated with a prolonged course of RDS and the development of bronchopulmonary dysplasia. To diagnose a PDA, echocardiography or even cardiac catheterization may be required. An electrocardiogram may show some indications associated with PDAs, but is too nonspecific to be of diagnostic value. A renal ultrasound and liver enzyme studies would not help identify the presence of a PDA.

142. Correct answer—C.

Indomethacin at a 0.1 to 0.3 mg/kg dose is used to pharmacologically close a patent ductus arteriosus in the neonate. The dose may be repeated, but the medication is not given by constant infusion. Prostaglandin E_1 is used to maintain the patency of a ductus arteriosus, not to close it.

143. Correct answer—C.

Patterns of pathological aeration associated with meconium aspiration include atelectasis, overexpansion from air trapping, air leaks, increase in expiratory resistance, and increase in functional residual capacity. Atelectasis occurs because of total small airway obstruction. Overexpansion of other areas is related to partial small airway obstruction and the ball-valve phenomenon, which allows air to enter but not leave the small airways and alveoli. This creates an overall increase in functional residual capacity in most cases. Air leaks commonly occur.

144. Correct answer—B.

Because choanal atresia is associated with congenital cardiac defects in 50% to 70% of cases, an echocardiogram is indicated to rule out cardiac malformations.

145. Correct answer—D.

Indomethacin or surgical intervention to close a patent ductus arteriosus may help reduce the risk of developing bronchopulmonary dysplasia in the infant with pulmonary disease. The development of chronic lung disease in neonates is associated with long-term positive pressure ventilation at high pressure support, especially with PEEP levels greater than 8 cm H_2O, peak pressures greater than 30 cm H_2O, an FiO_2 greater than 0.5, the presence of a patent ductus arteriosus, and excessive maintenance fluid therapy of more than the usual 60 to 100 mL/kg/day.

146. Correct answer—D.

Nutritional support is critical in infants with bronchopulmonary dysplasia because there is an increase in oxygen consumption related to the work of breathing. Nutritional support prevents fractures and bone demineralization related to malnutrition, prevents infection, and meets the needs of increased metabolic demand. It is important in responding to an increase in metabolic demand, but does not actually create an increase in metabolic demand.

CHAPTER 3

Endocrinology Care Problems

Passkeys

PEDIATRIC-SPECIFIC PRINCIPLES

ACUTE HYPOGLYCEMIA

- Infants are particularly susceptible to hypoglycemia as a result of their high glucose needs and low glucose stores. See boxes for risk factors for hypoglycemia in the neonate, causes of hypoglycemia in the neonate and signs and symptoms of hypoglycemia in the neonate.

- Hypoglycemia may been seen in severe stress states as a result of depletion or inability to produce glucose.

- Hypoglycemia, hyperglycemia, and glucosuria may be early signs of sepsis. See Table 3-1 for signs and symptoms of altered glucose metabolism in the newborn.

- Hypoglycemia severely affects cardiac function by acting as a depressant.

- Correction of hypoglycemia includes 1 to 2 mL/kg of 25% glucose solution. A constant source of glucose then needs to be made available—2 to 4 mL/kg/hr of D_5W should prevent hypoglycemia.

- Boluses of glucose are less desirable in maintaining a constant serum glucose level. A constant infusion is more effective.

DIABETES INSIPIDUS (DI)

- Diabetes insipidus (DI) can result from either a lack of antidiuretic hormone (ADH), which is neurogenic in origin, or a decreased renal response to ADH, which is nephrogenic in origin. See box for risk factors for the development of DI.

- ADH, also called vasopressin, is made by the hypothalamus.

- Insufficient amounts of ADH cause the kidneys to fail to reabsorb large amounts of water from the filtrate as it is formed. Therefore, severe hypovolemia occurs as a result of copious urine output.

- Large amounts of urine output and fluid loss result in severe hypovolemia, hemoconcentration, hypernatremia, and other electrolyte imbalances.

- Urine output in DI has a very low specific gravity, sodium content, and osmolality. Serum osmolality and sodium concentration are high.

Risk Factors for Neonatal Hypoglycemia

Maternal Factors

Maternal diabetes

Toxemia

Use of beta-adrenergic agents

Glucose infusion during labor and delivery

Intrauterine Factors

Placental insufficiency

Intrauterine infection

Miscellaneous

Hypothermia

Stress

Congenital heart disease

Respiratory distress syndrome

Adrenal hemorrhage

Polycythemia

Rh hemolytic disease

Central nervous system disease

Sepsis

Galactosemia

Causes of Hypoglycemia in the Neonate

Premature birth

Intrauterine growth retardation

Associated with:

- congenital cardiac defects
- central nervous system disease
- sepsis

Maternal ingestion of:

- beta-adrenergic blocking agents
- insulin
- oral hypoglycemic agents
- narcotics

Asphyxia

Galactosemia

Stress

Hypothermia

Acute illness

Signs and Symptoms of Hypoglycemia in the Neonate

Neurologic	**Respiratory**
Twitching	Cyanosis
Lethargy	Apnea
Hypotonia	Rapid, irregular respirations
Apathy	**Gastrointestinal**
Jitteriness	Poor feeding
Convulsions	**Miscellaneous**
Coma	Diaphoresis
Tremors	Weak cry
Twitching	High-pitched cry

Table 3-1
Signs and Symptoms of Altered Glucose Metabolism

Alteration	Signs and Symptoms
Hypoglycemia	Hunger Tremors Jitteriness Diaphrosis Alterations in consciousness Lethargy Seizures Hypotonia in infants Apnea in infants
Hyperglycemia	Thirst Increased urine output Fatigue May be asymptomatic in infants
Ketoacidosis	Rapid, deep breathing Nausea Vomiting Acetone breath

Risk Factors for the Development of Diabetes Insipidus

Neurologic

Head injury

Cranial surgery

Meningitis

Encephalitis

Neoplasms

Leukemia

Craniopharyngioma

Nephrologic

Polycystic disease

Pyelonephritis

Obstructive uropathy

Pharmacologic Agents

Phenytoin

Demeclocycline

Miscellaneous Causes

Sickle cell disease

Protein starvation

- Management focuses on rapid and aggressive fluid replacement and administration of Pitressin (vasopressin).
- At least two large intravenous lines need to be placed to manage fluid therapy.
- Vasopressin can be given intravenously (IV), intramuscularly (IM), or subcutaneously (SQ).
- Desmopressin acetate (dDAVP) is a synthetic type of vasopressin that can be given in a nasal spray (best absorption) or intravenously.

SYNDROME OF INAPPROPRIATE ANTIDIURETIC HORMONE (SIADH)

- Syndrome of inappropriate antidiuretic hormone (SIADH) can develop in association with head injuries, respiratory infections, neurosurgery, malignancies, anesthesia, hemorrhage, encephalitis, meningitis, increased intracranial pressure, subarachnoid hemorrhage, pulmonary hypertension, mitral valve repairs, and tumors. See box for risk factors for the development of SIADH.
- Antidiuretic hormone works on the collecting ducts of the kidneys to retain water. The higher the levels of ADH, the lower the urine output and the higher the body's water content.

Risk Factors for Syndrome of Inappropriate Antidiuretic Hormone (SIADH)

Fluid Loss

Trauma

Hemorrhage

Dehydration

Neurologic Disorders

Meningitis

Encephalitis

Hydrocephalus

Head trauma

Subarachnoid hemorrhage

Brain tumor

Coma

Gastrointestinal Disorders

Splanchnic sequestration

Cirrhosis

Pulmonary Disorders

Pneumonia

Pulmonary hypertension

Positive pressure ventilation in neonates

Cardiovascular Disorders

Repair of mitral stenosis

Miscellaneous

Carcinoma

Pain

Anxiety

Medications

Morphine

Antineoplastic agents

Barbiturates

Carbamazepine

Acetylcholine

Epinephrine

Norepinephrine

- SIADH is characterized by decreased urine output, hypervolemia, urine hyperosmolality, serum hypoosmolality, hyponatremia, and increased urine sodium content.

- Signs and symptoms of SIADH include neurologic manifestations such as irritability, lethargy, and seizures; gastrointestinal symptoms of anorexia, abdominal cramping, nausea, and diarrhea; and pitting edema over the sternum.

- A rough estimation of the serum osmolality can be determined by using the following equation: serum sodium level × 2 = serum osmolality. A normal range is 270 to 290 mOsm/L.

- Constant neurologic assessment is critical as a result of the risk of developing cerebral edema.
- Management includes careful recording of urine output and restricted fluid intake.
- Hypertonic saline can be used (2 to 4 mg/kg of 3% NaCl) along with lasix (1 mg/kg) to treat hyponatremia and hypervolemia.

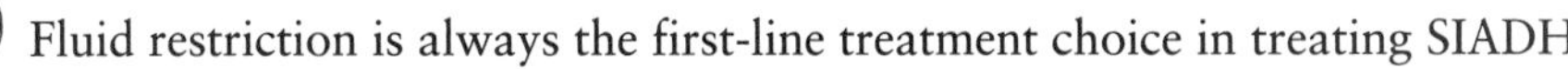

- Fluid restriction is always the first-line treatment choice in treating SIADH.
- See Table 3-2 for comparison of DI and SIADH.

DIABETIC KETOACIDOSIS (DKA)

- Diabetic ketoacidosis (DKA) develops when there is inadequate insulin for the body to utilize glucose. The body is forced to use fats as an energy source, forming acetoacetic acids. These in turn are converted into ketones. Metabolic acids accumulate resulting in acidosis.
- Respiratory compensation for metabolic acidosis results in Kussmaul breathing—deep, labored, rapid breaths to flow off CO_2, a respiratory acid.
- Serum glucose levels are high from the failure of insulin to move glucose into the cells, but also from the body's attempt to make glucose available to the cells by gluconeogenesis and glycogenolysis.

Table 3-2

Comparison of Laboratory Findings in Syndrome of Inappropriate Antidiuretic Hormone (SIADH) and Diabetes Insipidus (DI)

Assessment Data	SIADH	DI
Urine		
Specific gravity	>1.020	<1.005
Osmolality	>500 mOsm/kg of urine	<250 mOsm/kg of urine
Urine output	<1 mL/kg/hr	>3 mL/kg/hr
Sodium	>60 mEq/L	<40 mEq/L
Serum		
Osmolality	<275 mOsm/kg of serum	>305 mOsm/kg of serum
Sodium	<130 mEq/L	>150 mEq/L

- Elevated serum glucose levels increase the serum osmolality resulting in a diuresis—usually when the serum level is at or above 180 mg/dL. Sodium and potassium are lost in the urine in large amounts.

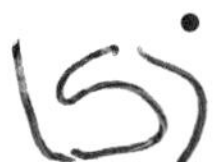

- Signs and symptoms of DKA include polydipsia, polyphagia, polyuria, weight loss, acidosis, hyponatremia, tachypnea, low serum bicarbonate, slightly elevated blood urea nitrogen (BUN) level, vomiting, abdominal pain, and lethargy.

- Treatment includes fluid replacement (solutions that do not contain glucose until the serum level is <300 mg/dL), potassium supplementation, and insulin.

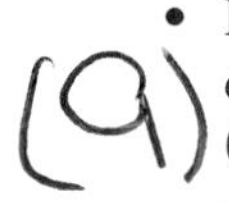

- Insulin 0.5 to 2.0 U/kg is given, half intravenously and half subcutaneously. A constant infusion may be used giving 0.1 U/kg intravenous push (IVP) and then 0.1 U/kg/hr until a serum glucose level of 250 mg/dL is reached. Then management changes to subcutaneous administration.

- The treatment goal includes not allowing a drop in the serum glucose level of greater than 100 mg/dL/hr.

- Watch carefully for cerebral edema during fluid resuscitation and insulin treatment.

NEONATAL-SPECIFIC PRINCIPLES

INBORN ERRORS OF METABOLISM (IEMS)

- Inborn errors of metabolism (IEMs) are inherited disorders caused by either a deficiency or an absence of a substance that is critical to metabolism. Most often the effected substance is an enzyme and results in problems with fat, carbohydrate, or protein metabolism. See Fig. 3-1 for normal metabolic pathways and how they can be altered with inborn errors of metabolism.

- The term *substrate* refers to the material that an enzyme is supposed to act upon to form a secondary product. When the enzyme is absent or insufficient, the substrate accumulates and the necessary product of the metabolic pathway is never formed.

CONGENITAL HYPOTHYROIDISM (CH)

- Congenital hypothyroidism (CH) may result from an enzyme defect in the synthesis of thyroxine.

- Screening at birth for CH is mandatory in most areas.

- CH is often seen in association with Down syndrome.

- See Table 3-3 for signs and symptoms of CH and other inborn errors of metabolism.

- CH may lead to growth and mental retardation.

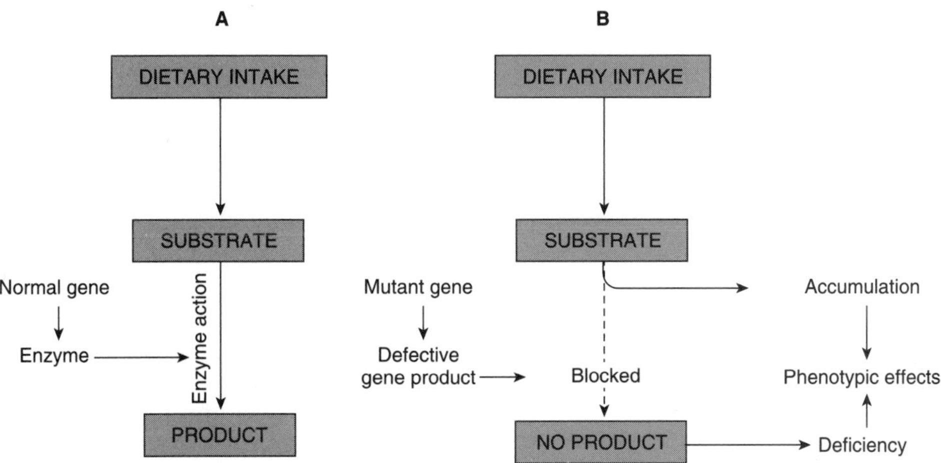

Fig. 3-1 Metabolic pathway. **A,** Normal metabolic pathway. **B,** Effect of defective gene action. (From Wong DL: Whaley and Wong's nursing care of infants and childrens, ed 5, St Louis, 1995, Mosby.)

PHENYLKETONURIA (PKU)

- Phenylketonuria (PKU) is a disorder of protein metabolism, specifically the amino acid phenylalanine.

- The major effects of PKU are on the central nervous system and can result quickly in mental retardation.

- The Guthrie blood test is performed on all newborns in most states to detect PKU.

- See Table 3-3 for signs and symptoms of PKU and other inborn errors of metabolism.

GALACTOSEMIA

- Galactosemia is a disorder of carbohydrate metabolism making the infant unable to convert galactose to glucose.

- Signs and symptoms result primarily from effects on the central nervous system. (See Table 3-3.)

INFANTS OF DIABETIC MOTHERS (IDMS)

- Maternal hyperglycemia early in pregnancy can have a teratogenic effect on the fetus. In the last two trimesters, abnormal growth (large for gestational age) and late surfactant production occur. An increase in prematurity, growth retardation, fetal death, respiratory distress syndrome, and polycythemia is seen.

Table 3-3
Inborn Errors of Metabolism

Disorders	Causes	Assessment Findings	Management
Congenital Hypothyroidism	Enzyme defect in thyroxine synthesis Down syndrome Poor development of the thyroid gland Maternal use of antithyroid drugs	Usually negative assessment findings until after 6 weeks of age Unconjugated hyperbilirubinemia Large tongue Flat nose Swollen eyelids Cold, mottled skin Coarse, dry hair Hypotonia Hyporeflexia Bradycardia Hypothermia Anemia Hypotension	Thyroid replacement therapy—synthetic levothyroxine sodium beginning at 10 mcg/kg Regular measurement of hormone levels
Phenylketonuria	Inability to metabolize the amino acid phenylalanine as a result of an absence of phenylalanine hydroxylase	Failure to thrive Hyperactivity Vomiting	Control the amount of phenylalanine in the diet Special milk substitutes Maintain serum levels of phenylalanine at 2-8 mg/dL
Galactosemia	Disorder of carbohydrate metabolism	Failure to thrive Jaundice Diarrhea Hepatosplenomegaly Lethargy Hypotonia Cataracts	Delete all milk and milk products—including breast milk Lactose-free formulas Soy-based formulas

Signs and Symptoms of Infants of Diabetic Mothers

Large for gestational age	Hyperglycemia
Large placenta and umbilical cord at birth	Hypoglycemia
May be normal or small for gestational age if the mother has vascular complications from diabetes	Hypocalcemia
Congenital anomalies	Polycythemia

- Infants of well-controlled diabetic mothers exhibit fewer signs and symptoms. See box for signs and symptoms of infants and diabetic mothers.
- During the last two trimesters, fetal serum glucose is dependent upon (though slightly less than) maternal glucose levels.
- Maternal hyperglycemia causes hypertrophy of the pancreatic islet cells and excessive insulin production by the fetus.
- Shortly after birth, neonatal glucose levels fall severely (within 4 hours) because the maternal source of glucose has been removed, but the neonate's pancreas secretion of insulin remains high. Acute hypoglycemia results.
- Infants of diabetic mothers are very large for gestational age (LGA) because they are subjected prenatally to high insulin levels which are growth promoting.
- Management goals of IDMs include electrolyte balance and feeding within the first hour of life.

ACUTE HYPOGLYCEMIA

- Infants are particularly susceptible to hypoglycemia as a result of their high glucose needs and low glucose stores. See earlier boxes on risk factors, causes, and signs and symptoms of hypoglycemia in the neonate, pp. 169-170.

Acute hypoglycemia is generally defined as follows:
- Low birth weight infants: <25 mg/dL
- The first 3 days of life: <35 mg/dL
- After 3 days: <45 mg/dL

- Hypoglycemia can results from poor glucose or fat stores, endocrine disorders, increased utilization, and other causes.

- Signs and symptoms of hypoglycemia may be general such as hypotonia and poor feeding to more life-threatening manifestations including jitteriness, seizures, and apnea.

- Treatment may include oral feedings of 10% glucose solutions or intravenous (IV) infusions. Initial IV treatment includes a push of 1 mL/kg of 25% dextrose solution. A maintenance intravenous rate may be used of 5 to 7 mg/kg/min to keep the serum glucose level between 45 and 120 mg/dL.

- If glucose infusions are abruptly stopped, rebound hypoglycemia can result.

Questions

PEDIATRIC-SPECIFIC QUESTIONS

Case Study

A 10-year-old boy has been admitted to the intensive care unit following a head injury from a skateboarding accident. He has a urine output of 11 mL/kg/hr, a urine specific gravity of 1.003, a serum osmolality of 326 mOsm/kg, and a serum sodium of 163 mEq/L. Questions 1 to 3 refer to this case study.

1. Which of the following signs and symptoms would the critical care nurse expect to find during assessment of this child?
A. Bounding pulses, tachycardia, seizures, and cyanosis
B. Stupor, hypertension, mottling of extremities
C. Weak and thready pulse, hypotension, pale extremities
D. Tachycardia, hypertension, thirst, equivocal pulses

2. What would be the most *immediate* priority in treating this patient?
A. Restoration of intravascular fluid volume
B. Administration of dDAVP
C. Administration of anticonvulsant pharmacologic agents
D. Restoration of normal serum sodium levels

3. An appropriate nursing diagnosis for this patient is:
A. Potential for fluid volume excess related to inadequate secretion of antidiuretic hormone
B. Potential for hypothermia related to excess fluid loss
C. Altered tissue perfusion: peripheral related to decreased circulating volume
D. Potential fluid volume deficit related to increased urinary output

4. Antidiuretic hormone has what mechanism of action?
A. Causes an active retention of sodium which results in a passive retention of water
B. Decreases the permeability of the glomerulus so that less filtrate is formed
C. Increases the permeability of the collecting ducts so that more water is reabsorbed
D. Decreases sodium retention which increases urinary output

5. Which of the following statements regarding diabetic ketoacidosis is *true?*
  A. An increase in urine output results primarily from an increase in oral intake
  B. Ketoacidosis is often associated with hyponatremia and hyperkalemia
  C. The patient in DKA has an increase in respiratory acids (pCO_2)
  D. The seizure threshold is increased so stimulation should be minimized

6. After 2 hours of fluid resuscitation for severe DKA, a 14-year-old patient offers each of the following complaints. Which one of these would signal the most critical potential complication?
  A. Nausea
  B. Thirst
  C. Incontinence
  D. Headache

7. A child with which diagnosis is at greatest risk for developing hypoglycemia?
  A. Acute renal failure
  B. Hepatitis
  C. Respiratory distress syndrome
  D. Cerebral edema

8. A 15-year-old girl develops SIADH following neurosurgery. Her serum sodium level is 128 mEq/L, serum osmolality is 256 mOsm/L, urine specific gravity is 1.022, and urine output is 1.0 mL/kg/hr. Which of the following would be the treatment of choice?
  A. Fluid restriction to 50% of maintenance requirements
  B. Administration of 3 mL/kg of 3% NaCl solution
  C. Lasix 3 mg/kg
  D. Administration of hypertonic saline and diuretics

9. Which of the following is the preferred route of administration of insulin in the child with DKA?
  A. Intravenous
  B. Subcutaneous
  C. Intramuscular
  D. Intraarterial

Case Study

A 16-year-old girl has been admitted to the intensive care unit for treatment of diabetic ketoacidosis. Questions 10 to 12 refer to this case study.

---

10. Which of the following laboratory results would the critical care nurse anticipate?
A. Serum glucose level greater than 400 mg/dL
B. Serum pH greater than 7.5
C. Serum glucose level greater than 500 mg/dL
D. Serum pH less than 7.3

11. The nurse caring for this patient plans to evaluate the effectiveness of IV insulin therapy by knowing that the half-life of intravenous insulin is closest to:
A. 60 minutes
B. 30 minutes
C. 15 minutes
D. 5 minutes

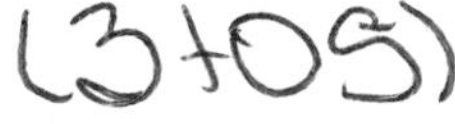

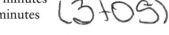

12. Before discontinuing intravenous insulin therapy to treat this patient's DKA, the critical care nurse would expect to administer:
A. A bolus dose of intravenous insulin to maintain lower serum glucose levels
B. A dose of subcutaneous insulin to prevent a lapse of insulin therapy
C. A bolus dose of 50% dextrose solution to prevent hypoglycemia
D. A continuous infusion of 10% dextrose solution to prevent hypoglycemia

13. In a critically ill child, the new finding of glucosuria without a history of diabetes mellitus is most likely directly related to:
A. Pancreatitis
B. Infection
C. Hypoinsulinemia
D. Electrolyte imbalance

14. Which of the following signs and symptoms would the critical care nurse recognize as a possible indication of hypoglycemia in an infant?
A. Increase in urine output
B. Increase in demand feeding
C. Irritability
D. Thirst

15. All of the following are risk factors for hypoglycemia in critically ill children *except*:
A. Increased circulating catecholamines
B. Decreased glucose stores
C. Inadequate dietary intake of substrates
D. Decreased insulin production

Case Study

An 18-month-old male infant is admitted to the PICU following a Fontan procedure for a single ventricle. He is intubated and on a positive pressure ventilator. After the first 16 hours, he begins to develop a decrease in urine output, an increase in his right atrial pressure (RAP), and an increase in his left atrial pressure (LAP). His urine output has decreased to 0.5 mL/hr with an increase in urine sodium and urine osmolality. Questions 16 and 17 refer to this case study.

16. The nurse suspects this patient most likely has developed:
A. Chronic renal failure
B. Syndrome of inappropriate antidiuretic hormone (SIADH)
C. Diabetes insipidus (DI)
D. Hypothyroidism

17. Which of the following nursing diagnoses would be the most appropriate for this patient?
A. Fluid volume excess
B. Altered tissue perfusion: renal
C. Ineffective breathing pattern
D. Impaired gas exchange

18. After discontinuing hyperalimentation, the critical care nurse would be alert to the development of which of the following?
A. Irritability, fatigue, nausea
B. Fatigue, thirst, increased urine output
C. Nausea, vomiting, hyperpnea
D. Tremors, diaphoresis, irritability

19. Which of the following forms of insulin is used in the early treatment of a child in DKA?
A. Regular
B. Semi-lente
C. Lente
D. Ultra-lente

20. Which of the following intravenous solutions would be used in a patient with DKA once the serum glucose level has fallen below 200 mg/dL but the ketones remain elevated?
A. 0.9% saline
B. 0.45% saline
C. 5% dextrose solution
D. Ringer's lactate

(do not have glucose)

21. All of the following are risk factors for the development of diabetes insipidus *except*:
A. Pyelonephritis
B. Sickle cell disease
C. Leukemia
D. Congestive heart failure

22. The nurse would expect the urine specific gravity of a patient with DI to be in the range of:
A. 1.001 to 1.005
B. 1.006 to 1.010
C. 1.011 to 1.015
D. 1.016 to 1.020

23. All of the following may be desired patient outcomes for an 8-year-old child with diabetes insipidus *except*:
A. Heart rate of 95 beats per minute at rest
B. Central venous pressure (CVP) of 12 mm Hg
C. Blood pressure of 110/60
D. Blood urea nitrogen (BUN) level of 15

24. Which of the following laboratory values would the critical care nurse expect in a patient with SIADH?
A. Urine sodium concentration greater than 30 mEq/L
B. Serum sodium level greater than 145 mEq/L
C. Serum osmolality level greater than 290 mOsm/kg
D. Serum creatinine of 1.5 mg/dL

25. The critical care nurse would identify the SIADH patient at severe risk for seizures and cerebral edema by all of the following symptoms *except*:
A. Lethargy
B. Hyperthermia
C. Hypothermia
D. Abnormal reflexes

NEONATAL-SPECIFIC QUESTIONS

26. An infant admitted to the NICU for hypoglycemia has been stabilized on intravenous glucose infusions. Which of the following principles will guide the critical care nurse's interventions when discontinuing IV glucose therapy? After blood glucose levels have stabilized,
A. The infusion may be discontinued
B. The infusion rate may be decreased by 75%
C. The infusion may be slowly weaned
D. The solution may be replaced by normal saline

27. All of the following are risk factors for the development of hypoglycemia in the neonate *except*:
A. Maternal diabetes
B. Asphyxia
C. Congenital heart disease
D. Congenital hypothyroidism

28. Galactosemia is an inborn error of metabolism of:
A. Fat
B. Protein
C. Carbohydrates
D. Fructose

Case Study

A full term 2450 gram infant of a diabetic mother (IDM) is admitted to the neonatal intensive care unit (NICU) for observation following low glucose levels.

Questions 29 to 31 refer to this case study.

---

29. In caring for a full term infant of a diabetic mother in the first 24 hours of life, the critical care nurse recognizes hypoglycemia as a serum glucose level less than:
A. 25 mg/dL
B. 35 mg/dL
C. 45 mg/dL
D. 55 mg/dL

30. Which of the following signs and symptoms would the critical care nurse be alert to as a possible complication in caring for an IDM?
A. Chvostek's sign
B. Cullen's sign
C. Kehr's sign
D. Cushing's sign

31. Besides frequent monitoring of the serum glucose levels, what other laboratory values would need to be frequently monitored in the infant?
A. Sodium
B. Bilirubin
C. Creatinine
D. Amylase

32. The preferred oral feedings during the first hours of life for this infant may include all of the following *except:*
A. Galactose fluids
B. Breast milk
C. Infant formula
D. Glucose fluids

33. A potential nursing diagnosis for the neonate with hypoglycemia is *least* likely to include:
A. Decreased cardiac output
B. Altered tissue perfusion: peripheral
C. Ineffective breathing pattern
D. Altered nutrition: less than body requirements

34. Phenylketonuria (PKU) requires dietary restrictions that may include:
A. Low iron formulas
B. Breast milk
C. Soy based formula
D. Lactose-free formulas

35. A patient outcome for the neonate with PKU includes maintenance of a serum phenylalanine level:
A. Less than 1 mg/dL
B. 2 to 8 mg/dL
C. 10 to 15 mg/dL
D. 16 to 21 mg/dL

36. Galactosemia, which is uncontrolled, can result in all of the following *except:*
A. Mental retardation
B. Cirrhosis of the liver
C. Retinopathy
D. Cataracts

Case Study

An neonate is admitted to the NICU directly from the delivery room because he is bradycardic, hypothermic, and shows poor reflex activity. He is admitted with a tentative diagnosis of congenital hypothyroidism. Questions 37 and 38 refer to this case study.

---

37. During the admission assessment, the critical care nurse would anticipate the following findings *except:*
A. Thin, patchy hair pattern
B. Narrow pulse pressure
C. Abdominal distension
D. Cold, dry skin

38. Laboratory findings to confirm the diagnosis in this neonate would be:
A. Elevated protein-bound iodine
B. High free thyroxine levels
C. Low T_4 and high TSH levels
D. Increased thyroxine levels

39. Hypoglycemia in infants of diabetic mothers is a result of:
A. Hyperinsulinemia
B. Decreased substrate stores
C. Decreased substrate intake
D. Decreased metabolic activity

40. Decreased levels of serotonin in infants with PKU place them at an increased risk for:
A. Bleeding
B. Bowel obstruction
C. Renal failure
D. Apnea

41. Hypoglycemia in the hypothermic newborn results from:
A. Decreased substrate stores
B. Increased substrate use
C. Hyperinsulinemia
D. Islet cell dysplasia

42. Symptoms of hypoglycemia in the neonate most dramatically affect which body system?
A. Gastrointestinal
B. Immunological
C. Renal
D. Neurological

43. Initial treatment of the symptomatic neonate with hypoglycemia would include:
A. 1 mL/kg of 5% dextrose solution
B. 1 mL/kg of 25% dextrose solution
C. 5 mL/kg of 10% dextrose solution
D. 1 mL/kg of 50% dextrose solution

44. A positive patient outcome for the neonate with hypoglycemia would be maintenance of blood glucose levels:
A. Greater than 100 mg/dL
B. 75 to 125 mg/dL
C. 100 to 150 mg/dL
D. 45 to 120 mg/dL

45. An infant is found to have a blood glucose level of 15 mg/dL by reagent strip and laboratory confirmation. The critical care nurse should *first* give a:

A. 10% glucose solution orally
B. 50% glucose solution bolus
C. 75% dextrose solution by constant IV infusion
D. 25% dextrose solution bolus

46. A 10-hour-old 4.2 kg infant of a diabetic mother is observed to be lethargic, have poor muscle tone, and be feeding poorly. The *first* action the critical care nurse should take is:

A. Perform a heelstick and measure the glucose level by reagent strip
B. Administer 4 ml of 25% dextrose solution
C. Send a serum sample to the laboratory to determine serum glucose level
D. Increase the intravenous infusion of 5% dextrose solution to 25 mL/hr

Answers

PEDIATRIC-SPECIFIC ANSWERS

1. **Correct answer—C.**
   Signs and symptoms of advanced diabetes insipidus include hypotension, weak and thready pulses, mottled or pale extremities, alterations in mentation, tachycardia, thirst, and possible seizures related to hypernatremia. Hypertension might be seen in early stages of hypovolemia related to DI, but a urine output of 11 cc/kg/hr is a severe loss of body fluids which would rapidly lead to hypovolemic shock. Cyanosis is usually seen with ventilation or shunting abnormalities and would not be associated with DI.

2. **Correct answer—A.**
   The most immediate priority in a patient with DI would be to restore intravascular fluid volume to treat hypovolemic shock and ensure adequate organ and tissue perfusion. Administration of dDAVP is important in preventing further fluid loss, but without restoration of the large amount of intravascular volume, it would be of limited value. Hypernatremia may put this patient at risk for seizures, but restoration of fluid volume will help lower the serum sodium level and probably ameliorate the need for anticonvulsant therapy.

3. **Correct answer—C.**
   This patient with DI has an excessive amount of urinary output which quickly will deplete his circulating volume. He has an actual, not potential, fluid volume deficit related to excess urinary output that has depleted his circulatory volume and resulted in poor peripheral perfusion. Dehydration is often associated with *hyper*thermia.

4. **Correct answer—C.**
   Antidiuretic hormone increases the permeability of the collecting ducts so that more water is reabsorbed by the peritubular vascular system. The net result is an increase in reabsorption of water and an increase in intravascular fluid volume. ADH does *not* act on sodium. Decreased filtrate formation related to a change in the permeability of the glomeruli occurs with glomerulonephritis, diabetic nephritis, and other kidney diseases which can lead to acute or chronic renal failure. Sodium regulation is accomplished by aldosterone.

5. **Correct answer—B.**
   Diabetic ketoacidosis often results in hyperkalemia related to metabolic acidosis and hyponatremia from polyuria. As hydrogen ions (positive charges) increase in the serum, they shift into the cells to try to equalize. As positive charges (H+) move into the cells, other positive charges (K+) must move out to equalize. Even though total body potassium may have been lost in the urine, serum levels remain

high or normal. Serum sodium levels are low because of excessive urinary output resulting from the osmotic effect of high serum glucose levels. An increase in oral intake of fluids results from the osmotic diuresis and increased urinary output associated with hyperglycemia. The patient in DKA has a decrease in respiratory acids (pCO_2) compensate for metabolic acidosis. Kussmaul breathing—fast, deep, labored breaths—help blow off pCO_2 and decrease respiratory acids to offset the increase in metabolic acids. Acidosis has a depressive, not a stimulative, effect on the central nervous system. As the acidosis is corrected, however, the potassium level will fall, and intravenous potassium supplements will be needed.

6. Correct answer—D.
Fluid resuscitation for DKA can lead to cerebral edema as intravenous solutions leave the intravascular space and enter dehydrated cells. Swelling of cells may occur, with symptoms and complications most severe when they affect brain cells encased in the noncompliant skull. Nausea and thirst often accompany DKA. Difficulty maintaining urinary continence may occur related to increased urinary output, increased intravascular fluid volume and fluid resuscitation, and environmental limitations on normal voiding patterns in the pediatric intensive care unit (PICU).

7. Correct answer—B.
A child with liver dysfunction is at greatest risk for developing hypoglycemia because of the liver's role in maintaining normal glucose levels. The liver performs such critical functions as storing glycogen and gluconeogenesis. A generalized stress response associated with severe illness and other organ dysfunction can lead to hypoglycemia, but a patient with liver dysfunction is at greatest risk.

8. Correct answer—A.
Despite the low serum sodium level and serum osmolality, the treatment of choice for SIADH, which is not complicated by severe hyponatremia and seizures, is fluid restriction. Restriction to 30% to 75% of fluid maintenance requirements may be effective in treating SIADH. Administration of hypertonic saline and diuretics is limited to patients with severe symptoms such as seizures and cerebral edema.

9. Correct answer—A.
The intravenous route is preferred in patients with DKA because its utilization is more predictable. The subcutaneous route often may be absorbed inconsistently, especially if the DKA is associated with poor peripheral perfusion. Insulin would not be administered intraarterially or intramuscularly.

10. Correct answer—D.
In diabetic ketoacidosis, the pH is less than 7.3 and the serum glucose level is greater than 300 mg/dL. The serum bicarbonate level is less than 15 mEq/L and serum total ketones are greater than 3 mM/L. Serum potassium is often elevated and serum sodium levels are usually low.

11. Correct answer—D.

The half-life of intravenous insulin is approximately 3 to 5 minutes.

12. Correct answer—B.

Because subcutaneous administration of regular insulin has a slower onset of action (approximately 30 minutes) and regular insulin has a short half-life, a potential for a lapse in insulin coverage can occur. Administration of insulin subcutaneously before discontinuing a continuous insulin infusion avoids this problem with lack of insulin coverage. A bolus of intravenous insulin would not be as useful because the half-life is too short to provide adequate coverage time. A bolus of 50% intravenous dextrose solution is indicated only if severe hypoglycemia occurs. Infusion of 5% dextrose solution is indicated once serum glucose levels approach normal, but continued high ketone levels require further insulin therapy.

13. Correct answer—B.

Newly developed glucosuria without a history of diabetes mellitus is often an early finding of infection in a critically ill child. Any critically ill child is at risk for developing infection. Symptoms of pancreatitis may often include hyperglycemia, but other more specific signs and symptoms such as severe abdominal pain, elevated white blood cell counts, and changes in serum lipase or amylase levels are also reliable indicators. Hypoinsulinemia is associated with diabetes mellitus. Electrolyte imbalances often accompany, but are not a primary cause of, hyperglycemia.

14. Correct answer—C.

Signs and symptoms of hypoglycemia in an infant include irritability, jitteriness, poor feeding, lethargy, hypotonia, high-pitched cry, diaphoresis, hypothermia, seizures, tachypnea, cyanosis, pallor, apnea, and arrest. An increase in urine output and thirst are associated with the osmotic diuretic effect of hyperglycemia.

15. Correct answer—D.

Risk factors for hypoglycemia include increased circulating catecholamines from stress, decreased glucose stores from inadequate dietary intake of substrates or increased utilization, and liver disease. Decreased insulin production would result in *hyper*glycemia.

16. Correct answer—B.

Syndrome of inappropriate antidiuretic hormone (SIADH) is a disorder of the body's ability to excrete water. Excessive amounts of ADH can be secreted in response to such stimuli as pulmonary disease, congestive heart failure, increased left atrial pressure, positive pressure ventilation, chemotherapy, tumors, and many medications. See box on pg. 170 for a list of conditions associated with SIADH. This patient could be at risk for acute renal failure related to acute tubular necrosis but not chronic renal failure, which is the result of end-stage renal diseases. Diabetes insipidus is associated with massive urinary output, not a drop in output. Hypothyroidism is not associated with an acute drop in urinary output.

17. Correct answer—A.
The inappropriate release of antidiuretic hormone directly causes an increase in fluid volume. Renal perfusion is not compromised, but the kidney's ability to excrete water is impaired because of the action of ADH. If fluid volume excess becomes excessive, this patient is at risk for impaired gas exchange related to pulmonary edema. Breathing patterns should not be directly affected.

18. Correct answer—D.
After discontinuing hyperalimentation, patients are at risk for developing hypoglycemia. Because hyperalimentation solution is high in glucose, patients are accustomed to an increased production of insulin. See Table 3-1 for signs and symptoms of hypoglycemia, hyperglycemia, and ketoacidosis.

19. Correct answer—A.
Regular insulin is used to treat DKA because of its rapid onset and short half-life. These features, along with an intravenous route, allow the most control in bringing down glucose and ketone levels quickly and safely. The Lente, Semilente, and Ultra-lente cannot be given intravenously, and have a longer time for onset and longer half-life. These features make it more difficult to bring down glucose and ketone levels quickly while preventing overcorrection, which can result in hypoglycemia.

20. Correct answer— C.
In DKA, serum glucose levels usually normalize more quickly than ketone levels. In order to prevent hypoglycemia while insulin is still being used to treat elevated ketone levels, a 5% dextrose-containing solution is used. Saline and ringer's lactate solutions do not contain glucose to prevent hypoglycemia.

21. Correct answer—D.
Risk factors for the development of DI include neurological causes, infections, vascular abnormalities, renal disease, and pharmacological agents. See box on p. 169 for specific etiologies. Congestive heart failure is a risk factor for developing SIADH.

22. Correct answer—A.
Diabetes insipidus is a disorder of either ADH production or effectiveness which results in the secretion of large amounts of very dilute urine. The specific gravity for urine in a patient with DI would be expected to be in the range of 1.001 to 1.005.

23. Correct answer—B.
In treating diabetes insipidus, the patient must be constantly evaluated for continued hypovolemia related to polyuria or inadequate fluid resuscitation as well

as hypervolemia related to excessive fluid resuscitation. A central venous pressure (CVP) of 12 is elevated, suggesting hypervolemia from too much intravenous fluids. A heart rate of 95 beats per minute and a blood pressure of 110/60 are normal for an 8-year-old child, indicating that the patient probably is normovolemic. Tachycardia would indicate either hypervolemia or hypovolemia. A BUN of 15 is also normal. In hypovolemia, this would be elevated from hemoconcentration which increases serum values, and decreased in hypervolemia from hemodilution which decreases serum values.

24. Correct answer—A.
SIADH is a disorder resulting from excess antidiuretic hormone. Water retention occurs which lowers serum laboratory values and tends to raise urine concentrations of electrolytes. A urine sodium concentration greater than 30 mEq/L would be expected in SIADH because of the decreased elimination of water, causing a concentration of eliminated electrolytes in the urine. Decreased serum sodium levels below 135 mEq/L, decreased serum osmolality below 270 mOsm/kg, and a serum creatinine below 1.0 mg/dL would be expected from dilution related to water retention.

25. Correct answer—B.
A patient with SIADH is at risk for developing seizures and cerebral edema with severe hyponatremia. Hyperthermia is associated with *hyper*natremia. Signs and symptoms of hyponatremia include lethargy, hypothermia, abnormal reflexes, abdominal cramping, diarrhea, hypotension, tachycardia, anxiety, and cold, diaphoretic skin.

NEONATAL-SPECIFIC ANSWERS

26. Correct answer—C.
Once an infant has been stabilized on intravenous glucose infusions, the infusion may be slowly weaned while the critical care nurse frequently checks serum glucose levels. The infusion should not be abruptly discontinued or decreased because it may cause rebound hypoglycemia. The solution should not be replaced with normal saline or other nonglucose-containing solutions because this also may lead to hypoglycemia.

27. Correct answer—D.
Congenital hypothyroidism is not typically associated with hypoglycemia. Risk factors for hypoglycemia do include maternal and intrauterine factors, as well as other disorders. See box on p. 167 for a list of risk factors for neonatal hypoglycemia.

28. Correct answer—C.
Galactosemia is an inborn error of metabolism of carbohydrates. Lactose in the diet, specifically milk and other lactose-containing formulas, should be broken

down into galactose, which in turn is metabolized by an enzyme formed in the liver into glucose. Because the hepatic enzyme *galactose-1-phosphate uridine transferase (UDP-galactose transferase)* is not present, the metabolism of lactose ends at the formation of galactose-1-phosphate which affects the nervous system, liver, and eyes.

29. Correct answer—B.
Hypoglycemia in the first 72 hours of life is generally defined as a serum glucose level less than 35 mg/dL. After the first 72 hours of life, hypoglycemia is determined by a glucose level less than 45 mg/dL. For a preterm low birth weight infant, hypoglycemia is recognized as less than 25 mg/dL.

30. Correct answer—A.
Infants of diabetic mothers are at risk for hypocalcemia, hyperbilirubinemia, and respiratory distress syndrome. Chvosstek's sign is seen in hypocalcemia and is a spasm of the facial nerve elicited by tapping the face near the parotid gland. Cullen's sign is discoloration around the umbilicus indicating a retroperitoneal bleed. Kehr's sign is pain in the left shoulder elicited by pressing on the left supper quadrant of the abdomen. It indicates damage to the spleen. Cushing's reflex (or triad) indicates increased intracranial pressure and includes an elevation in systolic blood pressure, slow and irregular respirations, and bradycardia.

31. Correct answer—B.
IDMs are at risk for hyperbilirubinemia, necessitating frequent evaluation of the serum bilirubin levels during the neonatal period. Renal function at birth is not affected by maternal diabetes, so the serum creatinine should be normal. Amylase is a pancreatic enzyme, but is not abnormal in IDMs. Serum sodium levels also are not affected by maternal diabetes.

32. Correct answer—D.
Infants of diabetic mothers are particularly sensitive to serum glucose levels. By administering glucose-containing solutions, the infant is at high risk for rebound hypoglycemia. The oral feedings of choice, therefore, include breast milk, infant formulas, or solutions that contain nonglucose sugars such as galactose.

33. Correct answer—D.
Altered nutrition: less than body requirements refers to an inability to ingest or digest food or absorb nutrients. Hypoglycemia in the newborn is generally not related to inadequate intake, but rather alterations and instability in metabolic functioning. Hypoglycemia can lead to a decrease in cardiac output, decreased peripheral perfusion, and even apnea and respiratory arrest.

34. Correct answer—B.
Breast milk is naturally low in phenylalanine, the amino acid that is unable to be metabolized in PKU. With careful monitoring of serum PKU levels, infants may be able to receive all or part of their dietary intake as breast milk. Special milk

substitutes low in phenylalanine are also available. Soy formulas, low iron formulas, as well as lactose-free formulas all contain phenylalanine in quantities too high for an infant with PKU.

35. Correct answer—B.
For an infant with PKU, an acceptable serum PKU level is 2 to 8 mg/dL. Brain damage generally occurs if levels rise above 10 to 15 mg/dL.

36. Correct answer—C.
Galactosemia, which is uncontrolled, can result in mental retardation, jaundice, cirrhosis, hepatosplenomegaly, and cataracts within the first weeks to months of life.

37. Correct answer—A.
Signs and symptoms of congenital hypothyroidism include coarse, dry hair, narrow pulse pressure, hypotension, bradycardia, anemia, wide cranial sutures, puffy eyelids, large tongue, abdominal distension, cold, dry skin, and flat nasal bridge.

38. Correct answer—C.
Laboratory findings to confirm the diagnosis of congenital hypothyroidism include a low T_4 level, high TSH level, decreased protein-bound iodine level, low free thyroxine level, and decreased thyroxine level.

39. Correct answer—A.
Hypoglycemia in infants of diabetic mothers is a result of hyperinsulinemia. Exposure to high serum glucose levels throughout fetal life causes the pancreas of an IDM to be overactive, resulting in hypoglycemia. Generally there is not a decrease in stores or intake of substrates. Decreased metabolic activity would not result in hypoglycemia because less glucose would be required.

40. Correct answer—A.
Infants with PKU and decreased levels of serotonin are at risk for bleeding disorders. Serotonin is released by platelets and plays an important role in aggregating platelets during the clotting process as well as causing vasoconstriction. Bowel obstruction, renal failure, and apnea are not directly linked to PKU.

41. Correct answer—B.
Hypoglycemia in the hypothermic newborn results from increased use of glucose. Glucose is metabolized in large amounts to try to raise the body temperature. Even in the presence of adequate substrates (substances capable of converting to glucose or glucose itself) stores, the demands of hypothermia can quickly outstrip immediately available supplies. Hyperinsulinemia and islet cell dysplasia are associated with infants of diabetic mothers.

42. Correct answer—D.

The brain depends heavily upon glucose as its energy source making it particularly susceptible to dysfunction with hypoglycemia. See box on p. 168 for systemic signs and symptoms of hypoglycemia.

43. Correct answer—B.

Initial treatment of the symptomatic neonate with hypoglycemia would include 1 mL/kg of 25% dextrose solution. Dextrose solutions of 5% and 10% would be unlikely to achieve a prompt and therapeutic effect in a symptomatic neonate. A 50% solution is too concentrated for use in neonates.

44. Correct answer—D.

The goal for serum glucose levels when treating neonates with hypoglycemia is to maintain the serum glucose level between 45 and 120 mg/dL. A level below 45 mg/dL is recognized as hypoglycemic. Levels greater than 125 mg/dL constitute hyperglycemia in a term infant.

45. Correct answer—D.

A confirmed glucose level of 15 mg/dL is extremely low and needs to be corrected immediately. A 25% dextrose solution bolus at 1 mL/kg would be the first action in attempting to restore normal serum glucose levels. Oral solutions are not always effective and in this case would take too long to be effective. A constant IV infusion of a 5% dextrose solution would be inadequate to meet the needs of an infant with severe hypoglycemia and 50% glucose solutions are too concentrated for use in neonates.

46. Correct answer—A.

An infant showing signs and symptoms of hypoglycemia needs to have immediate evaluation of the glucose level. A heelstick and measurement by reagent strip provide a quick and reliable method of screening. A sample may also be sent to the laboratory for confirmation, but the delay in receiving results should not delay identification by screening methods and early intervention. Administration of 4 mL of 25% dextrose solution should only be done when the serum glucose level is known by either a screening method or laboratory confirmation. Increasing the 5% dextrose solution rate is not likely to provide enough glucose to treat a symptomatic infant.

CHAPTER 4

Hematology and Immunology Care Problems

Passkeys

GENERAL PRINCIPLES OF HEMATOLOGY AND IMMUNOLOGY

- The partial thromboplastin time (PTT) and prothrombin time (PT) normally are prolonged in the neonate until approximately 1 month of age.
- Vitamin K deficiencies are common in the neonatal period and are manifested by prolonged PT and PTT.
- 2,3-diphosphoglycerate (2,3-DPG) is an intracellular red blood cell factor responsible for determining hemoglobin's affinity for oxygen (how tightly oxygen binds to hemoglobin). Decreased 2,3-DPG causes hemoglobin to hold onto oxygen, shifting the oxyhemoglobin dissociation curve to the left. Banked blood has decreased levels of 2,3-DPG resulting in blood volume with impaired oxygen delivery ability.
- Neonates and premature infants have hemoglobin that already possesses a high oxygen affinity. Transfusion of banked blood low in 2,3-DPG only makes it more difficult for oxygen to be released from the red blood cell, causing tissue hypoxia.
- IgG represents the largest proportion of antibodies and is the only one to cross the placenta. IgG attacks bacteria, viruses, protozoa, and toxins.
- IgM is responsible for antibodies to nonself ABO blood types and also helps kill bacteria.
- IgA is found in breast milk and offers immunity only by coating the gastrointestinal tract, not by absorption. IgA works against viruses.
- T cells are involved in cellular immunity. They are responsible for autoimmune diseases and organ transplant rejection.
- B cells are involved in humoral immunity (antibodies). See Fig. 4-1 for a schemata of the immune system.

DISSEMINATED INTRAVASCULAR COAGULATION

- Disseminated intravascular coagulation (DIC) is a disorder involving abnormal clotting that manifests as bleeding. It is *not* a *primary* bleeding disorder. DIC always results as a complication of other disorders. See Table 4-1 for common hematology disorders.

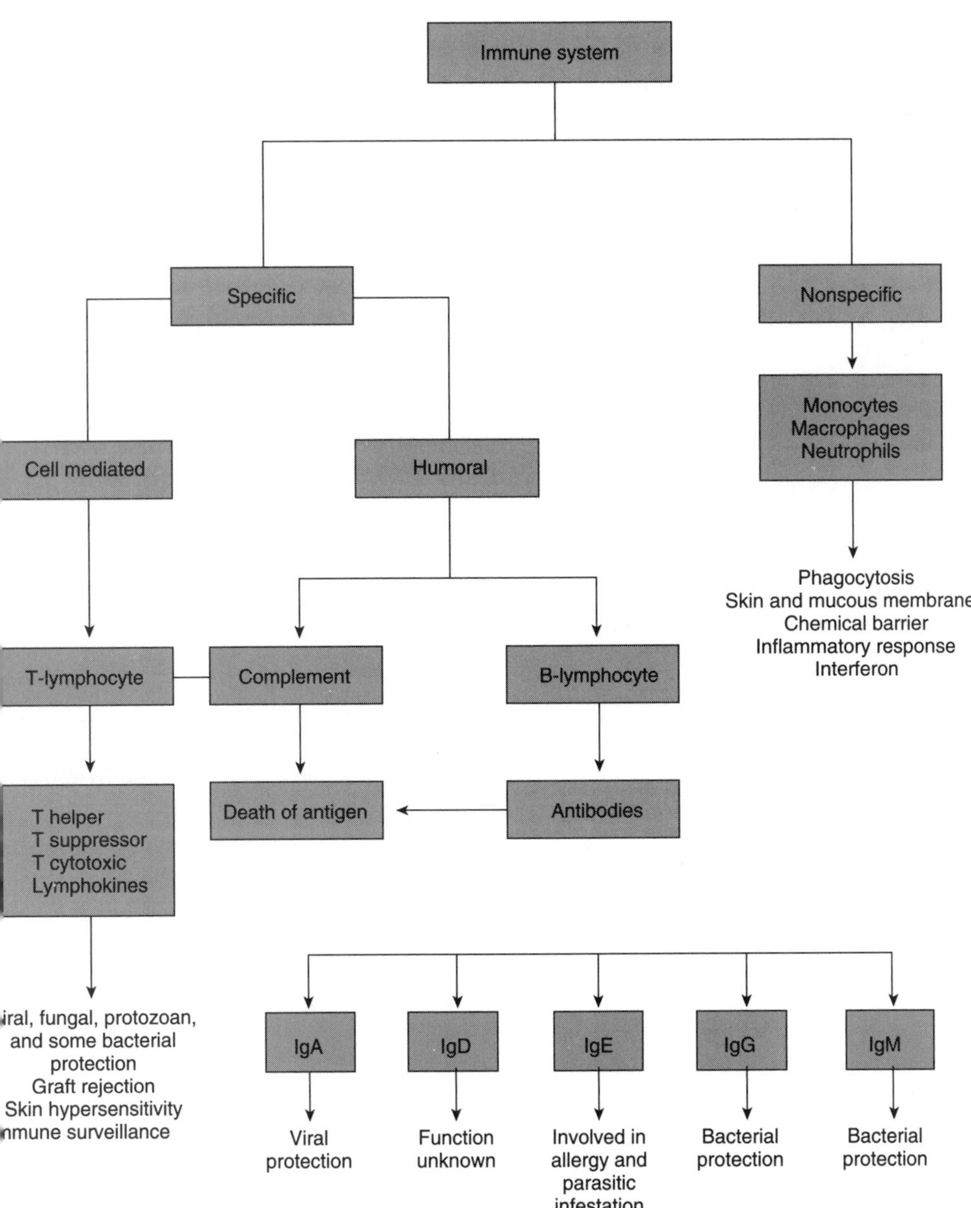

Fig. 4-1 Components of the immune system. (From Wong DL: Whaley and Wong's nursing care of infants and children, ed 5, St Louis, 1995, Mosby.)

Table 4-1
Hematology and Immunology Disorders

Disorder	Causes	Assessment Findings	Management
Disseminated intravascular coagulation	Sepsis Shock Snake bites Obstetrical emergencies and complications Thermal injuries Head injury Fat or pulmonary emboli Anoxia Necrotizing enterocolitis Viral or protozoal infections Organ transplant rejection Freshwater drowning Poisoning Transfusion reaction	Signs and symptoms related to bleeding or clotting, which occludes blood flow to all body systems Pallor Tachycardia Hypotension Bleeding from body orifices and injection or puncture sites Petechiae Ecchymosis Hematuria Melena Increased abdominal girth Headache Epistaxis Gangrene Prolonged prothrombin time and partial thromboplastin time Increased thromboplastin time Decreased platelet count Decreased fibrinogen levels Increased fibrin split products	Treat primary cause Treat shock, hypoxemia, acidosis, sepsis, and other systemic conditions Platelet transfusions of 1 unit/5 kg body weight for infants and children to keep count above 60,000/mL Clotting factor replacement of fresh frozen plasma at 10 mL/kg of body weight for infants and 10-15 mL/kg of body weight for children Cryoprecipitates are administered to elevate fibrinogen levels Exchange transfusions Heparinization: 50-100 units of heparin/kg loading dose accompanied by 10-20 units/kg/hr infusion
Idiopathic thrombocytopenia purpura	Passively acquired ITP: Maternal history or ITP or systemic lupus	Hematomas Ecchymosis Bleeding from orifices or puncture sites	Supportive treatment Prednisone Intravenous immune gamma globulin Methylprednisone

Table 4-1
Hematology and Immunology Disorders—cont'd

Disorder	Causes	Assessment Findings	Management
Idiopathic thrombocytopenia purpura—cont'd	Erythematosus Actively acquired ITP: Drug related (especially heparin) Autoimmune diseases Viral infections	Epistaxis Hematuria Melena Decreased hematocrit and hemoglobin Shock Decreased platelet count Alterations in neurological function	Platelet transfusions Exchange transfusions Splenectomy
Hyperbilirubinemia	Increased red blood cell destruction: Prematurity Hemolytic disease of the newborn Internal hemorrhage Impairments of transport of indirect bilirubin: Hypo-albuminemia Acidosis Hypoxia Impairment of bilirubin excretion: Liver disease Biliary atresia Other causes: Associated with breastfeeding Bacterial infection Physiologic jaundice	Elevated indirect and total bilirubin levels Jaundice Brown urine Pruritus Clay-colored stools Kerricterus Elevated total and indirect bilirubin levels Jaundice Kernicterus Low serum albumin levels Elevations of total and indirect bilirubin levels with liver disease Elevations of total and direct bilirubin levels with biliary disease Jaundice Elevations in total and unconjugated bilirubin levels	Treatment includes phototherapy for indirect hyperbilirubinemia Exchange transfusions Administration of albumin Avoid medications that bind to albumin Hydration

Continued.

Table 4-1
Hematology and Immunology Disorders—cont'd

Disorder	Causes	Assessment Findings	Management
Hyperbilirubinemia —cont'd		Increase in all levels with bacterial infection Increase in total and indirect bilirubin levels with physiologic jaundice	
Hemophilia	Most commonly transmitted genetically Many cases may be gene mutation without family history	Bleeding of gums Severe bruising in response to minor trauma Subcutaneous and intramuscular hemorrhages Hemarthrosis Hematuria Bleeding in virtually any organ system or tissue Prolonged PTT Prolonged whole blood clotting time Prolonged prothrombin time	Prevent injury! Avoid injections and deep intravenous sites Avoid nonsteroidal antiinflammatory drugs which inhibit platelet function Use of cryoprecipitates and fresh frozen plasma carries less of a risk of HIV and hepatitis transmission
Acquired immune deficiency syndrome (AIDS)	Infection with the HIV virus: Perinatal transmission from HIV+ mother Through sexual abuse From blood or blood products From breast milk	May have no symptoms and be HIV+ Encephalophathy Developmental delays Presence of opportunistic infections Lymphadenopathy	Universal precautions May require monthly gamma globulin therapy AZT Aerosolized antiprotozoal for pneumocystis carinii Do not use live virual vaccines with HIV+ children or family members

Table 4-1
Hematology and Immunology Disorders—cont'd

Disorder	Causes	Assessment Findings	Management
Sickle cell disease	Genetically transmitted Crises are precipitated by hypoxemia, dehydration, and acidosis	Pain Anemia Fever Signs and symptoms of hypoperfusion and vascular occlusion in any organ system or tissue	Fluid therapy at twice maintenance requirements Correction of acidosis and hypoxemia Partial exchange transfusions Blood transfusions to correct anemia Support of affected organ systems and tissues
Rh incompatibility	Rh– mother with an Rh+ fetus	Anemia Elevated reticulocyte count and nucleated red blood cells Increased total and indirect bilirubin levels Hepatosplenomegaly Hydrops fetalis Positive direct Coomb's test Stillbirth Jaundice	Preventative: Administer anti-D human gamma globulin (RhoGAM) to mother following the delivery or abortion of an Rh+ fetus or infant Partial and full exchange transfusion Phototheraphy to treat hyperbilirubinemia
ABO incompatibility	O blood type mother with A or B blood type fetus A blood type mother with B or AB blood type fetus	Elevated total and indirect bilirubin levels Anemia Jaundice	Exchange transfusion Transfusion to treat anemia Phototherapy to treat hyperbilirubinemia

Continued.

Table 4-1
Hematology and Immunology Disorders—cont'd

Disorder	Causes	Assessment Findings	Management
ABO incompatibility—cont'd	B blood type mother with A or AB blood type fetus	Increase in reticulocyte count and nucleated red blood cells Microspherocytes and spherocytes are found in peripheral blood smear Mother's serum has anti-A and anti-B IgG antibodies Slightly positive direct Coomb's test Positive indirect Coomb's test	

- The pathophysiology of DIC involves the formation of microclots throughout the body through accelerated clotting in the microcirculation, potentially interrupting and compromising any organ system. Consumption of clotting factors in the microcirculation results in bleeding disorders.

- In DIC, factors V and VIII, as well as fibrinogen and platelets, are abnormally consumed in clotting mechanism. This results in a *consumptive coagulopathy*. See Fig. 4-2 for the normal clotting pathway.

- Excessive amounts of thrombin are formed in a patient with DIC. Excessive thrombin levels cause further clotting by promoting platelet aggregation.

- Precipitating pathology associated with DIC includes shock, sepsis, obstetrical emergencies and complications, hemolytic processes, head injury, burns, organ transplant rejection, fat and pulmonary emboli, anoxia, snake bites, and freshwater drowning.

- Clotting factors, fibrinogen, and platelets are decreased in DIC. Partial thromboplastin time (PTT), prothrombin time (PT), and fibrin split products are increased. See Table 4-2 for a list of a various clotting factors and their role in the clotting cascade.

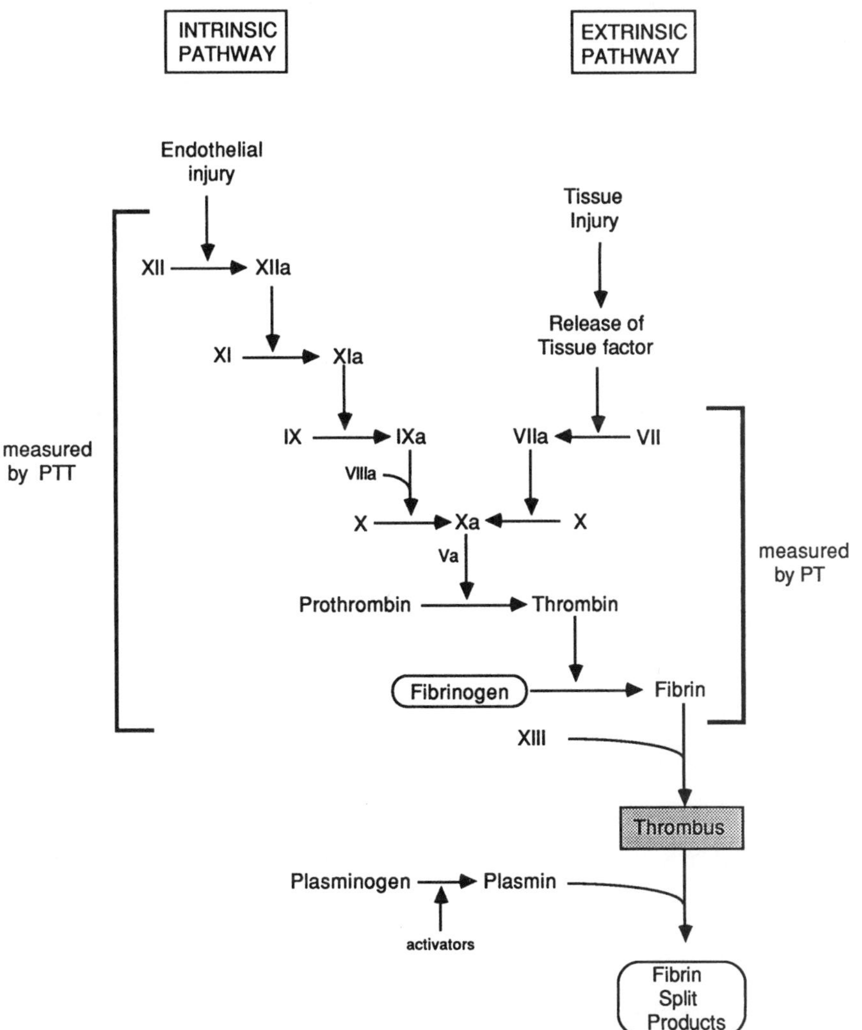

Fig. 4-2 Clotting cascade. (From Hazinski MF: Nursing care of the critically ill child, ed 2, St Louis, 1992, Mosby.)

- Fibrin split products or fibrin degradation products (FDP), are themselves anticoagulants. When these results from breakdown of massive clot formation, further bleeding is promoted. See Table 4-3 for laboratory diagnostic test findings in DIC.
- Cryoprecipitate is used to replenish fibrinogen levels and also contains clotting factors VIII and XIII.
- Fresh frozen plasma contains clotting factors, but *not* platelets.

Table 4-2
Coagulation Factors

Factor	Pathway
I: Fibrinogen	Common pathway
II: Prothrombin	Common pathway
III: Tissue thromboplastin	Extrinsic pathway
IV: Calcium	All pathways
V: Proaccelerin	Common pathway
VII: Proconvertin	Extrinsic pathway
VIII: Antihemophilic factor	Intrinsic pathway
IX: Christmas factor	Intrinsic pathway
X: Stuart factor	Common pathway
XI: Plasma thromboplastin antecedent	Intrinsic pathway
XII: Hageman factor	Intrinsic pathway
XIII: Fibrin stabilizing factor	Common pathway

IDIOPATHIC THROMBOCYTOPENIA PURPURA

- Idiopathic thrombocytopenia purpura (ITP) is a thrombocytopenia related to an autoimmune disease. Antibodies reduce the platelets' life span, which are destroyed in the spleen. (See Table 4-1.)
- Maternal ITP can affect the infant by passage of maternal antibodies (IgG antiplatelet antibodies) across the placenta. These maternal antibodies attack and destroy the infant's platelets causing an immune related thrombocytopenia.
- If identified prenatally, cesarean section is the delivery of choice for a neonate with ITP because thrombocytopenia in the fetus during labor and delivery carries a high morbidity and mortality.
- Either maternal lupus erythematosus or idiopathic thrombocytopenia purpura may cause acquired ITP in the neonate.

Table 4-3
Laboratory Results in DIC

Laboratory Test	Results in DIC
Prothrombin time	Prolonged
Partial thromboplastin time	Prolonged
Thromboplastin time	Prolonged
Platelet count	Decreased
Red blood cell count	Decreased
Hematocrit	Decreased
Fibrinogen levels	Decreased
Fibrin split products	Increased

- Decreased platelet counts in the neonatal period may last for weeks. Transfusions of platelets are minimally useful as a result of the presence of antiplatelet antibodies that quickly destroy freshly transfused platelets.

- Serious bleeding usually does not occur after the first week of life in acquired ITP, even if thrombocytopenia persists longer.

- Infants with ITP from maternal passage of antibodies manifest with petechiae and low platelet counts, less than 10,000/mm^3.

- Treatment of passively acquired ITP consists of intravenous immune gamma globulin at 0.4g/kg/dose, which can be repeated in 24 hours.

- Prednisone and exchange transfusions followed by platelet transfusions have also been used to treat passively acquired ITP.

- ITP may be an acute, self-limiting disease in children. Drugs such as heparin, and viral infections such as measles, mumps, and chicken pox may cause an acute course of ITP.

- Signs of bleeding associated with ITP may be seen in all body systems and be severe enough to result in shock.

- Platelet counts under 20,000/mm^3 may be associated with spontaneous bleeding. Intracranial hemorrhage may occur with counts as low as 5000/mm^3.

HYPERBILIRUBINEMIA

- Metabolism of bilirubin occurs in the liver and spleen as old red blood cells are broken down. Bilirubin comes from the breakdown of the heme portion of hemoglobin. (See Table 4-1.)
- Bilirubin in the plasma binds with albumin. This binding is affected by plasma pH and medications.
- Before bilirubin goes to the liver to be processed, it is in an unconjugated form (measured as the indirect or unconjugated bilirubin).
- After being processed in the liver, bilirubin becomes conjugated (measured as the direct or conjugated bilirubin).
- The gastrointestinal system of the newborn can convert conjugated bilirubin back into unconjugated bilirubin that may be reabsorbed, increasing the serum bilirubin level.
- The short life span of a neonatal red blood cell adds to the bilirubin level by increasing the amount of RBC destruction and therefore bilirubin, which must be metabolized and eliminated.
- Decreased serum albumin places the infant at risk for developing kernicterus, toxic levels of bilirubin. Because bilirubin is bound to albumin, if albumin levels are low, the serum (unconjugated) bilirubin level may reach toxic levels. See box below for signs and symptoms of kernicterus.
- Causes of hyperbilirubinemia can be divided into three categories (1) increased red blood cell destruction, (2) impaired transport of unconjugated bilirubin (increased total and indirect or unconjugated bilirubin levels), or (3) problems with bilirubin elimination (increased total and direct or conjugated bilirubin levels).

Signs and Symptoms of Kernicterus

Early Signs	Late Signs
Irritability	Irritable cry
Lethargy	Rigid extension of arms and legs
Decreased activity level	Opisthotonus
Poor feeding	Seizures
	Internal hemorrhages

- Jaundice describes the clinical findings of yellowing of the sclera, skin, mucous membranes, and other tissues. Urine become brown. The higher the level of unconjugated serum bilirubin, the greater the likelihood of developing kernicterus. Clinically, jaundice usually becomes apparent at serum levels of total bilirubin, which are greater than 3.0 mg/dL.

- High levels of unconjugated, not conjugated, bilirubin pose the threat of brain damage.

- Kernicterus is the presence of yellow pigment in the brain (basal ganglia) in the form of unconjugated bilirubin. This may result in encephalopathy and permanent brain damage.

- Phototherapy lights must be turned off while blood samples are obtained for serum bilirubin levels. The phototherapy lights can actually decrease levels of the sampled blood in the tube leading to a falsely low report. See Table 4-4 for adverse reactions associated with phototherapy.

- Liver disease and accompanying hypoalbuminemia may cause hyperbilirubinemia.

- Dehydration interferes with the elimination of conjugated (direct) bilirubin.

- Avoid drugs that bind with albumin. These drugs decrease the available binding sites for unconjugated bilirubin and lead to higher total and indirect bilirubin levels. Diazepam, gentamicin, furosemide, and digoxin are some medications that bind with albumin.

PEDIATRIC-SPECIFIC PRINCIPLES

ORGAN TRANSPLANTATION

Immunosuppression:

- T cells are primarily responsible for transplanted organ rejection.

- Immunosuppressive therapy may include one or more of the following medications: methylprednisolone, cyclosporin A, azathioprine, and FK-506.

- To treat rejection episodes, boluses of methylprednisolone or hydrocortisone may be used. Antilymphocyte monoclonal antibody (OKT_3) and antilymphocyte globulin (ALG) therapy may also be used to treat rejection.

- Cyclosporin is nephrotoxic and may cause a decrease in urine output. Hypertension and hemolytic uremic syndrome are other potential problems associated with cyclosporin. Serum cyclosporin levels should be monitored closely and dosage adjusted accordingly.

Table 4-4
Adverse Reactions Associated with Phototherapy

Adverse Reaction	Pathophysiology	Nursing Intervention
Retinal injury	Unknown, but demonstrated in animal studies	Cover eyes during therapy
Hypothermia	From radiant heat loss	Monitor temperature continuously
Hyperthermia	From heat of lamps especially when incubators or servocontrolled units are used	Monitor temperature continuously
Dehydration	From insensible water loss	Weigh twice a day or more frequently as needed Strict intake and output Intravenous fluids as needed
Loose bowel movements	Increased bowel motility	Carefully assess fluid balance and prevent skin breakdown
Lactose intolerance	Presence of reducing substances	Use of lactulose-free formulas
Thrombocytopenia	Decreased platelet lifespan	Observe for signs of bleeding
Bronze baby syndrome	Retention of bilirubin breakdown products	Discontinuance of phototherapy as needed
Tanning	Increased melanin production	Don't use oils or lotions Decrease or discontinue phototherapy
Hypocalcemia	Effects on albumin associated with therapy for hyperbilirubinemia	Use of a cap on the head may help decrease incidence Assess electrolyte levels frequently

Kidney:

- Potential postoperative complications include renal failure secondary to acute tubular necrosis, renal vascular artery obstruction, renal vein thrombosis, decreased renal blood flowing during surgical procedure, hypotensive episodes, and rejection.
- Signs of acute rejection occur within 2 to 10 days of transplantation and include fever, abdominal tenderness over the graft, hypertension, oliguria, weight gain, proteinuria, and a decrease in white cell count.
- Cyclosporin is not usually used in the immediate postoperative period for renal transplant patients because of its nephrotoxic effects. It is introduced into the immunosuppressive regimen after adequate renal function has been well established.

Liver:

- Bleeding is a significant and common postoperative complication following liver transplantation; therefore, heparin should not be added to any flush solutions for the postoperative liver transplant patient.
- Hypertension is a common postoperative complication following liver transplantation.
- Low dose dopamine therapy (1 to 4 mcg/kg/min) may be used to improve hepatic blood flow.
- Neurological function is an important reliable indicator of liver graft function. Alterations in or decreased levels of consciousness are serious indicators of postoperative liver transplant complications.
- If liver function is failing, drainage from the T tube in the bile duct will decrease and become pale in color.
- Signs of liver transplant rejection include increase in SGOT, SGPT (AST, ALT), LDH; bleeding; hypoglycemia; electrolyte imbalances; right upper quadrant or flank pain; and jaundice.
- Rejection is most likely to occur 4 to 10 days after surgery.

Heart:

- Rejection is best confirmed by right heart endomyocardial biopsy.
- Bleeding is a significant postoperative complication in heart transplantation related to liver dysfunction secondary to congestive heart failure preoperatively.

- Signs and symptoms of rejection include fever, tachycardia, dyspnea, congestive heart failure, dysrhythmia, and myocardial dysfunction by echocardiogram.

- Right ventricular failure posttransplantation must be observed for if pulmonary hypertension was present before the transplant.

- The transplanted heart does not have autonomic innervation that normally affects heart rate and cardiac output. To increase these in the transplanted heart, dobutamine may be needed.

HEMOPHILIA

- Hemophilia is a disorder of hemostasis where one or more clotting factors is deficient. (See Table 4-1.)

- Hemophilia A (classic hemophilia or factor VIII deficiency) and hemophilia B (Christmas disease or factor IX deficiency) are the most common forms.

- Bleeding can occur anywhere in the body as a result of trauma or normal activity, or spontaneously. For example, swollen joints with tingling and warmth can indicate bleeding into a joint.

- The partial thromboplastin time (PTT) and prothrombin time (PT) are increased in factor VIII deficiency. Both are used to monitor response to transfusions of factor VIII concentrates.

- When indicated, factor VIII infusions are administered *immediately* and all subsequent doses must be given on time.

- Intramuscular injections and femoral or subclavian venipunctures must be avoided. Only antecubital, external jugular, or other superficial veins can be used safely.

- Bleeding in neonates with hemophilia often is not manifested in the early weeks of life except with circumcision, joint bleeding, heel sticks, or other trauma.

CONGENITAL IMMUNOSUPPRESSION

- Primary immunodeficiencies occur as a result of genetic or congenital conditions.

- X-linked gammaglobulinemia is a B lymphocyte abnormality.

- DiGeorge syndrome is associated with an absent thymus and parathyroids. These children have T cell deficiencies and calcium imbalances.

- Combined immune deficiency is the absence or insufficiency of both B and T lymphocytes.

ACQUIRED IMMUNOSUPPRESSION

- Acquired immunosuppression may be permanent or temporary and related to such causes as medications, radiation, age, stress, malnutrition, human immunodeficiency virus (HIV), trauma, splenectomy, and surgery.

- Human immunodeficiency virus (HIV) is a retrovirus that attacks T cells. (See Table 4-1.)

- In HIV infection, helper T cells (T4, CD4, inducer cells) become less numerous than suppressor T cells (T8, CD8, cytotoxic lymphocytes) resulting in the immune system being turned off.

- A T4/T8 ratio of less than 1.0 signals immunodeficiency indicative of HIV infection.

- *Pneumocystis carinii* pneumonia (PCP) is an important opportunistic infection associated with HIV.

SICKLE CELL CRISIS

- Sickle cell disease is an inherited disorder that, in this country, primarily affects individuals of African or less often Mediterranean, Hispanic, and Middle Eastern descent. (See Table 4-1.)

- Sickle cell disease is a hemoglobinopathy that results in hemolytic anemia and organ dysfunction from vascular occlusion by clumping sickled cells.

- The tendency for a red blood cell to sickle is associated with dehydration, hypoxemia, and acidosis.

- Sickle cell disease is usually not apparent before 4 months of age because of the presence of fetal hemoglobin, which is not capable of sickling.

- All body systems and tissues can potentially be affected by sickling, leading to poor perfusion, thrombosis, and even necrosis of tissues and organs. See Fig. 4-3 for tissue effects of sickle cell disease.

- Treatment is aimed at prevention of crises by avoiding dehydration and hypoxemia.

- A sickle cell crisis usually manifests with severe pain and low grade fever. The specific organ or body area involved shows signs and symptoms of hypoperfusion, vascular occlusion, and tissue ischemia.

- In young children (6 months to 2 years), dactylitis may be the first indication of sickle cell disease. Painful swelling is seen in the hands and feet from obstruction

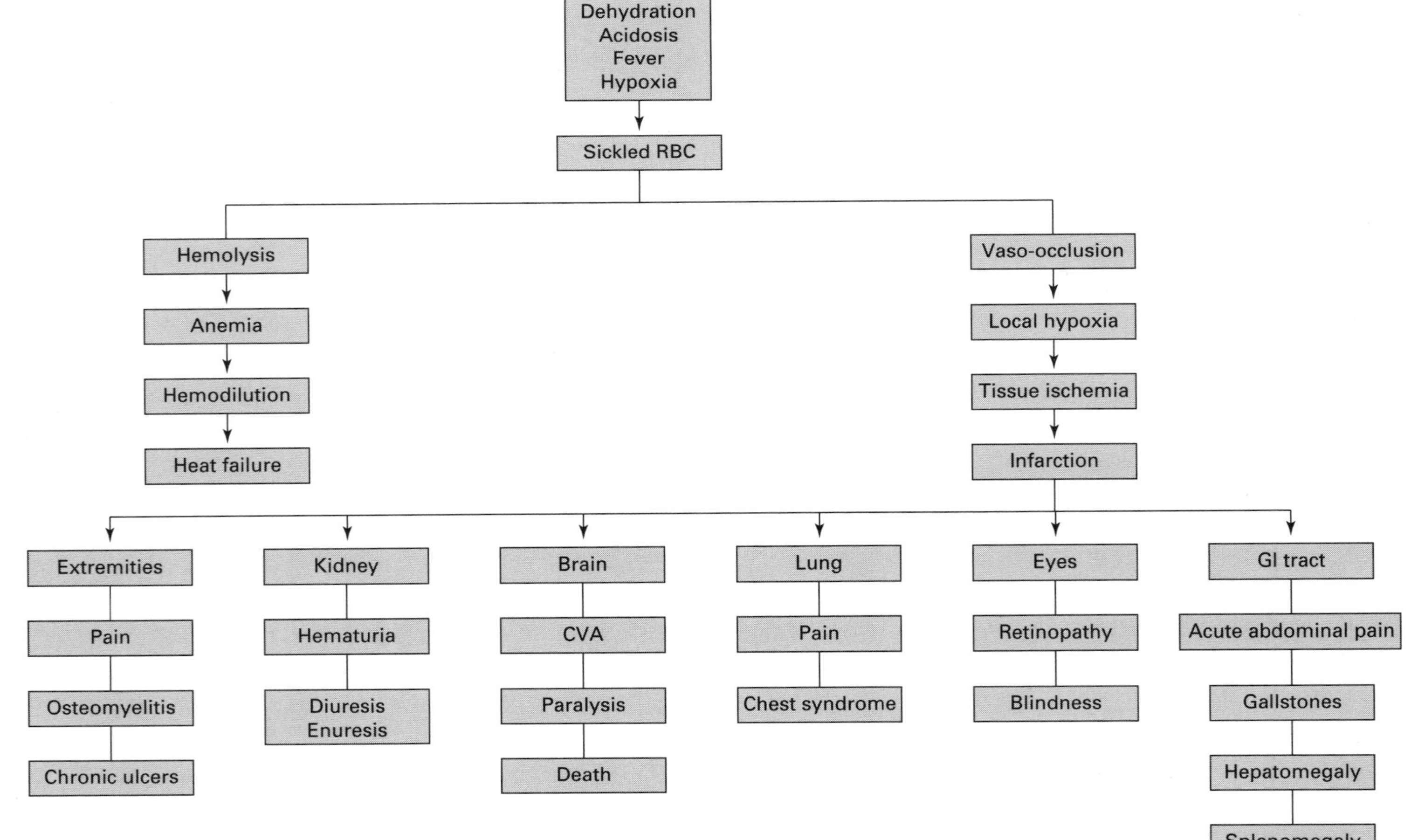

Fig. 4-3 Tissue effects of sickle cell anemia. (From Wong DL: Whaley and Wong's nursing care of infants and children, ed 5,

of blood flow to the bones. This is less commonly seen in older children and adults because the vessels increase in size with growth enough that occlusion becomes less common.

- Cerebrovascular accidents are a frequently seen problem. In younger children, the CVA is related to thrombosis, in older children and adults, the CVA is more commonly hemorrhagic.

- Acute splenic sequestration occurs when the splenic vein becomes occluded and a large proportion of the circulating volume of blood becomes trapped in the spleen. Splenomegaly, anemia, hypovolemia, and shock may be severe enough to be fatal.

- Priapism (painful, involuntary erection) may occur because blood from sickled cell becomes trapped in the cavernous sinuses.

- Sickle cell crises are managed by bed rest to decrease oxygen demand and consumption, fluid and electrolyte therapy, analgesics for pain, partial exchange transfusions, and treatment of anemia.

NEONATAL-SPECIFIC PRINCIPLES

RH INCOMPATIBILITY

- Difficulty in incompatibility between the mother and fetus occurs when the mother is Rh- and the fetus or neonate is Rh+. (See Table 4-1.)

- Maternal sensitization usually occurs during the delivery or abortion of her first Rh+ infant. The first Rh+ infant is usually not adversely affected.

- Rh hemolytic disease can be prevented by administering anti-D human gamma globulin (RhoGAM) to mothers following the birth or abortion of an Rh+ fetus or neonate.

- In affected fetuses, the maternal antibodies (IgG) to Rh+ blood attack the fetus and cause hemolysis. The fetus compensates by increasing the rate of RBC production resulting in the premature release and circulation of immature RBCs. See Fig. 4-4 for isoimmunization model in utero.

- Severe cases of erythroblastosis fetalis may result in hydrops fetalis or death.

- The presence of antibodies against Rh- blood in the neonate can be confirmed by the direct Coomb's test.

- The two major problems associated with neonates born in Rh- sensitized pregnancies are hemolysis resulting in hyperbilirubinemia and the potential for brain damage.

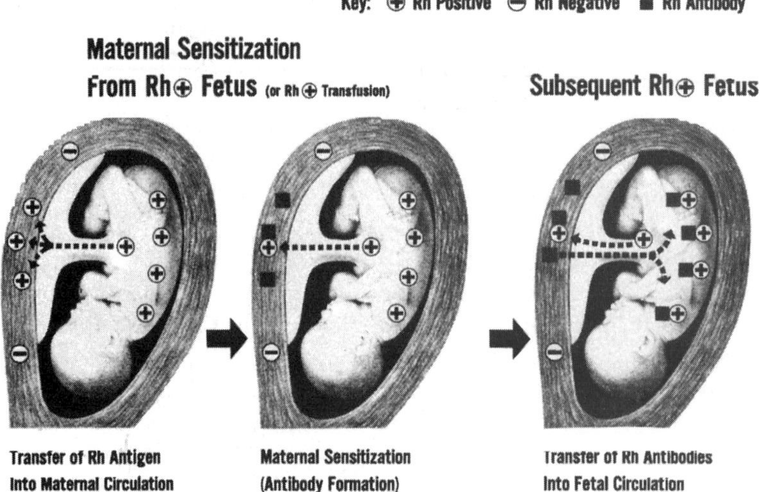

Fig. 4-4 Isoimmunization in utero. (From Merenstein GB and Gardner SL: Handbook of neonatal intensive care, ed 3, St Louis, 1993, Mosby.) (Courtesy of Ross Laboratories, Columbus, Ohio.)

Table 4-5
Compatibility of Blood Types Among Donors and Recipients

Blood Type	May Receive Blood From	May Donate Blood To
A+	A+, O+, A–, O-	A+, AB+
A-	A–, O-	A–, AB–, A+, AB+
B+	B+, O+, B–, O-	B+, AB+
B–	B–, O–	B–, AB–
O+	O+, O–	O+, A+, B+, AB+
O-	O–	O+, O–, A+, A–, B+, B–, AB+, AB-
AB+	A+, B+, O+, A–, B–, O–	AB+
AB-	A–, B–, O–, AB–	AB–, AB+

ABO INCOMPATIBILITY

- ABO hemolytic disease occurs in about 3% of pregnancies where the mother's blood type is incompatible with the fetus's blood type and maternal antibodies form, crossing the placenta and attacking and destroying fetal red blood cells. (See Table 4-1.)

- The direct Coomb's test is often falsely negative or only slightly reactive.

- A positive direct Coomb's test in ABO incompatibility usually indicates critical hemolytic disease.

- The indirect Coomb's test measures neonatal antibodies against adult A or B blood groups. It is more reliable in detecting ABO hemolytic disease in the newborn.

- See Table 4-5 on page 214 for blood type incompatibilities when donating and transfusing blood.

Questions

GENERAL HEMATOLOGY AND IMMUNOLOGY CARE QUESTIONS

Case Study

During the nursing assessment, a 28-hour-old neonate is found to have generalized petechiae and oozing from a heelstick site. The infant is afebrile, sucking well, and is alert and active when awake. There is a maternal history of systemic lupus erythematosus. Blood is drawn for a complete blood count with differential. Some of the results are as follows:

RBC: 2.8 million/mm^3
Hemoglobin: 12 g/dL
Hematocrit: 36%
White blood count: 6,100/mm^3
Platelet count: 10,000/mm^3

Questions 1 and 2 refer to this case study.

1. Which of the following laboratory values would the nurse also expect to be abnormal?
   A. Prothrombin time (PT)
   B. Partial thromboplastin time (PTT)
   C. Prothrombin consumption test
   D. Bleeding time

2. This infant is found to have a platelet count of 22,000/mm^3, bleeding from heel sticks, and generalized petechiae. Which of the following treatments would have the highest priority for this infant?
   A. Transfusion of platelets
   B. Intravenous immune gamma globulin
   C. Heparin therapy
   D. Exchange transfusion

3. A 10-day-old infant with a history of meconium aspiration has developed disseminated intravascular coagulation. Which of the following therapies would be a *priority* in treating DIC in this infant?
   A. Heparin therapy to reverse diffuse systemic clotting
   B. Transfusion of clotting factors to correct depleted levels
   C. Aggressive respiratory therapy to correct hypoxemia and acidosis
   D. Transfusion of platelets to correct depleted levels

4. Which of the following medications increases a patient's risk of developing hyperbilirubinemia?
A. Digoxin
B. Ampicillin
C. Dopamine
D. Dobutamine

5. All of the following are physiologic reasons for the development of hyperbilirubinemia in the newborn *except:*
A. Decreased life span of red blood cells
B. Decreased conjugating ability of the liver
C. Higher concentration of erythrocytes
D. Decreased fecal excretion

6. A 3-day-old infant is jaundiced and has the following blood chemistry results:
Direct (conjugated) bilirubin: 1.1 mg/dL
Indirect (unconjugated) bilirubin: 21.3 mg/dL
Total bilirubin: 22.4 mg/dL
Hemoglobin: 23 g/dL
Which of these results places the neonate at the *greatest* risk for developing kernicterus?
A. Direct bilirubin level
B. Indirect bilirubin level
C. Total bilirubin level
D. Hemoglobin

7. A 5-day-old full term neonate is found to be jaundiced and have a dangerously elevated total bilirubin level. During an exchange transfusion to treat severe hyperbilirubinemia, for which of the following would the critical care nurse be observant as potential complications?
I. Chvostek's sign
II. Cardiac dysrhythmia
III. Hypoglycemia
IV. Bronze baby syndrome
A. I, II, IV
B. II, III, IV
C. I, III, IV
D. I, II, III

8. Which of the following antibodies can cross the placenta?
A. IgG
B. IgA
C. IgE
D. IgM

(CON'T)

9. T lymphocytes are responsible for:
A. Suppressing the immune response
B. Producing antibodies
C. Manufacturing gamma globulin
D. Anamnestic response

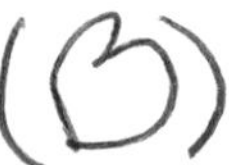

Case Study

Over the last 4 hours of caring for a septic patient, the nurse notes the oozing of blood from the intravenous sites and the development of petechiae over the trunk. Blood is drawn for testing. Some of the results are as follows:
Platelet count: 121,000/mm^3
Erythrocyte count: 3.8 million/mm^3
Hematocrit: 36%
Partial thromboplastin time: 41 seconds
Prothrombin time: 18 seconds
Fibrinogen level: 140 mg/dL

Questions 10 and 11 refer to this case study.

---

10. Based on these results and the patient's history, the nurse recognizes the patient is most at risk for:
A. Idiopathic thrombocytopenia purpura
B. Disseminated intravascular coagulation
C. Aplastic anemia
D. Nonimmune hemolytic anemia

11. The nurse would expect this patient's treatment plan to potentially include all of the following therapies *except*?
A. Administration of platelets
B. Infusion of fresh frozen plasma
C. Intravenous antibiotics
D. Prothrombin complex concentrates

12. The following results are reported from the laboratory on a critically ill patient:
Red blood cell count: 5.0 million/mm^3
White blood cell count: 20,000/mm^3
Hemoglobin: 13 g/dL
Hematocrit: 40%
Platelets: 135,000/mm^3
Which of the following results is abnormal in this neonate?
A. Red blood cell count
B. White blood cell count
C. Hemoglobin
D. Platelet count

13. Idiopathic thrombocytopenia purpura (ITP) is most often found in infants of mothers with:
A. Systemic lupus erythematosus
B. Diabetes mellitus
C. Toxemia of pregnancy
D. Disseminated intravascular coagulation

14. Which of the following laboratory values places a patient at the most risk for bleeding?
A. Decreased albumin
B. Decreased magnesium
C. Increased calcium
D. Decreased potassium

15. Which of the following is true of idiopathic thrombocytopenia purpura?
A. Bleeding is increased as a result of absence of clotting factor VIII
B. Consumptive clotting results in excessive bleeding
C. Bleeding occurs because platelets are not produced
D. Bleeding occurs because platelets are rapidly destroyed

16. Which of the following statements about transfusions of packed red blood cells (RBCs) and whole blood is correct?
A. Whole blood offers less of a risk of HIV transmission
B. Whole blood raises the hematocrit more efficiently
C. Packed RBCs offer less of a risk of hepatitis transmission
D. Packed RBCs increase the risk of congestive heart failure

17. When treating a critically ill patient with a bleeding disorder, which of the following does the nurse need to be aware is *not* contained in fresh frozen plasma?
A. Factor VIII
B. Platelets
C. Fibrinogen
D. Thrombin

18. Which of the following does *not* need to be typed and cross matched before administration?
A. Platelets
B. Fresh frozen plasma
C. Albumin
D. Packed red cells

19. All of the following are potential complications related to administration of stored blood *except*:
A. Hypocalcemia
B. Hypokalemia
C. Bleeding
D. Acidosis

20. Patients with asplenia syndrome are at an increased risk for:
A. Hemorrhage
B. Infection
C. Hemolysis
D. Thrombocytopenia

21. Red blood cells that have no antigenic material on the outer membrane belong to which blood group?
A. A
B. B
C. AB
D. O

22. A 2.2 kg infant whose blood type is A+ is undergoing a cardiac catheterization. Blood loss sufficient to require transfusion during the procedure is anticipated. Which of the following blood group types can be used as donor blood?
A. O+
B. AB-
C. B+
D. B-

23. Phagocytosis is an important immune function. Which of the following cells are *not* phagocytes?
A. Neutrophils
B. Monocytes
C. Lymphocytes
D. Macrophages

24. The passage of IgG antibodies across the placenta or through breast milk to a fetus or neonate is an example of what type of immunity?
A. Active acquired
B. Passive acquired
C. Natural
D. Innate

25. A patient with a congenitally absent or deficient thymus gland would be expected to exhibit which of the following?
A. Bleeding disorders
B. Aplastic anemia
C. Immunodeficiency
D. Hemolytic reactions

26. Which of the following organ systems is most critical to ensure adequate amounts of clotting factors?
A. Liver
B. Kidneys
C. Bone marrow
D. Spleen

27. A patient with an absent spleen has a decreased ability to form which of the following?
A. Clotting factors
B. Antibodies
C. Neutrophils
D. Reticulocytes

28. In which site are up to one-third of all available platelets stored?
A. Liver
B. Spleen
C. Lungs
D. Bone marrow

29. Which of the following cells are *least* capable of phagocytic activity?
A. Monocytes
B. Macrophages
C. Eosinophils
D. Basophils

30. In a patient with severe neutropenia, which of the following would be signs and symptoms of wound infections?
A. An increase in white blood cell count, fever
B. Irritability, hypothermia, anorexia
C. Fever, purulent drainage
D. Erythema, tenderness, exudate

PEDIATRIC-SPECIFIC QUESTIONS

31. Many factors promote sickling in sickle cell anemia. Which of the following factors *does not* promote sickling?
A. Hypoxemia
B. Dehydration
C. Alkalosis
D. Hypothermia

32. Which of the following is an example of cellular-mediated immune response?
A. Rejection of transplanted organ
B. ABO blood group incompatibilities
C. Rh blood group incompatibilities
D. IgM attack on bacteria in the blood

33. A 16-year-old boy develops a decrease in urine output 5 days following renal transplantation. Which of the following signs and symptoms would help confirm a diagnosis of renal transplant rejection rather than a diagnosis of acute tubular necrosis?
A. Weight gain, rise in blood urea nitrogen, abdominal tenderness
B. Weight gain, rise in serum creatinine and blood urea nitrogen
C. Elevated serum potassium, flank pain, generalized edema
D. Anorexia, nausea, decreased white blood cell function

34. The critical care nurse would question an order for which of the following immunosuppressive drugs in the first day following renal transplantation?
A. Cyclosporin
B. Azathioprine
C. Prednisone
D. Cyclophosphamide

35. Which of the following clotting factors is responsible for the most common form of hemophilia?
A. Factor IX
B. Fibrinogen
C. Factor VIII
D. Factor VII

Case Study

A 9-year-old boy with hemophilia A has been admitted following a bicycle accident. He was wearing a helmet, but assessment shows grossly ecchymotic areas over his legs, knees, elbows, and palms of his hands. His knees are swollen and range of motion is decreased. Questions 36 to 38 refer to this case study.

---

36. To control the bleeding, which of the following should the critical care nurse plan to do?
A. Administer a bolus dose of factor IX concentrate
B. Administer a continuous infusion of factor VIII
C. Administer platelets
D. Administer fresh frozen plasma

37. To measure the effectiveness of replacement therapy, which of the following laboratory values would the critical care nurse monitor in this patient?
A. Prothrombin time
B. Partial thromboplastin time
C. Fibrin split product levels
D. Fibrinogen levels

38. This patient has significant swelling and pain in his knees. The critical care nurse would anticipate all of the following steps to address his alteration in comfort *except*?
A. Immediate administration of factor replacements
B. Ibuprofen
C. Elastic wraps to his knees
D. Indomethacin

39. For the critically ill child with hemophilia, which of the following provides the best vascular access for administration of large amounts of fluids and blood or blood products as well as hemodynamic monitoring?
A. Internal jugular vein
B. Femoral vein
C. Subclavian vein
D. External jugular vein

40. In severe, acute hemorrhage associated with hemophilia, administration of which of the following would be of the highest priority?
A. Whole blood
B. Concentrated clotting factors
C. Fresh frozen plasma
D. Packed red blood cells

Case Study

A 7-year-old girl is admitted to the intensive care unit from the emergency room. Her parents brought her to the hospital because her epistaxis wouldn't stop at home. They deny any trauma, and say the bleeding began while she was blowing her nose. Further physical examination shows an unusual amount of bruising over her hips, legs, and arms. She admitted to bleeding gums the last 2 days while she brushed her teeth. Her parents deny any chronic illness and report only that she recovered from chicken pox approximately 10 days ago. Several bleeding and clotting studies are ordered. Some of the results are as follows:

Tourniquet test: positive: 3+
PT, PTT: normal
Fibrinogen level: normal
Platelet count: 19,500 mm^3/dL

Questions 41 to 43 refer to this case study.

---

41. Based on her history, examination, and lab results, which of the following diagnoses does the critical care nurse suspect?
A. Disseminated intravascular coagulation
B. Henoch-Schonlein purpura
C. Sickle cell disease
D. Idiopathic thrombocytopenia purpura

42. Which of the following therapies would the critical care nurse anticipate administering?
   A. Clotting factor concentrate
   B. Fresh frozen plasma
   C. Corticosteroids
   D. Salicylates

43. Which of the following additional assessment findings would the critical care nurse find most significant?
   A. Headache
   B. Hematuria
   C. Melena
   D. Petechiae

44. A 10-month-old infant has been admitted to the pediatric intensive care unit following a liver transplantation. Which of the complications listed below, all of which are associated with liver transplantation, is *least* likely to indicate rejection?
   A. Hypertension
   B. Elevated liver enzymes
   C. Decreased bile production
   D. Fever

45. A 15-year-old boy is admitted to the PICU following a motor vehicle accident in which he was a passenger. His injuries include chest and abdominal trauma. He has been intubated, and is mechanically ventilated. To maintain adequate arterial blood gases, he requires high peak inspiratory pressures as well as a positive end expiratory pressure of 12. Five days after admission some of his laboratory values are as follows:
   Na+: 135 mEq/L
   K+: 3.1 mEq/L
   Cl-: 99 mEq/L
   Hct: 30%
   Hgb: 10.8 g/dL
   PT: 21.1 sec
   Activated PTT: 43 sec
   Fibrin split products: 112 mcg/mL
   Based on this information, when assessing the patient, with which of the following findings would the critical care nurse be most concerned?
   A. Tented T waves on the ECG
   B. Chvostek's sign
   C. Slowed capillary refill
   D. Increased abdominal girth

46. The anemia of sickle cell disease results primarily from:
A. Decreased production of red blood cells
B. Increased production of reticulocytes
C. Hemolysis of erythrocytes
D. Bone marrow suppression

Case Study

A 6-year-old child has been admitted to the PICU with a sickle cell crisis. The history includes six prior PICU admissions for sickle cell disease. Initial assessment reveals a nonpalpable spleen, hepatomegaly, fever, abdominal pain, and mild hematuria.

Questions 47 to 49 refer to this case study.

---

47. For which of the following is this patient at the greatest risk?
A. Infection
B. Respiratory distress syndrome
C. Disseminated intravascular coagulation
D. Consumptive coagulopathy

48. Eight hours after admission, this child develops left-sided weakness and a dilated, sluggishly reactive right pupil. The critical care nurse should first prepare the child for:
A. Blood transfusion
B. CAT scan to diagnose the neurological deficit
C. Administration of streptokinase or TPA
D. Administration of heparin

49. Which of the following nursing diagnoses is most appropriate for this patient?
A. Impaired gas exchange
B. High risk for infection
C. Altered peripheral tissue perfusion
D. Ineffective breathing pattern

50. Which of the following is contraindicated in all posttransplant liver patients?
A. Saline instillation before suctioning
B. Heparinized flush solutions
C. Irrigation of the nasogastric tube
D. Rectal temperatures

51. Which of the following laboratory results would alert the nurse to the possible diagnosis of acquired human immunodeficiency syndrome?
A. Decreased WBC
B. Decreased T_4 levels
C. Decreased IgG levels
D. Decreased T_5 levels

52. When administering blood to a 12-year-old patient with internal hemorrhaging, the critical care nurse notes the patient has a temperature of 101.1°F (38.4°C), nausea, vomiting, headache, and shaking chills. Which of the following actions would the critical care nurse do first?

A. Administer antihistamines to counteract the allergic reaction and observe for dyspnea
B. Insert a Foley catheter to obtain a urine sample for hematuria and measure output
C. Slow the transfusion to keep an open rate and notify the physician
D. Stop the transfusion immediately, keep the IV patent, and notify the physician

NEONATAL-SPECIFIC QUESTIONS

53. All of the following conditions can cause hemolytic anemias in the newborn *except*:

A. Rh incompatibility
B. ABO incompatibility
C. Diamond-Blakfan anemia
D. Bacterial sepsis

54. Which of the following tests is *most* helpful in determining Rh hemolytic disease in the newborn?

A. Total bilirubin level
B. Indirect Coomb's test
C. Hemoglobin
D. Indirect bilirubin level

55. All of the following are possible complications of Rh incompatibility in the newborn *except*:

A. Hydrops fetalis
B. Brain damage
C. Hepatic failure
D. Shock

56. Which of the following is an indication for an exchange transfusion to treat Rh incompatibility in the full term newborn?

A. Indirect bilirubin level greater than 20 mg/dL
B. Cord hemoglobin of 14 g/dL
C. Total bilirubin level greater than 20 mg/dL
D. Positive direct Coomb's test

57. Which of the following nursing interventions will produce a more reliable peripheral measurement of the hematocrit?

A. Placing a blood pressure cuff around the upper arm, inflating to the systolic pressure and waiting 1 minute
B. Placing the extremity in a dependent position to encourage venous engorgement
C. Wrapping the extremity in a warm pack to increase circulation to the area
D. Manually milking the extremity to encourage arterial flow and venous congestion

58. A neonate has an indirect bilirubin level of 21 mg/dL at 26 hours of age, an increased reticulocyte count, and microspherocytes and spherocytes seen in the infant's peripheral blood smear. The infant is diagnosed with ABO hemolytic disease. Which of the following interventions should receive the highest priority?

A. Transfuse the infant at 15 mg/kg of whole blood
B. Administer ferrous sulfate 6 mg/kg/day
C. Infuse 2 mL/kg of packed red cells
D. Prepare for an exchange transfusion

59. Which of the following blood types would be used for transfusion in a neonate with ABO hemolytic disease?

A. A blood group type
B. B blood group type
C. AB blood group type
D. O blood group type

60. When parents are used as directed donors for their neonates, which of the following statements is most advisable to avoid serious adverse effects?

A. All parentally donated blood should be irradiated
B. Fathers may donate platelets but not red cells
C. Mothers can safely donate plasma but not red cells
D. Fathers may donate red cells only

61. An infant undergoing phototherapy for hyperbilirubinemia is at most risk for:

A. Hyperkalemia
B. Dehydration
C. Hypoalbuminemia
D. Hypervolemia

62. The critical care nurse would observe a neonate undergoing phototherapy for all of the following adverse reactions related to this treatment *except*:

A. Hyperthermia
B. Hypothermia
C. Thrombocytopenia
D. Leukocytosis

63. A 3-day-old infant is demonstrating signs and symptoms of hyperbilirubinemia. Which of the following symptoms would *not* indicate the development of kernicterus?
A. Poor sucking
B. High-pitched cry
C. Hypertonia (hypo)
D. Presence of a Moro reflex

64. Which of the following replacement therapies is the *most* appropriate for a neonate undergoing exchange transfusion for Rh hemolytic disease?
A. Freshly donated red blood cells
B. Banked red blood cells
C. Albumin
D. 10% dextrose solution

65. Orders for phototherapy have just been written on a neonate with hyperbilirubinemia. The critical care nurse should prepare the infant by:
A. Removing all clothing except the diaper to protect the genital area
B. Removing all clothing including the diaper to maximally expose the skin
C. Removing all clothing except the diaper and a small shirt to prevent hypothermia
D. Removing all clothing except a stocking cap to prevent heat loss

66. All of the following are risk factors for disseminated intravascular coagulation in the neonate *except*:
A. Prematurity
B. Necrotizing enterocolitis
C. Meconium aspiration
D. Apnea

67. When observing the infant with hyperbilirubinemia, the critical care nurse would be most concerned with which of the following findings?
A. Dermal icterus
B. Irritable cry
C. Increased urine output
D. Loose stools

68. In a neonate who manifests jaundice within the first 24 hours after birth, which of the following is most likely responsible for the hyperbilirubinemia?
A. Sepsis
B. Isoimmunization
C. Physiologic jaundice
D. Breast milk jaundice

Answers

1. **Correct answer—D.**
These results indicate a platelet deficiency rather than consumptive process. With platelet deficiencies, the infants usually appear well. Consumptive processes such as disseminated intravascular coagulation are associated with infants who are symptomatically ill. The information along with a maternal history of SLE is consistent with idiopathic thrombocytopenia purpura (ITP). In ITP, antiplatelet antibodies from the mother pass across the placenta to the fetus and destroy fetal or neonatal platelets. Because platelet dysfunction is the mechanism involved in bleeding, the bleeding time, tourniquet test, and clot retraction test are expected to be abnormal. The whole blood clotting time, partial thromboplastin time, prothrombin time, and prothrombin consumption test are expected to be normal as these measure clotting factor abnormalities, not platelet deficiency.

2. **Correct answer—B.**
Idiopathic thrombocytopenia purpura is an immune-mediated platelet disorder. Maternal antibodies against platelets (IgG) cross the placenta and attack the fetal or neonatal platelets resulting in very low counts, even below 10,000/mm^3. This is a passively acquired immune disorder and usually lasts only days to weeks before the maternal circulating antibodies are cleared. In the absence of life-threatening bleeding such as an intracranial hemorrhage, these infants are treated with immune gamma globulin or prednisone therapy. Platelet transfusions are of limited value because the maternal antibodies destroy transfused platelets rapidly. Although heparin therapy may be indicated for bleeding associated with disseminated intravascular coagulation, its use would worsen ITP. An exchange transfusion is also usually limited to infants displaying significant bleeding.

3. **Correct answer—C.**
Disseminated intravascular coagulation is not a primary disease, but rather a complication or secondary condition. The priority in treating DIC is always directed at removing or correcting the precipitating factor in its development. For an infant with meconium aspiration, aggressive therapy to correct hypoxemia and acidosis would be the greatest priority in treating DIC. Other treatments such as heparin therapy to reverse diffuse systemic clotting, transfusion of clotting factors to correct depleted levels, transfusion of platelets to correct depleted levels, and partial exchange transfusions may be employed, but are secondary to treating the cause.

4. **Correct answer—A.**
Hyperbilirubinemia occurs with an increase in red blood cell destruction, a decrease in bilirubin elimination, or a decrease in binding of unconjugated

bilirubin with serum albumin. Many medications such as diazepam, gentamicin, furosemide, and digoxin are drugs that bind with albumin, therefore decreasing albumin binding sites available to bilirubin. These medications would increase the risk of hyperbilirubinemia.

5. **Correct answer—D.**
   The neonate has a higher concentration of red blood cells that have a decreased life span, creating more unconjugated bilirubin from the breakdown of hemoglobin. The liver of the neonate is also less able to conjugate bilirubin as a result of reduced production of glucuronyl transferase, a key factor in the conjugation of bilirubin. There is normally no decrease in the ability of the intestinal tract to eliminate bilirubin.

6. **Correct answer—B.**
   Kernicterus is a serious complication of hyperbilirubinemia resulting in potential and permanent brain damage. Bilirubin encephalopathy, or kernicterus, occurs when high serum levels of unconjugated bilirubin are able to cross into the brain, particularly the basal ganglia, cerebellum, and hippocampus. Unconjugated bilirubin is toxic to the cells of the central nervous system. Once damage occurs, it is irreversible. While the total bilirubin level is important, the best indicator for potential risk of kernicterus is the indirect or unconjugated bilirubin level. The unconjugated bilirubin is what poses the threat to central nervous system cells. High hemoglobin levels may lead to high unconjugated bilirubin levels through the breakdown of hemoglobin during the neonatal period, but they are not a reliable predictor of how high the indirect bilirubin levels may rise.

7. **Correct answer—D.**
   Potential complications of exchange transfusions include hypocalcemia (Chvostek's and Trousseau's signs), cardiac dysrhythmias, hypoglycemia, hypervolemia, hyperkalemia, acidosis, alkalosis, necrotizing enterocolitis, bleeding, thrombocytopenia, and thromboemboli. Bronze baby syndrome is seen as a potential complication of phototherapy to treat hyperbilirubinemia.

8. **Correct answer—A.**
   IgG is the only antibody that can cross the placenta. IgG if found mainly in the serum and interstitial fluid and is responsible for immunity against bacteria, viruses, bacterial toxins, and protozoa. IgA is found predominantly in the intestinal and respiratory tracts as well as breast milk. IgA is important in protecting mucous membranes from viral and bacterial pathogens. IgE is found in the serum and bodily secretions and is important in allergic responses. IgM is found in serum and is critical in fighting bacteria found in the blood.

9. **Correct answer—A.**
   T lymphocytes are responsible for immune functions such as suppressing and augmenting the immune response, cellular immunity, release of lymphokines,

"memory" to foreign antigens, and recognition of the body's own tissue. The B lymphocytes are responsible for immune functions such as producing antibodies (immunoglobulins), blood group types, and an anamnestic response (higher levels of antibodies after the first exposure to an antigen).

10. Correct answer—B.

Based on these results and the patient's history, the nurse recognizes the patient is most at risk for disseminated intravascular coagulation (DIC). DIC is never a primary disorder, but rather occurs as a complication of other major pathologies such as sepsis, hypoxia, acidosis, obstetrical emergencies, shock, head injuries, burns, rejection of transplanted organs, snake or other venomous bites, and drowning. Idiopathic thrombocytopenia purpura (ITP) is a platelet problem that also manifests as a bleeding disorder. ITP, however, is an immune-mediated thrombocytopenia and is usually seen in patients who are not initially acutely ill and are not secondary to illnesses such as sepsis. Aplastic anemia results from bone marrow depression and does not primarily manifest as a bleeding disorder. Nonimmune hemolytic anemias such as ABO and Rh incompatibilities would not have prolonged PT and PTT nor would platelet and fibrinogen levels be decreased.

11. Correct answer—D.

DIC is treated first by treating the cause or primary triggering condition. Antibiotics would be most important in treating this patient's sepsis. Administration of platelets and fresh frozen plasma would be important to replace platelets and clotting factors consumed during diffuse clotting. Exchange transfusions may also be used in infants to treat DIC. Prothrombin complex concentrates would not be used because these would promote further clotting.

12. Correct answer—C.

Normal laboratory values for the neonate include:
Red blood cell count: 4.0 to 6.8 million/mm^3
White blood cell count: 6000 to 30,000/mm^3
Hemoglobin: 14 to 23 g/dl
Hematocrit: 44 to 65%
Platelets: 130,000 to 350,000/mm^3
Neonates may generally have higher laboratory values related to erythrocytes as a result of the increased values during fetal life when increased oxygen carrying capacity was critical.

13. Correct answer—A.

Autoimmune diseases such as SLE in the mother form antiplatelet antibodies that can pass across the placenta and attack the fetus's platelets resulting in a thrombocytopenia. Of these conditions, only maternal SLE produces antiplatelet antibodies. This process may last up to several weeks until maternal circulating antiplatelet antibodies are eliminated from the neonatal circulation.

14. Correct answer—A.

Calcium is an important component in the clotting mechanism, but serum levels of calcium are dependent upon adequate albumin levels. If albumin levels are inadequate, calcium cannot function properly in its clotting role. Hypocalcemia would also be present with hypermagnesemia or hyperphosphatemia. Potassium has no direct effect on the intrinsic, extrinsic, or common clotting pathways.

15. Correct answer—D.

The pathologic process of idiopathic thrombocytopenia purpura involves bleeding from rapid platelet destruction and depletion. Clotting is inhibited by the absence of platelets. Clotting factor VIII causes bleeding in hemophilia. Inadequate production or manufacturing of platelets occurs in bone marrow suppression.

16. Correct answer—C.

Because packed RBCs are washed and theoretically do not contain serum or white blood cells, less of a risk of HIV and hepatitis transmission exists. Packed RBCs raise the hematocrit and hemoglobin more efficiently because more RBCs are contained per unit of packed cells than whole blood. Packed RBCs actually decrease the risk of congestive heart failure because fewer units need to be transfused to raise the hematocrit and hemoglobin.

17. Correct answer—B.

Fresh frozen plasma contains all the clotting factors necessary except platelets.

18. Correct answer—C.

Albumin does not need to be typed and cross matched before administration. Platelets, fresh frozen plasma, cryoprecipitates, whole blood, and packed red blood cells all must be typed and crossed before transfused.

19. Correct answer—B.

Potential complications related to administration of stored blood include hypocalcemia and metabolic acidosis from the sodium citrate used to preserve blood, hyperkalemia from cellular breakdown over storage time, and bleeding from deterioration of clotting factors and platelets.

20. Correct answer—B.

The spleen is an important organ involving humoral immunity and B lymphocyte functioning. The spleen removes old red blood cells and platelets, bacteria, and produces immunoglobulins. Therefore, a patient with an absent or underdeveloped spleen is at risk for infection.

21. Correct answer—D.

Red blood cells that have no antigenic material on the outer membrane belong to the O blood group. Other blood cells have A, B or A and B surface antigenic material that determine the blood type.

22. Correct answer—A.

The A blood group contains A antigens on the surface of its red blood cells and naturally occurring anti-B antibodies. Blood group O has no surface antigens on its red blood cells, but has naturally occurring anti-A and anti-B antibodies. Blood group B contains B antigens on the surface of its red blood cells and naturally occurring anti-A antibodies. Blood group AB has both A and B surface antigens and no anti-A or anti-B antibodies. Rh- blood groups have no Rh antigen, but form Rh antibodies when exposed to Rh+ blood. Rh+ blood groups do have an Rh antigen, but no antibodies to Rh. Therefore an A+ individual can receive blood from another A+ individual, an A- individual, an O+ individual, and an O- individual. (See Table 4-5.)

23. Correct answer—C.

Phagocytosis is performed by the granulocytes which include neutrophils, eosinophils, basophils, monocytes, and macrophages. Lymphocytes are the white blood cells involved in cellular and humoral immunity and include B lymphocytes and T lymphocytes.

24. Correct answer—B.

The passage of IgG antibodies across the placenta or through breast milk to a fetus or neonate is an example of passively acquired immunity. In passive immunity, the antibodies found are not formed by the fetus or neonate, but rather come from the mother. Therefore, this type of immunity is temporary. Injections of gamma globulin would be another example of passive immunity. Actively acquired immunity occurs when individuals actually manufacture their own antibodies in response to an illness or from immunization with live or attenuated vaccines. The antibodies present in actively acquired immunity are not temporary. The body is capable of making these antibodies. Natural immunity is species specific and is demonstrated by the fact that humans do not develop such animal diseases as canine distemper or heartworm. Innate immunity refers to immunity at birth which is related to natural immunity, heredity, sex, and race.

25. Correct answer—C.

The thymus gland is critical in the development of cell-mediated immunity. Bleeding disorders would be found in some liver diseases, congenital deficiencies of clotting factors, and thrombocytopenia. Aplastic anemia would be found in bone marrow suppression. Hemolytic reactions are commonly found in ABO and Rh blood group incompatibilities as well as other diseases. Because the thymus plays a crucial role in cell-mediated immunity, an individual with a congenitally absent or deficient thymus would exhibit signs and symptoms of immunodeficiency.

26. Correct answer—A.

The liver is responsible for manufacturing most clotting factors, including fibrinogen which are produced in the liver. Factor VIII is not produced in the liver. The kidneys play an important role in the stimulation of red blood cell production by manufacturing erythropoietin, but do not produce clotting factors. The bone marrow is the source of platelets, which are important components of clot formation, but platelets themselves are not classified as clotting factors. The spleen is important in the removal of old abnormal red blood cells from the circulation.

27. Correct answer—B.
A patient with an absent spleen has a decreased ability to form antibodies. The spleen is responsible for B lymphocyte function and humoral immunity. Clotting factors are formed in the liver. Neutrophils are formed in the bone marrow and are highly phagocytic cells. Reticulocytes are also found in the bone marrow and are early red blood cells.

28. Correct answer—B.
Up to one-third of all available platelets are stored in the spleen. While the liver makes clotting factors that are essential to hemostasis, it does not manufacture or store platelets. The bone marrow is the site of platelet production, but once mature, they are not stored there.

29. Correct answer—D.
Phagocytosis, or the engulfment and killing of bacteria, can be accomplished by monocytes, macrophages, eosinophils, and polymorphonuclear neutrophils. Basophils are important in preventing clot formation and allergic reactions.

30. Correct answer—B.
A patient with severe neutropenia is unable to mount a normal response to an infection. Signs and symptoms such as an inflammatory reaction, increased white blood cell count, or purulent drainage are largely absent. Nonspecific indicators of infection must be relied upon in the neutropenic patient such as fever, hypothermia, irritability, and anorexia.

PEDIATRIC-SPECIFIC ANSWERS

31. Correct answer—C.
Factors that promote sickling in sickle cell anemia include hypoxemia, dehydration, acidosis, hypothermia, and hyponatremia.

32. Correct answer—A.
Rejection of a transplanted organ is an example of cellular-mediated immune response. Graft-versus-host disease and autoimmune diseases are other examples of T lymphocyte-mediated reactions. ABO and Rh blood group incompatibilities and immune responses involving immunoglobulins (IgA, IgG, IgM, IgD, IgE) are examples of B lymphocyte-mediated reactions.

33. Correct answer—A.
Signs and symptoms of renal transplant rejection include those of renal failure and acute tubular necrosis because rejection leads to decreased renal function.

Signs of decreased renal function include anorexia, nausea, electrolyte imbalances, increased serum creatinine and blood urea nitrogen levels, decreased creatinine clearance, poor white cell and platelet function, oliguria, edema, weight gain, hypertension, and anemia. In transplant rejection, these and additional signs and symptoms specific to rejection are apparent as well. Because the kidney is transplanted into the lower abdominal region, abdominal tenderness over the graft site may be present. Fever may be another hallmark sign of rejection. Patients on cyclosporin, however, may be less likely to exhibit abdominal tenderness and fever.

34. Correct answer—A.
Because cyclosporin is nephrotoxic, it is usually not used in the immediate postoperative period until the danger of impaired renal function related to acute tubular necrosis has passed. Cyclosporin is usually begun only after the blood urea nitrogen and serum creatinine levels are at or near normal. Azathioprine, prednisone, and cyclophosphamide are all immunosuppressive drugs that may be used without danger or nephrotoxicity in the early posttransplant period.

35. Correct answer—C.
Hemophilia A accounts for about three-quarters of all cases of hemophilia. In this classic hemophilia, factor VIII is present, but does not function normally in promoting clot formation. Factor VIII is part of the intrinsic pathway activated by vessel injury. Factor IX is also part of the intrinsic pathway and causes hemophilia B or the Christmas disease, which accounts for far fewer forms of hemophilia. Factor VII is part of the extrinsic pathway. Neither of these clotting factors is responsible for the major forms of hemophilia. A deficiency of fibrinogen will result in clotting abnormalities, but is not part of the pathophysiology of hemophilia.

36. Correct answer—B.
To control significant bleeding in a patient with hemophilia A, either continuous infusion or multiple bolus dosing of factor VIII is required. This may be in the form of factor VIII concentrate or cryoprecipitate, which includes factors VIII and XIII and fibrinogen. Factor IX is not deficient in hemophilia A. Although platelets might become deficient with significant bleeding and restoration of clotting function, alone they will not correct the coagulopathy associated with hemophilia A. Fresh frozen plasma does contain factor VIII, but would require more quantity than factor concentrates to correct bleeding. (See Table 4-2.)

37. Correct answer—B.
The partial thromboplastin time (PTT) is used to monitor the effectiveness of factor replacement therapy. A PTT should be assessed immediately following infusion and throughout the critical period to ensure therapy is effective and not transitory. The prothrombin time measures the extrinsic system and factors V, VII, and X as well as oral anticoagulation therapy. The partial thromboplastin time is used to monitor the intrinsic pathway and all factors except factors VII and XIII and is also used to monitor heparin therapy. Fibrin split products are formed when clots are broken down and are particularly useful in diagnosing

disorders that involve increased clot formation such as disseminated intravascular coagulation (DIC). Fibrinogen levels (factor I) are useful in diagnosing DIC, inflammatory diseases, and congenital afibrinogenemia.

38. Correct answer—D.

Nonsteroidal antiinflammatory drugs such as indomethacin, aspirin, and phenylbutazone should not be used in patients with hemophilia because they interfere with platelet function and can exacerbate bleeding problems. Ibuprofen and acetaminophen, however, can be used safely. Elastic wraps to the knees along with ice packs can reduce swelling, bleeding, and pain. Factor replacement therapy should be initiated immediately to control bleeding, which will also reduce the pain and discomfort associated with hemarthrosis.

39. Correct answer—D.

For the critically ill child with hemophilia or any significant bleeding disorder, the best vascular access for administration of large amounts of fluids and blood or blood products as well as hemodynamic monitoring is a superficial vein such as the external jugular. The femoral, internal jugular, and subclavian veins are all deep and would not allow adequate observation of potential bleeding and hematoma formation.

40. Correct answer—B.

In severe, acute hemorrhage associated with hemophilia, administration of concentrated clotting factors would be the highest priority followed by blood and volume replacement. Without transfusion of clotting factors, bleeding would continue even in the presence of transfusions of whole blood or red blood cells and, therefore, would be of limited value. Fresh frozen plasma contains clotting factors and platelets, but a much larger volume is needed to deliver the required amount of clotting factor VIII to stop bleeding.

41. Correct answer—D.

Based on her history, examination, and lab results, idiopathic thrombocytopenia purpura (ITP) is the most likely diagnosis. ITP results in hemorrhage from antibody-directed destruction of thrombocytes. The mechanism is unknown, but believed to be immune related and often is seen following chicken pox, measles, upper respiratory tract infections, and other viral illnesses. Because platelet function is the primary pathology and there is no deficiency of clotting factors, tests that measure clotting factors such as the PT and PTT are usually normal. Disseminated intravascular coagulation is not a primary disease, but rather is seen in association with other major illness and both the PT and PTT would be prolonged in DIC. Henoch-Schonlein purpura is not associated with thrombocytopenia. Sickle cell disease is not usually associated with bleeding.

42. Correct answer—C.

Steroids and gamma globulin have been used to treat ITP because they have been shown to decrease the removal of sensitized platelets from the circulation and to increase production. Splenectomies have also been performed when severe, uncontrollable bleeding occurs because of the spleen's role in destroying sensitized platelets. Clotting factor concentrates and fresh frozen plasma would be indicated in hemophilia and other clotting factor disorders. Salicylates would be contraindicated because of aspirin's role in decreasing platelet adhesion.

43. Correct answer—A.
Although hematuria, melena, and petechiae all are clear indications of bleeding, a headache would receive the greatest priority of assessment and evaluation because it could signal an intracranial hemorrhage. Additional signs and symptoms of an intracranial hemorrhage would include alterations in level of consciousness, decreased sensory or motor functions, change in pupils, seizures, and irritability.

44. Correct answer—A.
Complications following liver transplantation are largely related to rejection, hepatic failure, and immunosuppressive therapy. Elevated enzymes and decreased bile production are related to decreased hepatic function either from a compromised graft or rejection. Fever more commonly is associated with rejection than hepatic failure. Hypertension is not an indication of hepatic failure or rejection, but rather is a side effect of cyclosporin therapy or hypervolemia.

45. Correct answer—D.
This patient's laboratory data show indications of disseminated intravascular coagulation because clotting times are prolonged and fibrin split products are elevated. Tall, tented T waves are associated with hyperkalemia, and this patient's potassium is low normal. Chvostek's sign is associated with hypocalcemia, and there is no evidence to suggest this. Slowed capillary refill may be related to decreased circulating volume or vasoconstriction. Increasing abdominal girth, especially with a history of abdominal injury, could indicate internal bleeding and would prompt the nurse to further collaborate with the physician or advanced practice nurse to assess and identify the cause. (See Table 4-3.)

46. Correct answer—A.
The anemia of sickle cell disease results from hemolysis related to the body's destruction of the sickled cells. Bone marrow suppression or decrease in the production of red blood cells in sickle cell disease occurs only with an aplastic crisis. The increase in reticulocytes (immature red cells) is a natural response to correct, not cause, the anemia from destruction of sickled cells.

47. Correct answer—A.
A child admitted to the PICU with a sickle cell crisis and a history that includes six prior PICU admissions for the same has serious, advanced disease. The initial assessment which revealed hepatomegaly, fever, abdominal pain, and mild hematuria would also be expected to reveal splenomegaly. The absence of this finding suggests that the spleen has fibrosed and is not functional. The loss of

splenic function makes this patient greatly at risk for infection. Although respiratory distress syndrome and disseminated intravascular coagulation (a consumptive coagulopathy) would be risks associated with severe critical illness, infection would present the more likely risk for this patient.

48. Correct answer—A.

A child with sickle cell disease and signs and symptoms of neurological deficit should receive immediate transfusion of blood to decrease the concentration of sickled cells. Streptokinase, TPA, and heparin are of no value because mechanical clumping of sickled cells is the pathology, not clotting. CAT scan, MRI testing, and angiography are indicated only after the child has been stabilized. Neurological signs in the presence of sickle cell disease are assumed to be a cerebrovascular accident and treated with transfusion immediately. Following immediate transfusion, a partial exchange transfusion to reduce the sickled hemoglobin levels to less than 30% is indicated.

49. Correct answer—C.

The most appropriate nursing diagnosis for this patient is altered peripheral tissue perfusion. As the sickled cells coagulate in small capillaries found in the peripheral tissues, they can occlude blood flow and cause ischemia and infarction.

50. Correct answer—B.

Heparinized flush solutions are contraindicated in the posttransplant liver patient because of the risk of coagulopathies. Pretransplant coagulopathies are usually present as a result of end-stage liver disease. In the immediate posttransplant period, coagulopathies continue until good hepatic function is established. Saline instillation before suctioning should not be done routinely, but is not contraindicated because of liver transplantation. Irrigation of the nasogastric tube may be done safely if required. There is no absolute contraindication to rectal temperatures, though the risk of bleeding related to the mucous membranes in the rectum should make the critical care nurse cautious.

51. Correct answer—B.

One of the laboratory tests most suggestive of AIDS is the T-helper/T-suppressor ratio. Levels of T-helper cells (T_4) are decreased and impair the body's ability to turn on and fight infection. These cells appear to be directly attacked by the HIV virus. While the WBCs may be decreased, this may occur in many conditions and is not specific enough to suggest AIDS. Decreased IgG levels are associated with B cell immunity problems and AIDS is a T cell immunity disease. Suppressor T cells, or T_5 cells, may actually be increased in AIDS and are responsible in part for the body's inability to turn on and fight infection.

52. Correct answer—D.

The first action the nurse would take would be to stop the transfusion immediately, keep the vein open with an infusion through the intravenous needle, and notify the physician or advanced practice nurse. Signs and symptoms of hemolytic transfusion reactions include fever, nausea, vomiting, headache, flank pain, hematuria, chest discomfort, shock, pain at the infusion site, and shaking chills. Antihistamines would be indicated for allergic reactions that include symptoms of itching, wheezing, laryngeal edema, and rash after the transfusion was stopped. A Foley catheter would be important in assessing renal function in a blood transfusion reaction, but would not be the first intervention. The transfusion must be stopped, not just slowed, to avoid more serious transfusion reaction symptoms.

NEONATAL-SPECIFIC ANSWERS

53. Correct answer—C.

Hemolytic anemias in the newborn can be caused by conditions such as Rh incompatibility, ABO incompatibility, bacterial sepsis, medications, congenital infections, disseminated intravascular coagulation, coarctation of the aorta, and renal artery stenosis. Diamond-Blakfan anemia is caused by a failure of bone marrow to produce red blood cells and is usually not apparent until the infant is 2 to 3 months old.

54. Correct answer—D.

Rh hemolytic disease in the newborn is best diagnosed through interpreting the results of the direct Coomb's test and indirect bilirubin levels. The hematocrit, hemoglobin, reticulocyte count, and nucleated red cell count are also helpful in diagnosing any hemolytic disease, but are not specific to Rh hemolytic anemia. The total bilirubin is less helpful than the indirect bilirubin level because it doesn't help interpret if the pathology stems from increased red cell destruction, liver disease, or biliary tract obstruction. The indirect Coomb's test is helpful in diagnosing ABO hemolytic anemia.

55. Correct answer—C.

Possible complications associated with Rh incompatibility in the newborn include hydrops fetalis, brain damage from hyperbilirubinemia, shock, still birth, and hepatosplenomegaly. Although jaundice is present, it results from increased RBC destruction and grossly elevated indirect bilirubin levels and does not involve hepatic failure.

56. Correct answer—A.

Exchange transfusions are used to treat Rh incompatibility if the cord hemoglobin is less than 12 g/dL; the indirect bilirubin level is greater 20 mg/dL; edema, hepatomegaly, splenomegaly, acidosis, or ascites are present; or the infant is in heart failure or shock. Total bilirubin levels are not as sensitive indicators and therefore are not used to base treatment therapy without the breakdown of direct and indirect values. Although the direct Coomb's test would be positive in Rh incompatibility, alone it does not tell the severity of the clinical symptoms and would be used only in diagnosis, not to determine therapy.

57. Correct answer—C.

Because peripheral measures of the hematocrit are often not very reliable as a result of stasis of blood, warming the extremity to increase circulation to the area improves the reliability of the hematocrit value obtained. Using a blood pressure cuff or dependent positioning is often helpful in identifying a vein for venipuncture, but would only contribute to venous stasis producing an even less reliable result.

58. Correct answer—D.

An ABO hemolytic reaction between the mother and infant will result in symptoms of hyperbilirubinemia, an increased reticulocyte count, a positive direct Coomb's test (weak), mild anemia, and microspherocytes and spherocytes seen in the infant's peripheral blood smear. Transfusion of whole blood or packed red blood cells is usually required an anemia from blood loss or Rh hemolytic disease, which results in more severe anemia. ABO incompatibilities usually results in milder anemias that are better treated by exchange transfusions that remove sensitized red blood cells thereby stopping the hemolytic process.

59. Correct answer—D.

Neonates with ABO hemolytic disease most often have mothers with O blood group type and are A, B, or AB blood group types themselves. Because maternal anti-A or anti-B antibodies are passed from the mother into the neonate's blood, O blood group type would be preferred for any transfusions the infant may need. By using O blood group type, the transfused blood would not be attacked by maternally passed anti-A and anti-B antibodies.

60. Correct answer—A.

There are many reasons why parents should not be directed donors for their own neonates or why precautions need to be taken. The risk of graft versus host disease is increased with blood donations from either parent. During the early period following the birth of an infant, maternal blood often carries antibodies against paternal red cells, platelets, leukocytes, and HLA antigens. Because these antigens may be present in the mother, they may have also been passed to the neonate making the use of paternal blood donations hazardous. Irradiation helps decrease the risk of adverse effects of parental donation by decreasing the antigenicity of the donated cells. Fathers should not be granulocyte, red cell, or platelet donors because of the possibility of maternal sensitization that can be passed to the fetus. Mothers should definitely not donate blood products containing plasma that would potentially carry antibodies. If parental donations are used, ideally mothers would donate washed, irradiated, red cells.

61. Correct answer—B.

An infant undergoing phototherapy for hyperbilirubinemia is at most risk for dehydration as a result of insensible water loss. Hyperkalemia is more likely to be seen with renal failure. Hypoalbuminemia worsens the clinical course of hyperbilirubinemia by providing less albumin binding sites for bilirubin.

62. Correct answer—D.
Adverse reactions resulting from phototherapy affect many body systems. (See Table 4-4.)

63. Correct answer—C.
Signs and symptoms of kernicterus include poor sucking, high-pitched cry, *hypo*tonia, a weak Moro reflex, vomiting, and seizures.

64. Correct answer—A.
Replacement therapies for a neonate undergoing exchange transfusion for Rh hemolytic disease would be freshly donated red blood cells. Banked red blood cells risk increasing the potassium from cellular deterioration. Adequate albumin levels are important in treating hyperbilirubinemia, but albumin alone is not a suitable exchange fluid because it does not replace red cells. A 10% dextrose solution also would not replace red blood cells.

65. Correct answer—B.
Phototherapy requires maximally exposed skin in order to have enough surface area to be effective. The genital area does not need to be protected from light, but a small covering such as a surgical mask may be used to control stool and urine. A diaper would not be left on because it covers too much skin surface area. Although prevention of hypothermia is important, clothing must be removed for phototherapy to be effective.

66. Correct answer—A.
Risk factors for disseminated intravascular coagulation in the neonate include necrotizing enterocolitis, meconium aspiration, apnea, respiratory distress syndrome, hypothermia, thrombosis, sepsis, asphyxia at birth, and pulmonary hemorrhage. The uncomplicated premature infant without other system problems is not at greater risk based solely on prematurity.

67. Correct answer—B.
The most severe consequence of hyperbilirubinemia is the development of kernicterus, or bilirubin encephalopathy. Dermal icterus would be expected in hyperbilirubinemia (yellow skin) and is not, by itself, a serious assessment finding. Increased urine output would not be related to hyperbilirubinemia, but a decreased output may be seen if the infant is undergoing phototherapy and has a fluid volume deficit related to increased insensible losses of water. Loose stools are another side effect of phototherapy. See box on p. 206 for signs and symptoms of kernicterus.

68. Correct answer—B.
A neonate who manifest jaundice within the first 24 hours after birth is most likely to have hemolytic disease of the newborn as a result of maternal-fetal blood incompatibilities. Isoimmunization, or Rh hemolytic disease of the newborn, and ABO incompatibility are two forms of maternal-fetal blood incompatibilities. Sepsis usually causes jaundice after 3 days, physiologic jaundice is not seen until after 24 hours, and breast mild jaundice is seen at 4 to 5 days.

CHAPTER 5

Neurology Care Problems

Passkeys

GENERAL PRINCIPLES OF NEUROLOGY
Neuroanatomy and Neurophysiology

- Remember "PAD" in order to remember the meninges of the brain. *P* is for pia mater, the innermost membrane. *A* is for arachnoid, the middle layer, and *D* is for dura mater, the outermost layer. They act as a covering or "pad" to protect the brain and spinal cord. See Fig. 5-1 for an illustration of the meninges of the brain.

- The pia mater is very vascular.

- The arachnoid layer is made up of spiderlike tissue. The space below the arachnoid layer and above the pia mater is the subarachnoid space. The subarachnoid space is filled with cerebrospinal fluid.

- The dura mater is made up of tough tissue that lines the skull cavity.

- Cerebrospinal fluid is constantly formed by the chorid plexus and reabsorbed by the arachnoid villae.

- Three main divisions of the brain include the cerebrum, the brainstem, and the cerebellum. See Table 5-1 for the functions of the main divisions of the brain.

- The posterior fontanelle closes at about 2 months of age. The anterior fontanelle closes at about 16 to 18 months of age. With an increase in ICP or cranial volume, however, the fontanelles can still separate up to age 12 years. See Fig. 5-2 for an illustration of the fontanelles.

- Basal ganglia are found in the cerebrum and regulate the extrapyramidal tracts—intentional movement. Kernicterus (high bilirubin levels in neonates) can damage these permanently and cause cerebral palsy.

- Cerebral perfusion pressure (CPP) = mean arterial pressure (MAP) – intracranial pressure (ICP). CPP = MAP – ICP

- Normal ICP = 4 to 15 mm Hg.

- CPP should be maintained above 50 mm Hg to ensure adequate cerebral perfusion. If less than 40 to 50 mm Hg pressure, ischemia of the brain can develop.

Autonomic Nervous System

- The autonomic nervous system (involuntary control: homeostatic functions) is comprised of the sympathetic and parasympathetic systems.

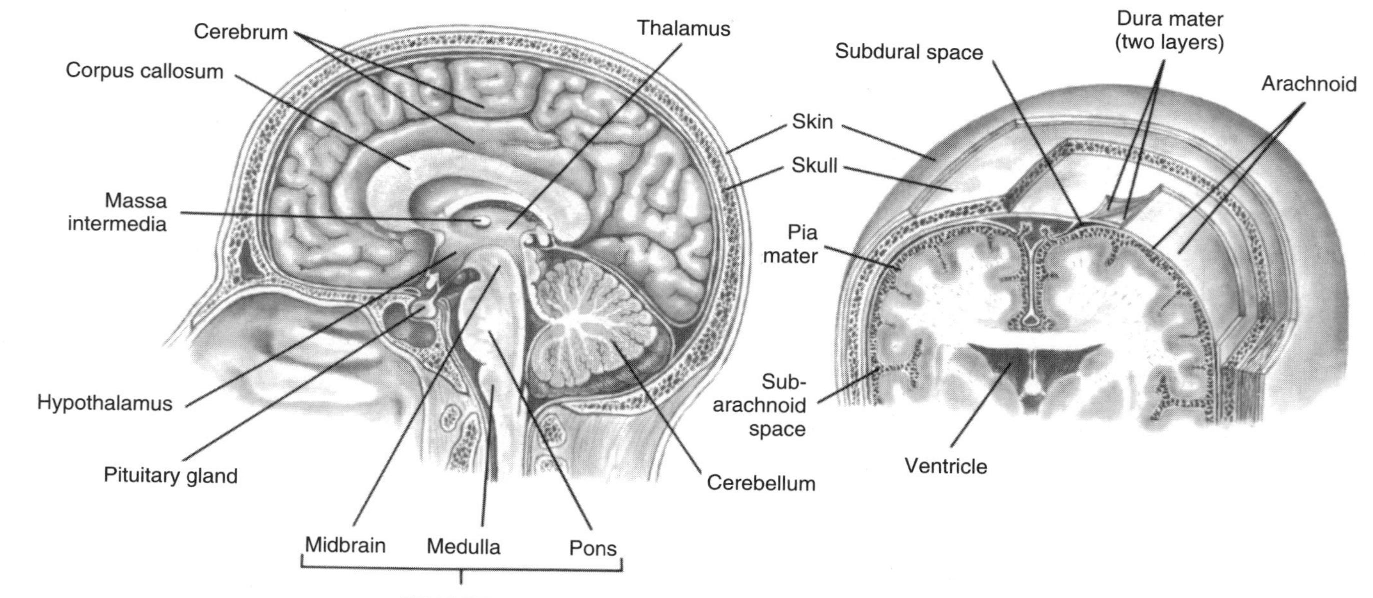

Fig. 5-1 Meninges of the brain. (From Thompson et al: Mosby's clinical nursing, ed 3, St Louis, 1993, Mosby.)

Table 5-1
Functions of the Main Divisions of the Brain

Major Area	Function
Cerebrum	Sensory and motor function
Frontal lobe	Contains the pyramidal tracts Voluntary motor activities Smell Memory Judgment Affect Personality
Parietal lobe	Sensory function Speech High level sensory function, such as stereogenesis
Occipital lobe	Vision Memory
Corpus callosum	Connects and integrates the two cerebral hemispheres
Limbic lobe	Moods Instincts Visceral response to moods and emotions
Basal ganglia	Integration of motor function Center for extrapyramidal tracts Controls much of posture Suppresses undesired or unnecessary muscle activity
Thalamus	Relays sensory input of taste, vision, and hearing to cerebral cortex
Hypothalamus	Regulates temperature Regulates food and water consumption May affect sleep, aggressive, and sexual behavior Important in autonomic nervous system responses Controls secretion by the posterior pituitary gland of antidiuretic hormone (ADH) and oxytocin Controls secretion by the anterior pituitary gland of thyroid-stimulating hormone (TSH), adrencorticotropic hormone (ACTH), growth hormone (GH), and other hormones

Table 5-1
Functions of the Main Divisions of the Brain—cont'd

Major Area	Function
Brain stem	Origin of most cranial nerves Contains three major divisions
Midbrain	Motor and sensory pathways Involved with vision and hearing Cranial nerves 3,4
Pons	Helps integrate the cerebral cortex with the cerebellum for motor function Motor and sensory pathways Cranial nerves 5,6,7,8
Medulla	Contains motor and sensory tracts Cranial nerves 8,9,10,11,12
Reticular activating system	Controls wakefulness and sleepiness
Respiratory and cardiac centers	Influence on respiratory and cardiac rates, rhythm, and function
Cerebellum	Responsible for balance, voluntary movement, and posture

- The sympathetic system controls those involuntary activities related to "fight or flight." In order to prepare the body to fight or flee danger, this system causes pupil dilatation, increased heart rate, increased blood pressure, bronchodilation, and increased circulation to major muscles. It decreases blood pressure, bronchodilation, and increased circulation to major muscles. It decreases blood flow to the gut and decreases bladder tone because these are not critical to saving life (adrenergic response).

- Drugs that mimic or cause sympathetic functions to occur are sympathomimetics (or adrenergic agonists) and anticholinergics. Atropine (anticholinergic) and dobutamine, phenylephrine, epinephrine, and methyldopa (adrenergic agonists) are a few examples.

- The parasympathetic system controls those involuntary activities associated with relaxing after danger has passed. Heart rate decreases, blood pressure lowers, pupils constrict, bronchioles constrict, bladder tone increases, and blood flow to the gut increases (cholinergic response).

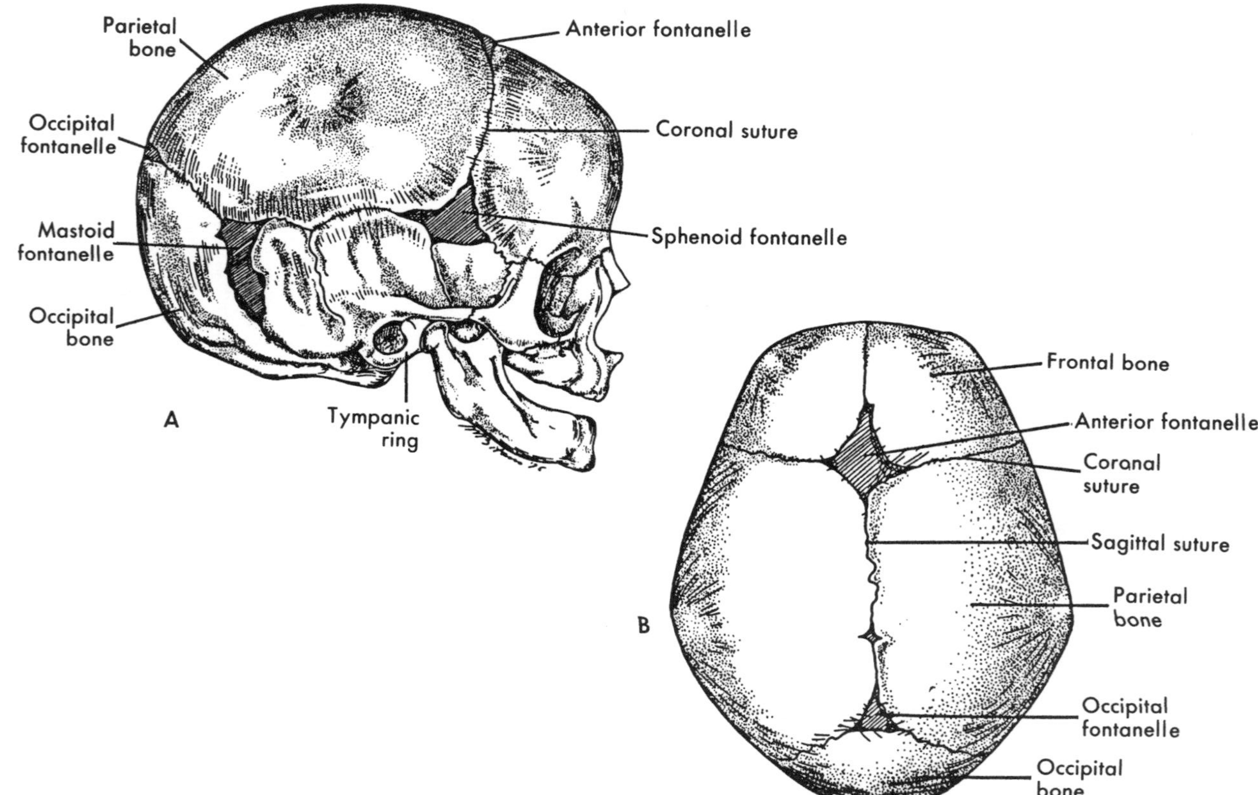

Fig. 5-2 Infant skull. **A,** Lateral view. **B,** Superior view. (From Conway BL: Pediatric neurological nursing, St Louis, 1977, Mosby.)

- Drugs that mimic or cause parasympathetic functions to occur are cholinergic, antiadrenergic, or beta-adrenergic blockers. Examples include propranolol, tolazoline, labetalol, and esmolol.
- Most drugs ending in *-lol* are beta-blockers.
- Special pediatric and infant Glasgow coma scales better assess these age groups. (See Table 5-2.)

ENCEPHALOPATHY

- See Table 5-3 for a summary of causes, findings, and management of various forms of encephalopathy.

Table 5-2
Modified Glasgow Coma Scale for Infants and Children

	Child	Infant	Score
Eye opening	Spontaneous	Spontaneous	4
	To verbal stimuli	To verbal stimuli	3
	To pain only	To pain only	2
	No response	No response	1
Verbal response	Oriented, appropriate	Coos and babbles	5
	Confused	Irritable cries	4
	Inappropriate words	Cries to pain	3
	Incomprehensible words or nonspecific sounds	Moans to pain	2
	No response	No response	1
Motor response	Obeys commands	Moves spontaneously and purposefully	6
	Localizes painful stimulus	Withdraws to touch	5
	Withdraws in response to pain	Withdraws in response to pain	4
	Flexion in response to pain	Decorticate posturing (abnormal flexion) in response to pain	3
	Extension in response to pain	Decerebrate posturing (abnormal extension) in response to pain	2
	No response	No response	1

From Hazinski MF: Nursing care of the critically ill child, ed 2, St Louis, 1992, Mosby.

Table 5-3
Metabolic Encephalopathy

Disorder	Causes	Assessment Findings	Management
Anoxia and hypoxia	Birth trauma Fat embolism Hypertension Thromboembolic events	Infants: Global dysfunction Irritability Decreased level of consciousness Seizures Children: Anxiety Impaired thinking Restlessness Combativeness Seizures	Correct the anoxia and hypoxia by addressing the cause
Hypoglycemia	Infants: Stress Maternal diabetes Infection Placental insufficiency Children: Endocrine abnormalities Pharmacological agents Liver disease Malnutrition Hyperinsulinemia	Infants: Jitteriness Apnea Cyanosis Hypotonia Seizures Children: Somnolence Decreased level of consciousness Seizures	Administration of glucose to normalize serum glucose levels Correction of precipitating causes
Pulmonary disease	Hypoxia Hypercarbia Acidosis Infections	Headache Decreased level of consciousness Coma Increased intracranial pressure Myoclonus Asterixis	Respiratory support to correct acidosis, hypoxemia, and hypercarbia

Table 5-3
Metabolic Encephalopathy—cont'd

Disorder	Causes	Assessment Findings	Management
Hepatic disease	Hepatitis Congenital liver disease	Altered level of consciousness Apathy Obtundation Asterixis Posturing	Cessation of protein intake Sterilization of the gastrointestinal tract Lactose administration
Renal disease	Uremia dysequilibrium syndrome	Decreased alertness and level of consciousness Delirium Hyperpnea Asterixis Seizures	Renal replacement therapies such as hemodialysis, peritoneal dialysis, continuous arterio-venous hemofiltration
Diabetes mellitus	Ketoacidosis Hypoglycemia	Dehydration Altered mentation Headache Seizures Coma	Treat elevated glucose and ketone levels Treat hypoglycemia
Thyroid disease	Hyperthyroidism	Anxiety Obtundation	Treatment of underlying hormone levels
	Hypothyroidism	Decreased mentation Coma	
Adrenal disease	Addison's disease	Delirious Flaccid weakness Poor reflexes Decreased level of consciousness	Normalization of cortisol levels

- Possible etioloties of encephalopathy can include lead poisoning, hypoxic events, hypertension, metabolic disorders, herpes, chicken pox, measles, or even vaccinations.

- Most forms of encephalopathy are generally characterized by a decreased level of consciousness, irritability, seizures, motor deficits, sensory impairments, headache, and hyperventilation. (See the following box.)

- Lumbar puncture in encephalopathy usually reveals normal CSF pressure, normal glucose levels, normal or slightly increased protein levels, and normal or increased cell counts. Gram stains and cultures are negative.

Signs and Symptoms of Various Forms of Encephalopathy

Hypoxic

Mild

- poor sucking
- irritability
- hyperalertness
- overactivity of the sympathetic system
- uninhibited reflexes

Moderate

- hypotonia
- poor reflexes
- stupor
- lethargy
- seizures

Severe

- flaccid muscle tone
- coma
- poor brainstem function
- seizures
- increased intracranial pressure
- multiorgan dysfunction

Hepatic

Tremors

Poor coordination

Muscle twitching

Asterixis

Decreased level of consciousness

Coma

Hypertensive

Headache

Elevated systemic arterial pressure

Decreased level of consciousness

Coma

Lead

Paralysis

Seizures

Blindness

Coma

- Encephalopathy can develop 48 to 72 hours after a fall in cardiac output.

- Treatment is supportive and directed at the cause, focusing especially on treating increased ICP.

- Reye's syndrome is one form of encephalopathy, including also fatty infiltration of the liver. Links have been found between viral illnesses and the use of aspirin.

- Liver enzymes are markedly elevated in Reye's syndrome, along with serum ammonia levels and prothrombin time (PT).

INCREASED INTRACRANIAL PRESSURE (ICP)

- Cerebral edema can be vasogenic (water and protein move into interstitial space), cytotoxic (intracellular edema), and interstitial or hydrocephalic (seen with hydrocephalus from increased pressure in the ventricles which forces CSF into the brain tissue). See Table 5-4 for a comparison of ICP monitoring systems.

- Treat an increase in ICP with diuresis and hyperventilation to decrease circulating blood volume within the brain. Decreased blood volume in the brain can help decrease intracranial pressure.

- Hyperventilation decreases ICP by causing vasoconstriction of cerebral arteries in response to decreased carbon dioxide levels. Maintain pCO_2 25 to 30 torr. This therapy is only effective for a short period of time. Keeping the pCO_2 <25 torr can cause severe vasoconstriction of the cerebral arteries and lead to hypoxia, cell death, and an increase in cerebral edema.

- Carbon dioxide is the most important factor in regulating cerebral blood flow. Increased pCO_2 levels cause vasodilation and further elevate the ICP through an increase in blood volume inside the cranial vault. Decreased pCO_2 levels cause vasoconstriction which can lower the ICP through a decrease in blood volume inside the head.

- Treat with diuretics such as mannitol (0.5 to 1 g/kg/dose), furosemide (1 mg/kg/dose q 4 to 6 hr) to reduce intracerebral volume. Carefully monitor serum osmolality levels.

- Hypoxia, infection, trauma, tumors, hydrocephalus, encephalopathy, and chronic pulmonary disease can all cause an increase in ICP.

- Maintain pO_2 >100 mm Hg to prevent hypoxia and provide optimal O_2 in patients with elevated ICP.

- Bulging or tense fontanelles signify an increased ICP.

Table 5-4
Comparison of ICP Monitoring Systems

	Fiber-Optic Catheter	Fluid-Filled with IVC Catheter or Bolt	Epidural Sensor
Placement	Subarachnoid, intraventricular, or intraparenchymal	Subarachnoid or intraventricular	Epidural only
CSF drainage	Able to drain with ventricular catheter while continuously monitoring ICP	Able to drain with ventricular catheter; if continuous ICP recording is performed, waveform will be dampened	No drainage capability
Infection risk	Lack of static fluid may reduce risk	Static fluid column with stopcocks, tubing, etc., may increase risk	Lack of static fluid system and intact dura may reduce risk
Waveform	Requires dedicated equipment that interfaces with bedside alarm system	Uses bedside monitor to display waveform and generate alarms	Requires dedicated equipment; does not interface with bedside monitor
Artifact	Minimal or none	May be present because of air, kinked tubing, patient movement, dampening	Minimal or none
Zero reference	Zeroing is performed *only prior* to insertion, cannot be verified after insertion	Repeated zero adjustment necessary	Factory set; cannot be checked after insertion
Transducer calibration	Factory set, no calibration required	Required before and during patient use	Factory set, no calibration required

Table 5-4
Comparison of ICP Monitoring Systems—cont'd

	Fiber-Optic Catheter	Fluid-Filled with IVC Catheter or Bolt	Epidural Sensor
Advantages	Excellent signal transmission and waveform reproduction Decreased risk of infection because it is a "dry" system Can be used in infants	Subarachnoid bolts are less invasive than intraventricular catheters and may be useful for monitoring with "moderate" head injuries; the bolt works well in the presence of cerebral edema IVC allows CSF drainage to manage ICP	Placement outside of dura decreases risk of infection Devices can be implanted for long-term monitoring
Disadvantages	The catheter is fragile, and the fiber-optic elements are easily damaged	The main disadvantage of all fluid-filled systems is the risk of infection. This is especially true with intraventricular catheters (IVCs) Subarachnoid bolts cannot be placed or stabilized in the thin skull of an infant IVC may lose monitoring capabilities if the ventricles become compressed by intracranial hypertension	The principal problem with epidural sensor is zero drift, which becomes significant after prolonged use. Other difficulties include hysteresis, inadequate frequency response, and temperature sensitivity

From Hazinski MF: Nursing care of the critically ill child, ed 2, St Louis, 1992, Mosby.

- Measure head circumference in infants as an indicator of increased ICP. Document trends.

- Barbiturates are used to treat an elevated ICP that is unresponsive to other treatments because they decrease cerebral metabolism and O_2 demands.

- Hypothermia and pharmacological paralysis may be used to decrease cerebral metabolism.

- Cushing's triad is a late sign and a medical emergency indicating increased ICP. The triad of symptoms is increased systolic BP, bradycardia, and slowed or irregular respirations.

- Promote cerebral venous drainage to decrease the ICP by elevating the head of the bed 30 degrees and keeping the head midline. Do *not* turn the head to the side. This can occlude venous drainage and increase ICP.

- An infant with elevated ICP is lethargic and has a high-pitched cry.

- Some nursing interventions, activities, and environmental factors that increase ICP include crying, suctioning, turning head, handling of any artificial airway or respiratory tubing, and coughing.

NEUROLOGICAL INFECTIOUS DISEASES

- Lumbar punctures are generally not indicated or must be performed with extreme caution in meningitis associated with increased ICP because decompression or release of acutely increased ICP can result in brain herniation and death.

- Lumbar punctures are done between the third and fourth lumbar space (below the fourth in infants). Position with knees and head flexed.

- Viral meningitis has a normal CSF glucose and protein level. Bacterial meningitis has a low CSF glucose level and high protein level.

- Bacterial meningitis is most often caused by *Hemphilus influenza, Streptococcus pneumoniae,* or *Neisseria meningitides.*

- Encephalitis often accompanies bacterial meningitis.

- Symptoms of meningitis may include photophobia, headache, nuchal rigidity (resistance of the neck to flexion), neck pain, pain with extension of the legs (Kernig's sign), and flexion of the neck causing hip and knee flexion (Brudzinski's sign).

- White blood cell count is higher in CSF of bacterial meningitis (>500 WBC/mm^2) than of viral (<500).

- Fluid intake should be reduced to control ICP.

- Potential complications of meningitis are syndrome of inappropriate antidiuretic hormone (SIADH) and diabetes insipidus (DI).

SEIZURES

Partial seizures (affects local parts of the brain):
- Jacksonian seizures: usually no loss of consciousness, focal motor seizures, seen with brain lesions, uncommon in children. Seizure activity spreads in an orderly progression to other areas.

- Psychomotor seizures: last minutes to hours, occur in any age group, appear to be bizarre behavior such as picking of clothes, chewing, staring, roaming. Originate in the motor area of the frontal lobe.

- Focal sensory seizures: paresthesia in various parts of the body.

Generalized seizures (affects large parts of the brain):
- Petit mal (absence) seizures are seen most often in patients 6 to 14 years of age (rarely before age 4) and are characterized by staring and twitching. Petit mal seizures generally last only 2 to 10 seconds. Seizure activity is manifested by a seeming unawareness of their surroundings.

- Myoclonic infantile spasms are seen most often at 3 to 8 months of age. These seizures are characterized by head bobbing or jerking, and opisthotonos; however, they can progress to generalized seizures.

- Myoclonic seizures are characterized by sudden, yet short contractions of either single muscles or muscle groups. They may occur in isolation or repetitively, and are not associated with loss of consciousness or a postictal state.

- Febrile seizures occur most often in children under 3 years of age, but can occur from 6 months to 6 years. Seizures occur because the threshold is lowered by temperatures greater than 101.8°F. Treatment includes use of antipyretics and phenobarbital or diazepam to both prevent and control seizures.

- Generalized tonic-clonic seizures previously were known as "grand mal" seizures. The tonic phase is characterized by loss of consciousness and eye rolling, with stiffening and contraction of the entire body. Apnea and cyanosis often occur during this stage. The clonic phase is when stiffness is replaced by jerking of muscles and relaxation, incontinence, and salivation. A postictal state occurs with tonic-clonic seizures. See box on p. 258 for emergency treatment.

- Treatment of seizures includes the following: asses seizures for vital information such as presence and type of aura, length of seizure, occurrence of incontinence,

Emergency Treatment—Seizures

Tonic-Clonic Seizure

During the Seizure

Time seizure episode.

Approach calmly.

If child is standing or seated, ease child down.

Place pillow or folded blanket under child's head. If no bedding is available, place own hands under child's head.

Loosen restrictive clothing.

Remove eyeglasses.

Clear area of any hazards or hard objects.

Allow seizure to end without interference.

If vomiting occurs, try to turn child to one side as a unit.

Do not:

- Attempt to restrain child or use force
- Put anything in child's mouth
- Give any food or liquids

After the Seizure

Time postictal period.

Check for breathing. Check position of head and tongue. Reposition if head is hyperextended. If breathing is not present, give rescue breathing and call emergency medical system (EMS).

Check out around mouth for evidence of burns or suspicious substances that might indicate poisoning.

Keep child on side.

Remain with child until full recovery.

Do not give food or liquids until fully alert and swallowing reflex has returned.

Call EMS when necessary.

Emergency Treatment—Seizures—cont'd

Look for medical identification and determine what factors occurred before onset of seizure and which may have been triggering factors.

Check head and body for possible injuries and fractures. Check inside of mouth to see if tongue or lips have been bitten.

Complex Partial Seizure

During the Seizure

Do not restrain unless in danger.

Remove harmful objects from path.

Redirect to safe area.

Do not agitate; instead, talk in calm, reassuring manner.

Do not expect child to follow instructions.

Watch to see if seizures generalizes.

After the Seizure

Stay with child and reassure until fully conscious.

Call Emergency Medical Service If:

Child stops breathing.

There is evidence of injury or youngster is diabetic or pregnant.

Seizure lasts for more than 5 minutes (unless duration of seizure is typically longer than 5 minutes).

Status epilepticus occurs.

Pupils are not equal after seizure.

Child vomits continuously 30 minutes after seizure had ended (sign of possible acute problem).

Child cannot be awakened and is unresponsive to pain after seizure has ended.

Seizure occurs in water (shock and aspiration may be delayed).

This is child's first seizure.

From Wong DL: Whaley and Wong's nursing care of infants and children, ed 5, St Louis, 1995, Mosby.

level of consciousness during and following seizure, respiratory effort, and behavior following seizure (postictal state). Protect from injury during and after seizure.

Pharmacological management of seizures

- Phenytoin is used to treat grand mal seizures, psychomotor seizures, and status epilepticus, and to prevent or treat seizures associated with neurosurgery.

- Therapeutic serum phenytoin levels are 10 to 20 mcg/mL. Toxic levels are 30 to 50 mcg/mL.

- The onset of phenytoin is 15 to 20 minutes, making it better suited for chronic maintenance or in status epilepticus when other first-line drugs have been ineffective.

- Phenytoin should *not* be mixed in dextrose solutions or with other medications.

- Diazepam is used in the initial treatment of seizures at a dose of 0.1 to 0.3 mg/kg by slow intravenous push. The rapid onset of minutes makes it effective, but the short half-life of 7 minutes may necessitate frequent redosing and use of another longer-acting anticonvulsant.

- Side effects of diazepam include hypotension, laryngospasm, respiratory depression, and arrest.

- Other phramacologic agents used to treat status epilepticus include lorazepam, phenobarbital, valproic acid, and paraldehyde. See Table 5-5 for common drugs used to control seizures.

HYDROCEPHALUS

- Causes of hydrocephalus include intrauterine infections, genetic X-linked defects, various cerebellar defects, blockage to CSF flow, ventricular inflammation, and overproduction of CSF.

- Hydrocephalus occurs from either an obstruction to the flow of cerebrospinal fluid (noncommunicating), an increase in production of CSF (excessive secretion), or decreased absorption of CSF (communicating).

- Infants will develop an increased head circumference with hydrocephalus.

- An increase in ICP will develop in all children with hydrocephaly.

- See box on pp. 264-265 for ventriculoperitoneal shunt care.

INTRACEREBRAL AND INTRAVENTRICULAR HEMORRHAGES

- Risk factors for intracerebral and intraventricular hemorrhages include hypernatremia, blood transfusions, shock, acidosis, seizures, and rapid volume expansion.

Table 5-5
Major Drugs Used for Control of Seizures

Drug	Therapeutic Dosage	Therapeutic Plasma Level	Seizure Type	Comments/Side Effects
Adrenocorticotropic hormone (ACTH, H.P. Acthar gel)	May range from 20 to 160 units		Infantile spasms, Lennox-Gastaut syndrome	Acts only on developing brain Given intramuscularly No standard length of therapy; usually a few weeks to several months *Side effects:* Cushingoid appearance, extreme irritability, hypertension, transient glycosuria
Carbamazepine (Tegretol)	10-15 mg/kg/day Half-life: 9-19 hr	4-12 mcg/mL	Secondary tonic-clonic Complex partial Simple partial	Relatively free from unwanted side effects: fewer sedative properties *Side effects:* Blurred vision, diplopia, drowsiness, vertigo, headache *Toxic effects:* Leukopenic aplastic anemia
Clonazepam (Klonopin)	0.05-0.20 mg/kg/day Half-life: 18-20 hr	20-80 mcg/mL	Absence Myoclonic	Usually given as adjunct to other antiepileptic drugs *Side effects:* Drowsiness ataxia, hyperactivity, agitation, slurred speech, double vision, increased salivation
Divalproex sodium, valproate, valproic acid (Depakote, Depakene)	20-60 mg/kg/day Half-life: 6-18 hr	50-150 mcg/mL	Myoclonic Absence Tonic-clonic Mixed seizure types Lennox-Gastaut syndrome	Potentiates action of phenobarbital and phenytion *Side effects:* Hair loss, tremor, elevated liver enzymes, irregular menses, increased appetite, nausea and vomiting (not as common with Depakote) *Toxic effect:* Hepatic toxicity

Continued.

Table 5-5

Major Drugs Used for Control of Seizures—cont'd

Drug	Therapeutic Dosage	Therapeutic Plasma Level	Seizure Type	Comments/Side Effects
Ethosuximide (Zarontin)	15-35 mg/kg/day Half-life: 24-72 hr	40-100 mcg/mL	Absence	Occasionally aggravates generalized seizures Administer with food *Side effects:* Nausea, gastric discomfort, anorexia, headache, drowsiness, dizziness
Felbamate (Felbatol)	15 mg/kg, increased to 30, 45,or 60 mg/kg as needed Half-life: 20-23 hr	Not established, but studies suggest 30-100 mcg/mL	Lennox-Gastaut syndrome	Not affected by food Monitor weight Give in early morning to reduce insomnia Interacts with other antiepileptic drugs (i.e., increases phenytoin and valproic acid levels and decreases carbamazapine levels) Side effects increased when given with other antiepileptic drugs *Side effects:* Anorexia, nausea, vomiting, insomnia, headache, weight loss *Toxic effect:* Aplastic anemia
Phenobarbital (Luminal)	4-6 mg/kg/day Half-life: 53-104 hr	10-40 mcg/mL	Tonic-clonic	May interfere with concentration and motor speed May cause vitamin D and folic acid deficiencies *Side effects:* Drowsiness, irritability, hyperactivity, skin rash, mild ataxia, hyperpyrexia, diminished cognitive performance

Table 5-5
Major Drugs Used for Control of Seizures—cont'd

Drug	Therapeutic Dosage	Therapeutic Plasma Level	Seizure Type	Comments/Side Effects
Phenytoin (Dilantin)	5-10 mg/kg/day Half-life: 7-22 hr	10-20 mcg/mL	Tonic-clonic Complex partial Simple partial	May cause behavioral disturbances in children May aggravate absence and myoclonic seizures *Side effects:* Gum hyperplasia, hirsutism, ataxia, nystagmus, diplopia, anorexia, nausea, nervousness, folate deficiency *Toxic effects:* Stevens-Johnson syndrome (erythema multiforme), thrombocytopenia
Primidone (Mysoline)	12-25 mg/kg/day Half-life: 3-12 hr	5-12 mcg/mL	Tonic-clonic Complex partial Simple partial	Effective with phenobarbital in mixed-type seizure patterns *Side effects:* Drowsiness, ataxia, diplopia

From Wong DL: Whaley and Wong's nursing care of infants and children, ed 5, St Louis, 1995, Mosby.

- Intracerebral hemorrhages result in acute neurological deterioration as a result of a rapid rise in ICP and damage to brain tissue.
- Computerized tomography (CT) scan or angiography are diagnostic studies of choice.
- Wherever possible and indicated, cerebral hematomas are evacuated to reduce the ICP.
- Periventricular-intraventricular hemorrhages are generally confined to preterm infants and generally occur in the first few hours to days of life. See Fig. 5-3 for an illustration of the grading of intraventricular hemorrhages.
- Signs and symptoms of intraventricular hemorrhage include change in level of consciousness, shock, acidosis, anemia, seizures, bradycardia, and apnea.
- Ultrasonography is the diagnostic test of choice in diagnosing an intraventricular hemorrhage in the neonate.

Ventriculoperitoneal Shunt

Purpose: To drain excess cerebrospinal fluid (CFS) from the ventricles into the peritoneum to relieve intracranial pressure, prevent further damage to the brain, and promote optimal outcome.

I. Positioning
   A. Place on unaffected side (may position on shunt side with "donut" over operative site once incision has healed). Keep head of bed flat—no more than 15 to 30 degrees to prevent too-rapid fluid loss.
   B. Support head carefully when moving infant.
   C. Turn q 2 h from unaffected side of head to back.

II. Shunt site
   A. Use strict aseptic technique when changing dressing.
   B. Pump shunt if and only as directed by neurosurgeon.
   C. Observe for fluid leakage around pump.

III. Observe and document all intake and output. Watch for symptoms of excessive drainage of CSF:
   A. Sunken fontanel
   B. Increased urine output
   C. Increased sodium loss

IV. Observe, document, and report any seizure activity or paresis.

V. Observe for signs of ileus:
   A. Abdominal distention (serially measure abdominal girth)
   B. Absence of bowel sounds
   C. Loss of gastric content by emesis or through orogastric tube

VI. Perform range-of-motion exercises to all extremities.

VII. Observe and assess for symptoms of increased intracranial pressure (shunt failure):
   A. Increasing head circumference (measure daily)
   B. Full and/or tense fontanel

Ventriculoperitoneal Shunt—cont'd

C. Sutures palpably more separated

D. High-pitched, shrill cry

E. Irritability/sleeplessness

F. Vomiting

G. Poor feeding

H. Nystagmus

I. Sunset sign of eyes

J. Shiny scalp with distended vessels

K. Hypotonia/hypertonia

VIII. Observe and assess for signs of infection:

A. Redness or drainage at shunt site

B. Hypothermia/hyperthermia

C. Lethargy/irritability

D. Poor feeding/weight gain

E. Pallor

IX. Parent teaching

A. Teach parents and give written copy of signs and symptoms of increased intracranial pressure, infection, and dehydration.

B. Emphasize importance of notifying physician for any signs and symptoms.

C. Demonstrate and receive return demonstration of proper head positioning (at rest, lifting, and carrying).

D. Demonstrate and receive return demonstration of drug administration. Teach parents side effects of medications.

E. Emphasize importance of follow-up medical care for assessment and medication adjustment.

From Merenstein GB and Gardner SL: Handbook of neonatal intensive care, ed 3, St Louis, 1993, Mosby.

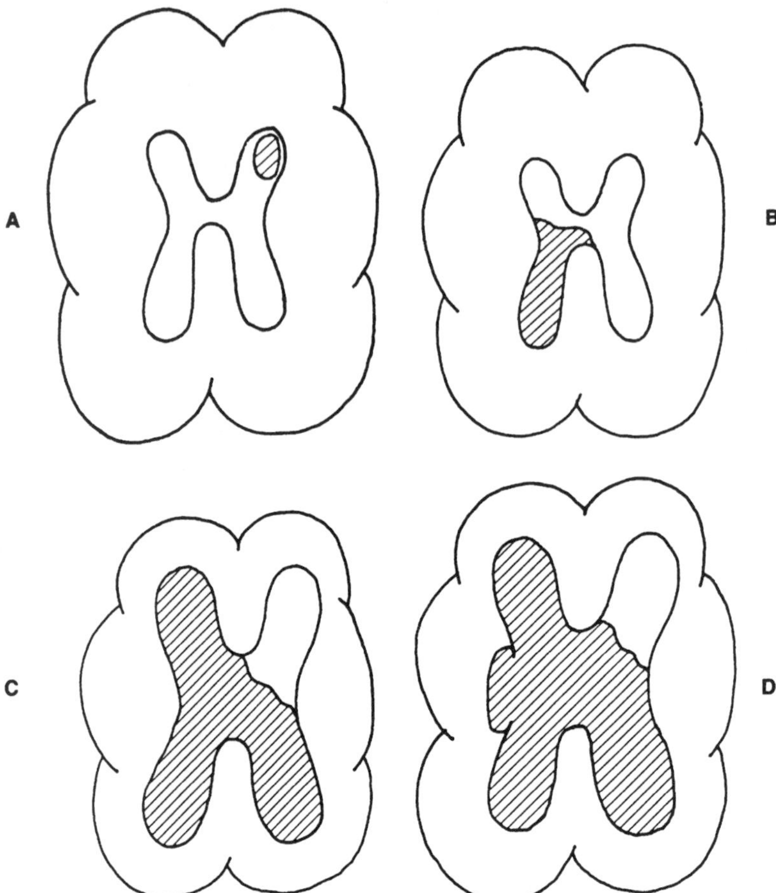

Fig. 5-3 Intraventricular hemorrhage. **A,** Grade I: subependymal hemorrhage only. **B,** Grade II: intraventricular hemorrhage without ventricular dilatation. **C,** Grade III: intraventricular hemorrhage with ventricular dilatation. **D,** Grade IV: intraventricular hemorrhage with parenchymal hemorrhage. (From Merenstein GB and Gardner SL: Handbook of neonatal intensive care, ed 3, St Louis, 1993, Mosby.)

- Hydrocephalus may develop as a complication following intraventricular hemorrhage.

SPINA BIFIDA AND MYELOMENINGOCELE

- Spina bifida and myelomeningocele occur as a result of failure in embryological development (approximately 3 to 6 weeks' gestation) for the neural tube to close properly, leading to neural tube defects (NTDs).

- Causative factors of NTDs may include exposure to radiation, maternal diabetes, vitamin deficiencies, and multifactorial inheritance.

- Spina bifida occulta occurs when any of the posterior arches of the spinous processes fail to close.
- Myelomeningoceles are defects in the meninges found in combination with spina bifida with pathology of the spinal cord and nerve roots. Neurological deficits are found below the level of the lesion.
- The amount of neurological deficit is dependent upon the level of the lesion.
- Most myelomeningoceles are found in the lumbar or lumbosacral areas.
- Clues to the presence of spina bifida include a patch of abnormal hair, a dimple, a hemangioma, or a lipoma over the lumbosacral area.
- Myleomeningoceles are very frequently associated with hydrocephalus.
- At birth, sensory function can be tested and used to accurately predict the degree of motor function later in life. Sensory function may, however, be present lower than motor function.
- If the motor-sensory level is L5-S1, ambulation is probably possible. If the defect is L3-L4, ambulation may be possible with braces and crutches. If the lesion is at L1-L2, the infant will have complete paraplegia.
- Generally the myelomeningocele should be closed surgically within 48 hours after birth.
- Hydronephrosis and neurogenic bladder need to be carefully evaluated throughout the neonatal period.
- Arnold-Chiari malformation is almost always found in spina bifida patients and results in hydrocephalus from CSF outflow obstruction. These patients commonly have central hypoventilation, apnea, reflux, weak sucking, aspiration, and laryngeal stridor.

PEDIATRIC-SPECIFIC PRINCIPLES

HEAD TRAUMA

- Goals of management include maintaining cerebral perfusion and preventing elevated intracranial pressure by intubating, hyperventilating, pain management, and pharmacological paralysis.
- Drainage from the ears and nose needs to be tested for CS fluid by testing for glucose.

- Concussion: blow to the head or shearing that results in relatively short loss of consciousness (seconds to hours) with no other associated neurological manifestation.

- Contusion: accompanied by bruising or local hemorrhage and edema of brain tissue. This also may be accompanied by loss of consciousness plus increased ICP. Seizure sequelae is common.

- Coup injury: involves the side of the brain that was directly struck.

- Contrecoup injury: involves the opposite side of the brain resulting from the brain "bouncing" inside the skull cavity.

- Skull fractures: usually result in underlying tissue injury such as vascular tears, edema, bruising. The types of skull fractures include:

  - Linear (simple) fracture: the bones broken remain in alignment and the meninges are not torn.
  - Depressed fracture: one or more pieces is indented damaging underlying brain tissue.
  - Compound fracture: scalp laceration and depressed fracture allow passage of contaminants from the scalp into the skull cavity.
  - Basilar fracture: a fracture in the posterior base of the skull. Contamination of CS fluid is common. May not be seen on x-ray. CT scan may be needed to diagnose. Signs and symptoms include battle sign (bruising behind the ears) and raccoon sign (periorbital bruising).

- Epidural hematoma: blood accumulates above the dura and is an arterial bleed (usually from the middle meningeal artery). Brief loss of consciousness is often followed by reawakening with lucidity and then rapid deterioration. Dilation of one pupil (ipsilateral to the injury) is most common. CT scan is the diagnostic test of choice. Remember: *e*pidural and *a*rtery both begin with vowels.

- Subdural hematoma: blood accumulates below the dura or between the dura and the arachnoid layers. This type of bleed can be acute, subacute, or chronic. Because subdural hematomas are venous, the bleeding can be slower. This type of injury is often seen with child abuse. Most lose consciousness and have ipsilateral pupil dilation, focal seizures, and contralateral hemiparesis. CT scan or angiography is the diagnostic test of choice. Remember: *s*ubdural and *v*enous both begin with consonants.

- Subarachnoid hemorrhage: rapid symptoms of increased ICP or seizures. Blood is very irritating and irritates the brain tissue directly, resulting in seizures. Highly suspicious of abuse or obvious trauma.

- Diffuse axonal injury (DAI) is a diffuse brain injury that includes mild concussions, cerebral concussions, and prolonged comas. DAI is classified as mild, moderate, or severe. Mild DAI produces a coma that lasts 6 to 24 hours and typically results in temporary deficits of memory and cognition, though permanent damage may occur. Moderate DAI results in a coma that lasts more than 24 hours and has little or no brainstem involvement. Severe DAI also results in a coma that lasts more than 24 hours, but also involves the brainstem and cerebrum.

SPINAL CORD INJURIES

- Spinal cord injuries are often associated with head injuries. Any infant or child with a head injury should also be assessed for a spinal cord injury.
- Children may manifest delayed symptoms in spinal cord injuries. Assessment must be frequent and ongoing.
- Spinal cord injury without radiological abnormality (SCIWORA) is common in children. X-rays may not show the presence of spinal cord injury.
- Steroids should be administered within the first 8 hours following injury to minimize neurological damage.
- Spinal fusion may be necessary when traction has not successfully stabilized a fracture or subluxation injury.

SPACE-OCCUPYING LESIONS

- Primary brain tumors are the most common form of cancer in children and adolescents. Most frequently they occur in children from 5 to 10 years of age.
- Classification is by location, degree of malignancy, and histologic features.
- Supratentorial tumors can occur in either cerebral hemisphere and above the tentorium cerebelli. The most common are astrocytoma and crainiopharyngioma.
- Infratentorial tumors occur in the brainstem and below the tentorial cerebelli. The most common types are medulloblastoma, astrocytoma, ependymomas, and brainstem gliomas.
- Up to 12 years of age, the skull can expand to help accommodate space-occupying lesions.
- Treatment includes managing ICP, surgical excision, radiation, and chemotherapy.

ARTERIOVENOUS (AV) MALFORMATION

- Arteriovenous (AV) malformations are direct connections between arteries (usually middle cerebral artery) and veins in the brain. An AV malformation results in high pressure, high volume flow through the veins causing them to become distended, sclerosed, and weakened.

- High volume flow into the veins can cause congestive heart failure from volume overload or stroke from rupture of weakened vein walls.

- Complications of AV malformations include congestive heart failure from increased venous return to the heart and intracranial hemorrhages from thin-walled, stressed veins.

NEONATAL-SPECIFIC PRINCIPLES

ANENCEPHALY

- Anencephaly is a congenital defect where there is no normal brain tissue above the brainstem and thalamus. Even these structures are often malformed. This is a neural tube defect that occurs as early as the third to fourth week of gestation.

- Because the brainstem is often intact and/or functional, anencephalic infants do not meet the criteria for brain death.

Questions

GENERAL NEUROLOGY CARE QUESTIONS

1. Cerebrospinal fluid is formed by the:
A. Choroid plexus
B. Cerebral ventricles
C. Arachnoid villae
D. Pia mater

2. Which of the following assessment findings in an infant is *not* indicative of an increase in intracranial pressure?
A. Lethargy
B. Bulging fontanels
C. Hypotension
D. Tachycardia

3. A patient has been admitted with a suspected intracranial bleed. Which of the following diagnostic tests would be *least* helpful in diagnosing this condition?
A. Cerebral blood flow studies
B. Computerized axial tomography
C. Lumbar puncture
D. Skull x-rays

Case Study

A patient is admitted to the critical care unit with a diagnosis of hypoxic-ischemic encephalopathy following a traumatic delivery. Questions 4 to 6 refer to this case study.

---

4. The *first* nursing priority would be to assess:
A. Pupillary reaction
B. Level of consciousness
C. Ability to maintain airway
D. Blood glucose level

5. The critical care nurse would recognize as signs and symptoms of mild hypoxic-ischemic encephalopathy all of the following *except*:
A. Irritability
B. Tachycardia
C. Hyperalertness
D. Hypotonia

6. This infant is intubated and mechanically ventilated. Besides providing optimal oxygenation, which of the following is also a benefit of mechanical ventilation in this type of infant?
A. Reduction of intracranial pressure
B. Prevention of seizure activity
C. Prevention of long-term complications
D. Reduction of hypocarbia

7. The mechanism of the development of hydrocephalus is most commonly related to:
A. Increased flow of cerebrospinal fluid
B. Increased resorption of cerebrospinal fluid
C. Obstructed flow of cerebrospinal fluid
D. Decreased production of cerebrospinal fluid

8. Which of the following infants is *least* likely to develop hypoxic-ischemic encephalopathy? An infant with:
A. Pulmonary atresia
B. Sepsis
C. Coarctation of the aorta
D. Persistent pulmonary hypertension

9. A neonate is admitted to the critical care unit following unexplained seizure activity. In planning this newborn's treatment, the critical care nurse recognizes the highest priority is given to:
A. Correcting metabolic imbalances
B. Administering prophylactic anticonvulsant therapy
C. Obtaining an EEG to identify focal site
D. Obtaining a lumbar puncture to rule out meningitis

10. A nurse observes shakiness in an infant. Which of the following interventions can help identify this activity as either tremors or seizures?
A. Stimulate sucking
B. Hold the infant's arms
C. Observe for nystagmus
D. Note change in consciousness

11. Which of the following explains the mechanism of most neonatal seizures?
A. Increase of inhibitory control
B. Loss of inhibitory control
C. Increase of excitatory centers
D. Loss of excitatory centers

Case Study

A 3-day-old infant is admitted to the critical care unit with a history of irritability, opisthotonos, stridor, and periods of apnea. Sucking has been poor and the nurse at transfer reveals to the critical care nurse that the neonate has also been difficult to console, and actually quiets better when left lying on his stomach. The critical care nurse's assessment reveals an increased head circumference, decreased gag reflex, and bulging fontanelles. The infant is diagnosed with hydrocephalus. Questions 12 to 14 refer to this case study.

---

12. Which of the following signs and symptoms would the critical care nurse recognize as indicating further serious deterioration in the infant's condition?
A. Lethargy
B. Lower extremity spasticity
C. Sluggish pupillary response
D. Emesis

13. The tests that are most helpful in diagnosing and evaluating hydrocephalus are:
I. Computerized axial tomography
II Skull x-rays
III. Ultrasound imaging
IV. Magnetic resonance imaging
A. I, II, and III
B. I, II, and IV
C. II and III
D. I and IV

14. Following placement of a ventriculoperitoneal shunt, the critical care nurse would recognize which of the following as a desired outcome?
A. Rapid return to a normal intracranial pressure (ICP)
B. Gag reflex with suctioning
C. Firm, round fontanels
D. Dilated scalp veins

15. Which of the following is *not* a likely potential complication of a ventriculoperitoneal shunt?
A. Subdural hematoma
B. Peritonitis
C. Intraventricular hemorrhage
D. Meningitis

16. A lumbar puncture is ordered for a full term infant with decreased level of responsiveness, irritability, hyperventilation, and seizure activity 1 hour before the test. The results were as follows:
CSF pressure: normal
White blood cell count: 4 cells/mm^3
Red blood cell count: 0 cells/mm^3
Protein: 53 mg/dL
Glucose: 54 mg/dL
Which of the following diagnoses is *most likely* based on these findings?
A. Encephalopathy
B. Viral meningitis
C. Bacterial meningitis
D. Intraventricular hemorrhage

17. A sympathomimetic drug would be expected to produce which of the following symptoms in addition to any desired effects?
A. Pupil constriction
B. Bronchodilation
C. Bradycardia
D. Increased bladder tone

18. Cushing's triad consists of which of the following clinical findings?
I. Widening pulse pressure
II. Bradycardia
III. Pupillary dilatation
IV. Bradypnea
A. I, II, and III
B. I, II, and IV
C. I, III, and IV
D. II, III, and IV

19. In caring for a patient with increased intracranial pressure, the critical care nurse places the patient in which optimal position?
A. Left lateral
B. Dorsal with the head turned to the right
C. Supine with the bed flat
D. Supine with the head of the bed elevated

20. In monitoring the therapeutic effect of phenytoin for seizures, the critical care nurses recognizes therapeutic serum levels as:
A. 5 to 10 mcg/dL
B. 10 to 25 mcg/dL
C. 25 to 40 mcg/dL
D. 40 to 55 mcg/dL

21. In caring for a patient who has received diazepam for acute seizure activity, the critical care nurse observes for which of the following adverse reactions?
A. Laryngospasm
B. Cushing's triad
C. Acute hypertension
D. Ventricular ectopy

22. For a patient with bacterial meningitis, how long is isolation indicated?
A. Until the organism is identified
B. Until antibiotics are initiated
C. Until antibiotics have been administered for 24 hours
D. Until 10 days of antibiotic therapy has been completed

23. Anencephalic neonates are *not* usually suitable organ donors because they frequently have:
A. An intact brainstem
B. Multiple anomalies affecting other organs
C. Congenital viral infections
D. No organ systems that function normally at birth

24. All of the following may be helpful in treating hydrocephalus that follows an intraventricular hemorrhage *except*:
A. Ventricular taps
B. Diuretic therapy
C. Serial lumbar taps
D. Fluid restriction

Case Study

A 26-hour-old neonate is admitted to the critical care unit with hypotension, cold and mottled skin, bradycardia, and a pH of 7.21. A lumbar tap reveals increased pressure, white blood cell count of 4 cell/mm^3, glucose of 55 mg/dL, and erythrocytes at 518 cells/mm^3. Questions 25 to 27 refer to this case study.

---

25. The assessment findings and results of the diagnostic tests suggest which neurological problem?
A. Hydrocephalus
B. Intraventricular hemorrhage
C. Intracerebral hematoma
D. Encephalitis

26. What diagnostic test would be *least* helpful in diagnosing this condition?
A. Ultrasonography
B. Skull x-rays
C. Magnetic resonance imaging
D. Computerized axial tomography

27. Which of the following interventions would be the *greatest* priority?
A. Correcting the acidosis
B. Sending cultures on the CSF
C. Initiating fluid and vasopressor support
D. Typing and cross matching for blood products

28. All of the following conditions have been found to further increase intracranial pressure *except*:
A. Hypoxemia
B. Acidosis
C. Hypercapnia
D. Hyperglycemia

29. The critical care nurse positions the patients undergoing a lumbar puncture in a side-lying knee-chest position to:
A. Facilitate access to the spinal canal
B. Restrain the patient and prevent movement
C. Decrease pain through comfort measures
D. Prevent injury to the spinal cord

30. The critical care nurse observes a patient with the neck and back arched and extremities severely extended. This position is called:
A. Decerebrate posturing
B. Decorticate posturing
C. Opisthotonos
D. Jacksonian seizure

31. An infant returns to the critical care unit following placement of a ventriculoperitoneal (VP) shunt. Which of the following positions are optimal for the infant?
I. Supine with the head aligned straight
II. Prone with the head turned to the unaffected side
III. On the affected side
IV. On the unaffected side
A. I or IV
B. I or II
C. I or III
D. II or IV

32. Which of the following nursing interventions would the critical care nurse find *least* helpful in monitoring for complications in an infant following surgical placement of a VP shunt?
A. Measurement of abdominal girth
B. Measurement of head circumference
C. Measurement of chest circumference
D. Measurement of emesis

33. Which of the following is the normal range of intracranial pressure?
A. 0 to 5 mm Hg
B. 5 to 10 mm Hg
C. 0 to 15 mm Hg
D. 10 to 25 mm Hg

34. During the care of an infant, the critical care nurse notes eye rolling and profuse diaphoresis accompanied by tachycardia. The nurse suspects the infant may be:
A. Experiencing a rapid increase in intracranial pressure
B. Exhibiting seizure activity
C. In supraventricular tachycardia
D. Hypoglycemic

35. The cerebral perfusion pressure (CPP) is calculated by:
A. CPP = systolic pressure – intracranial pressure
B. CPP = diastolic pressure – intracranial pressure
C. CPP = systolic pressure – diastolic pressure
D. CPP = mean arterial pressure – intracranial pressure

36. The critical care nurse observes a patient apparently beginning seizure activity. After assessing the airway, the *immediate* priority should be to:
A. Insert an artificial airway
B. Restrain the extremities to protect from injury
C. Observe the seizure activity
D. Administer diazepam

37. Which of the following is the most important factor regulating cerebral blood flow?
A. pO_2
B. pCO_2
C. Acidosis
D. Alkalosis

38. The cerebral perfusion pressure should be:
A. Less than 10 mm Hg
B. Greater than 5 cm H_2O
C. Equal to 50 to 200 mm H_2O
D. Greater than 50 mm Hg

39. Head circumference on an infant should be measured:
A. Directly over the orbits
B. Around the tragus of the ears
C. Above the supraorbital ridges
D. Over the base of the skull

40. Which of the following may be a contraindication to performing a lumbar puncture?
A. Increased intracranial pressure
B. Suspected infection
C. Intracranial hemorrhage
D. Following seizures

41. Barbiturates may be used to treat increased intracranial pressure because their primary effect is to:
A. Promote an oncotic diuresis
B. Decrease metabolic demand
C. Decrease muscular activity
D. Relieve pain

42. When morphine sulfate is used to sedate and/or relieve pain in a patient with increased intracranial pressure, to what would the critical nurse be particularly alert?
A. Level of consciousness
B. Depth of respirations
C. Pupillary response
D. Tachycardia

43. An infant is brought to the critical care unit for uncontrolled seizure activity. The pharmacological treatment of choice would be:
A. Diazepam 0.5 mg/kg
B. Phenobarbital 20 mg/kg
C. Phenytoin 5 mg/kg
D. Dextrose 200 mg/kg

Case Study

A 16-hour-old female infant is admitted to the critical care unit. Her diagnostic workup includes the following information.

pH:	7.21
pO_2:	41 torr
pCO_2:	35 torr
Base deficit:	-8
Blood arterial pressure:	52/43

The tentative diagnosis is sepsis. She received 30 cc/kg of fluids during resuscitative efforts in the emergency room. Questions 44 to 45 refer to this case study.

---

44. Based on these assessment findings, the critical care nurse recognizes that this infant is *most likely* also at risk for developing:
A. Intraventricular hemorrhage
B. Seizures
C. Hydrocephalus
D. Meningitis

45. An immediate nursing priority upon admission to the critical care unit would be:
A. Administer diuretic therapy for fluid overload
B. Administer sodium bicarbonate to correct acidosis
C. Begin vasopressive support to improve perfusion
D. Administer diuretics to decrease intracranial pressure

46. Hypoxic-ischemic encephalopathy is often accompanied by all of the following *except*:
A. Renal dysfunction
B. Necrotizing enterocolitis
C. Metabolic acidosis
D. Hydrocephalus

47. Which of the following symptoms would the critical care nurse recognize as a common sequelae of hypoxic-ischemic encephalopathy?
A. SIADH
B. Nonketotic hyperglycemia
C. Cardiomyopathy
D. Bronchopulmonary dysplasia

48. All of the following can increase intracranial pressure *except*:
A. Turning of the head to one side
B. Mechanical ventilation
C. Tension pneumothorax
D. Elevating the head of the bed

PEDIATRIC-SPECIFIC QUESTIONS

49. A patient in the critical care unit has a systolic pressure of 80 mm Hg, a diastolic pressure of 52 mm Hg, a pulse rate of 110 beats per minute, a respiratory rate of 30, and an intracranial pressure of 20 mm Hg. What is this patient's cerebral perfusion pressure?
A. 61 mm Hg
B. 41 mm Hg
C. 32 mm Hg
D. 66 mm Hg

Case Study

A patient is being admitted to the critical care unit from the emergency room. He was brought in by his parents because he had had a seizure 1 hour ago and fever, chills, and vomiting for 24 hours. Questions 50 to 52 refer to this case study.

50. When receiving a transfer report from the emergency room, the critical care nurse is told the patient is agitated and has a positive Brudzinski's sign. This sign indicates:
A. Increased intracranial pressure
B. Meningeal irritation
C. Encephalitis
D. Intraventricular hemorrhage

51. Based on these findings, the critical care nurse suspects the patient has:
A. Encephalitis
B. Meningitis
C. Intracerebral bleeding
D. Brain abscess

52. The nurse would also expect to find on physical examination which of the following findings:
A. Kernig's sign
B. Cullen's sign
C. Chvostek's sign
D. Trousseau's sign

53. A 7-year-old boy has been admitted to the critical care unit, with his parents at the bedside, following a bicycle-motor vehicle accident. As the nurse applies electrocardiogram electrodes to his chest, she explains the purpose and he responds by nodding and looking away. The nurse explains that blood must be drawn and asks his parents to leave the room. He continues to look away and offers no protest as his parents leave. The critical care nurse interprets this behavior as a child who possibly:
A. Is very cooperative and mature for his age
B. Is too frightened to protest
C. Has compromised neurological or cardiopulmonary function
D. Has a poor relationship with his parents

54. A 15-year-old boy is a patient following a head injury from a baseball. During the first hours after admission, he sleeps unless awakened, but can be aroused easily and is oriented. The critical care nurse correctly documents this condition as:
A. Semicomatose
B. Lethargy
C. Obtunded
D. Stuporus

55. An advantage of an intraventricular catheter in monitoring intracranial pressure over other methods includes:
A. Less invasiveness into the brain
B. Ability to inject medications
C. Reduced rate of infection
D. Ability to block leakage of CSF

56. After receiving a blow to the head, an 8-year-old girl is diagnosed with having an epidural bleed. This type of bleeding is usually associated with:
A. Arterial bleeding
B. Venous bleeding
C. Bleeding into the brain tissue
D. Intraventricular bleeding

57. When returning from neurosurgery, the critical care nurse would *first* assess:
A. Systemic perfusion
B. Orientation
C. Presence of reflexes
D. Pupillary response

58. A 5-year-old boy is admitted after being involved in a motor vehicle accident in which he did not wear a seat belt. He is complaining of numbness and tingling in his legs and feet, and has decreased sensation. His x-rays are normal and show no evidence of fractures or other abnormalities. The critical care nurse plans care to include:
A. Removing the cervical collar
B. Discontinuing log rolling to turn the patient
C. Administration of antianxiety medications
D. Continuation of spinal cord protective measures

59. Following complaints of headache, unexplained emesis, blurring vision, and change in ability to perform daily physical activities, a 13-year-old girl is admitted to the critical care unit with a diagnosis of astrocytoma. Following the initiation of antineoplastic therapy, the critical care nurse observes the patient closely for all of the following *except*:
A. Sepsis
B. Increased intracranial pressure
C. Hydrocephalus
D. Intraventricular hemorrhage

60. A 6-year-old male victim of a pedestrian-motor vehicle accident has shown no neurological deficits in his extremities during the 2 hours since his admission to the critical care unit. When planning his care, the critical care nurse writes nursing orders to continue with complete neurological assessments every hour. The best reason for this action is:

A. All the diagnostic tests have not been completed to rule out neurological injuries
B. Onset of neurological manifestations of injury are often delayed in children
C. Neurological assessments for sensation and pain are often unreliable in children of this age group
D. Neurological assessments are a poor indicator of neurological function and injury

NEONATAL-SPECIFIC QUESTIONS

61. Preterm infants are prone to intraventricular hemorrhages because they:

A. Frequently have clotting disorders
B. Are more likely to receive trauma to the head during delivery
C. Have more vascularization in the ventricular areas
D. Have higher intracranial pressures

62. A preterm infant is at greatest risk for an intraventricular hemorrhage at what age?

A. 1 to 3 days
B. 7 days
C. 30 days
D. 60 days

63. In preterm infants, the most common source of bleeding in an intraventricular hemorrhage is the:

A. Choroid plexus
B. Arachnoid villae
C. Germinal matrix
D. Meningeal artery

64. Neonatal seizures related to pyridoxine deficiency are related to a deficiency in:

A. Vitamin C
B. Iron
C. Magnesium
D. Vitamin B_6

Answers

GENERAL NEUROLOGY CARE ANSWERS

1. **Correct answer—A.**
Cerebrospinal fluid is continuously formed by the choroid plexus found in the ventricles of the brain. The arachnoid villae are responsible for absorbing cerebrospinal fluid, which prevents excess quantities. The pia mater is the innermost layer of the meninges.

2. **Correct answer—C.**
Hypotension is not a sign of increased intracranial pressure. Signs and symptoms of an increase in intracranial pressure in infants include lethargy, irritability, bradycardia, tachycardia, apnea, bulging fontanels, vomiting, and *hyper*tension.

3. **Correct answer—D.**
Skull x-rays would be least helpful in identifying an intracranial bleed because they poorly image soft tissue and do not image blood flow. They would be most useful in diagnosing skull fractures or other disorders of the bones in the skull. Computerized axial tomography is a very important test used to diagnose intracranial hemorrhages as well as tumors, hematomas, brain abscesses, hydrocephalus, and other conditions. Cerebral blood flow studies are also helpful in diagnosing intracranial hemorrhages by identifying areas of the brain not receiving blood flow or identifying hemorrhagic areas. A lumbar puncture may be useful if blood has entered the cerebrospinal fluid (CSF).

4. **Correct answer—C.**
The priority in assessing any critically ill patient follows the ABC rule—airway, breathing, and circulation. The first priority would be to establish the patient's ability to maintain a patent airway. Pupillary reaction and level of consciousness provide important information about the patient's neurological status. Determining the blood glucose level is also important because hypoglycemia may actually cause or contribute to neurological dysfunction. However, neither the neurological assessment nor the blood glucose determination would be the *first* priority in ensuring the patient's immediate safety.

5. **Correct answer—D.**
Signs and symptoms of mild hypoxic-ischemic encephalopathy would not include any symptoms as severe as hypotonia. See Table 5-3 for clinical manifestations of mild, moderate, and severe hypoxic-ischemic encephalopathy.

6. **Correct answer—A.**
Intubation of an infant with hypoxic-ischemic encephalopathy can help reduce intracranial pressure by controlling the levels of carbon dioxide. Through

hyperventilation, pCO_2 levels can be reduced, which in turn cause vasoconstriction in the brain, helping to reduce intracranial volume and pressure. Seizure activity is best controlled by controlling the underlying cause such as hypoxia or metabolic derangements. However, following a hypoxic-ischemic episode, adequate oxygenation alone may not prevent seizures that need to be further controlled with anticonvulsant therapy. Optimal oxygenation through intubation and mechanical ventilation can help prevent long-term complications associated with further hypoxemia, but cannot prevent complications from the neurological damage that has already occurred. Hypocarbia is the state in which mechanical ventilation seeks to achieve to reduce intracranial pressure. Reduction of hypocarbia would be counterproductive by increasing intracranial pressure through cerebral vasodilation.

7. Correct answer—C.

Decreased resorption of CSF (communicating hydrocephalus) and obstruction to flow of CSF (noncommunicating hydrocephalus) are the most common mechanisms of the development of hydrocephalus. While increased production of CSF rarely occurs, most cases of hydrocephalus result from an obstruction to the normal flow and circulation of CSF causing an accumulation of fluid and increased intracranial pressure. Obstruction of flow may result from congenital anomalies, inflammation, external blockage, and other causes. Increased resorption and decreased production of CSF would not cause hydrocephalus because there would not be an accumulation of CSF in these cases.

8. Correct answer—C.

Coarctation of the aorta results in a left-to-right cardiac shunt when the ductus arteriosus and atrial septum are open and, therefore, oxygenated systemic blood is maintained. In a left-to-right shunt, blood flow is shunted from the oxygenated systemic circulation (left side) to the unoxygenated pulmonary system (right side). Pulmonary blood flow is *increased,* not decreased, and there is no mixing of unoxygenated blood into the systemic circulation. Infants at risk for developing hypoxic-ischemic encephalopathy include those with severe cyanotic congenital cardiac disease such as pulmonary atresia (right-to-left shunt), those with respiratory failure, apnea, idiopathic respiratory distress syndrome (IRDS), persistent pulmonary hypertension (persistent fetal circulation), intrauterine asphyxia, and cardiovascular collapse secondary to sepsis or other causes.

9. Correct answer—A.

The highest priority in treating seizures is always treatment of the cause. Correcting metabolic imbalances such a hypoglycemia, and disturbances in electrolytes such as calcium, sodium, and magnesium are always the first priorities. Administering prophylactic anticonvulsant therapy is not indicated until a cause has been identified and treated whenever possible. While obtaining an EEG may be helpful, it does not reveal a diagnosis in many cases. Obtaining a lumbar puncture is important diagnostic information when a cause is not known, but treating a cause is still the first priority over diagnostic tests.

10. Correct answer—A.
By offering a pacifier or gloved finger to suck on, a nurse can help differentiate tremors from seizures. If the movement stops immediately with sucking, and starts when sucking ceases, the observed motor behavior is most likely tremors. If sucking has no effect, seizure activity is suspected. Holding the infant's arms will not provide any differential information. Nystagmus may be present with some seizure activity, but its absence does not rule out seizures. Finally, not all seizures are accompanied by a change in the level of consciousness.

11. Correct answer—B.
Most neonatal seizures result from a loss of inhibitory control. Rather than increased excitatory stimulation, it is most often a lack of inhibitory control that results in seizure activity. Seizure activity is often characterized by inappropriate repetitive behaviors.

12. Correct answer—D.
While all these symptoms are characteristic of hydrocephalus, emesis would signify the most severe deterioration. Emesis results when pressure has built up so much that even the lower brainstem area is affected. Lethargy, sluggish pupillary response, and lower extremity spasticity generally develop earlier and with less severe rises in pressure. Emesis may, however, occur early and quickly if the intracranial pressure rises quickly and severely.

13. Correct answer—D.
The test most helpful in diagnosing and evaluating hydrocephalus are computerized axial tomography (CT scan) and magnetic resonance imaging (MRI). These tests help identify and differentiate tissue densities and tissue from fluids. Skull x-rays would give little information about the size of the ventricles and whether they are engorged with CSF. While ultrasonography provides excellent imaging, the CT and MRI scans generally provide superior diagnostic information.

14. Correct answer—B.
A ventriculoperitoneal (VP) shunt is used to decrease hydrocephalus by providing a route for the accumulated fluid to escape. Gagging associated with suctioning is a positive finding following placement of a VP shunt because it demonstrates a reduction in intracranial pressure allowing brainstem reflexes to function normally. Despite the need to reduce intracranial pressure, a rapid reduction can result in subdural hematoma. Firm, round fontanels and dilated scalp veins usually indicate a persistently increased intracranial pressure (ICP).

15. Correct answer—C.
An intraventricular hemorrhage is usually associated with preterm infants and is not a complication of a VP shunt. Common complications associated with VP shunts include subdural hematoma from rapid reduction in ICP, peritonitis, meningitis, septicemia, ventriculitis, and an abdominal abscess.

16. Correct answer—A.

A lumbar puncture in an infant with encephalopathy generally produces normal findings such as these presented in this question. The CSF pressure is generally normal because there is no increase in CSF as would be found in hydrocephalus. The red blood cell count is essentially 0, whereas with an intraventricular bleed the red cell count would be high as a result of the presence of blood in the CSF. Both bacterial and viral meningitis would result in an elevation of the white blood cell count of CSF, with bacterial meningitis causing the largest increase. Protein and glucose levels would also be expected to be raised in bacterial meningitis. CSF pressure may rise in bacterial meningitis if the choroid plexes are obstructed by exudate.

17. Correct answer—B.

A sympathomimetic drug would be expected to produce bronchodilation, pupillary dilatation, tachycardia, increased blood pressure, decreased blood flow to the gut, and decreased bladder tone. By stimulating or mimicking the effect of the sympathetic nervous system, these drugs cause a "flight or fight" response in the body. Each of these manifestations assists the body by supporting only essential body functions for an emergency situation.

18. Correct answer—B.

Cushing's triad consists of a widening pulse pressure, bradycardia, and slow or irregular respirations. While pupillary dilatation is often associated with an increase in intracranial pressure, it is not part of Cushing's triad, a medical emergency indicating a severe increase in intracranial pressure.

19. Correct answer—D.

In order to help decrease intracranial pressure, cerebral venous drainage is promoted by placing the patient in a supine position with the head of the bed elevated and the head *not* turned to either side. By facilitating cerebral venous drainage, the intravascular volume of the brain is reduced, helping to reduce the ICP. Laying in a lateral position or turning the head can cause the neck to be malaligned and decrease the cerebral venous return. While supine is the optimal position, raising the head of the bed further optimizes venous drainage.

20. Correct answer—B.

The therapeutic serum level of phenytoin is 10 to 25 mcg/dL. Toxic levels are considered to be 30 to 50 mcg/dL.

21: Correct answer—A.

In caring for a patient who has received diazepam for acute seizure activity, the critical care nurse would observe for laryngospasm, hypotension, respiratory depression, and cardiopulmonary arrest. Cushing's triad is seen with increased intracranial pressure and would not be directly related to the use of diazepam. Cardiac dysrhythmias are potential adverse reactions to the use of phenytoin.

22. Correct answer—C.
Isolation is indicated for bacterial meningitis until antibiotics have been given for 24 hours. Isolation must be maintained until the antibiotics have been administered for a full 24 hours to ensure that the bacteria has been affected, but need not to be continued for the entire duration of pharmacologic therapy.

23. Correct answer—A.
Anencephalic neonates are generally not suitable organ donors because they frequently have in intact brainstem that allows then to breath spontaneously, withdraw to pain, swallow, and even suck. They do not typically have multiple anomalies but frequently have normal organ systems and functioning in all other areas. These newborns have no higher incidence of congenital infection than other neonates.

24. Correct answer—D.
Fluid restrictions are generally not helpful in treating hydrocephalus following an intraventricular hemorrhage. Hydrocephalus associated with intraventricular hemorrhages is believed to be related not to increased production of cerebrospinal fluid, but rather to blockage of the resorption mechanism by blood clots. Ventricular taps, diuretic therapy, and serial lumbar taps all may be used to control excessive cerebrospinal pressure.

25. Correct answer—B.
The assessment findings and results of the diagnostic tests suggest an intraventricular hemorrhage. The presence of a large number of erythrocytes (red blood cells are normally absent) indicates a bleed within the cerebrospinal fluid system. Hydrocephalus is an increase in cerebrospinal fluid, but does not include bleeding. An intracerebral hematoma is bleeding within the brain tissue itself and would not necessarily be associated with bleeding within the cerebrospinal fluid system. Encephalitis is an inflammation of brain tissue, but also is not associated with bleeding within the CSF.

26. Correct answer—B.
Skull x-rays would be least helpful in diagnosing an intraventricular bleed because of its relative insensitivity to visualizing soft tissues, vessels, and blood. Ultrasonography would probably be the diagnostic test of choice because it can be done quickly, at the bedside, and would not require sedation.

27. Correct answer—C.
The priorities in treating any critically ill patient are to establish an airway, ensure breathing, and facilitate adequate circulation. This neonate is showing signs of circulatory insufficiency that require intravascular volume support and vasopressor therapy. Correcting the acidosis and typing and cross matching for blood products are also important interventions, but adequate circulation must be established first. Sending the CSF for cultures is not the greatest priority for this diagnosis and in the resuscitative phase of treatment.

28. Correct answer—D.
Hyperglycemia can actually cause an oncotic diuresis resulting in intracellular dehydration of brain cells and decreased cranial volume. Intracranial pressure is increased by hypoxemia, acidosis, and hypercapnia because each of these conditions causes vasodilation of cerebral vessels in an attempt to increase oxygen delivery and remove excessive acids and carbon dioxide.

29. Correct answer—A.
The critical care nurse positions the patient undergoing a lumbar puncture in a side-lying knee-chest position to facilitate access to the spinal canal. A knee-chest position helps open the intravertebral spaces and allow easier access to the spinal canal. This position does not make it easier to restrain the patient's movements or decrease the patient's pain. A lumbar puncture is performed below the level of the spinal cord nerves, so injury to the spinal cord is avoided simply by performing the tap below L4.

30. Correct answer—C.
This position of the neck and back arched and extremities severely extended is called opisthotonos, which is seen in patients with severe increases in intracranial pressure.

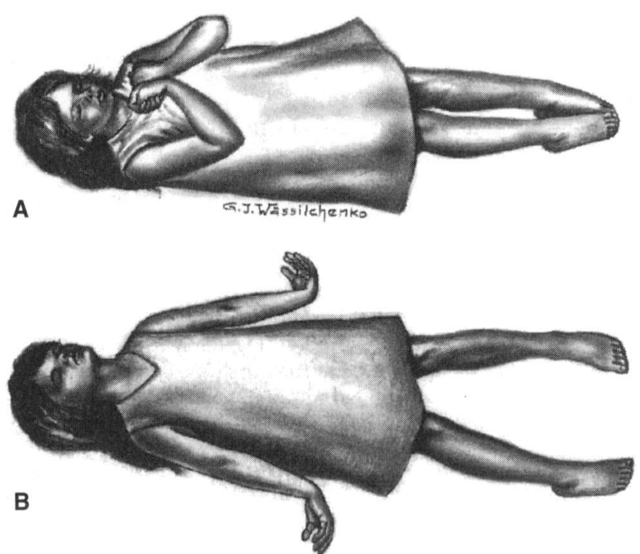

A, Decorticate posturing. **B,** Decerebrate posturing. (From Wong, 1995.)

31. Correct answer—A.
A postoperative infant with a ventriculoperitoneal shunt is most safely and effectively positioned in the supine position or laying laterally on the unaffected side. Laying on the affected side may be acceptable if a doughnut-shaped support is used to protect the site. Turning the head, which is generally required if

laying in the prone position, does not promote cerebral venous return and may contribute to increased intracranial pressure.

32. Correct answer—C.
Measurement of chest circumference to monitor for complications in an infant following surgical placement of a VP shunt would not be helpful because the infant has no risk of an increase or decrease in measurement. Assessment of the abdominal girth and measurement of any emesis is very helpful because these infants are at risk for ileus. Measurement of head circumference would give important information if the shunt were not functioning properly and a buildup of CSF occurred.

33. Correct answer—C.
The normal range of intracranial pressure is 0 to 15 mm Hg or 0 to 18 cm H_2O.

34. Correct answer—B.
Eye rolling and profuse diaphoresis accompanied by tachycardia may be indicative of seizure activity. Other often less obvious seizure activity may be accompanied by eye blinking, lip smacking, sucking, bicycling movements, swimming movements, and apnea.

35. Correct answer—D.
The cerebral perfusion pressure (CPP) is calculated by subtracting the intracranial pressure from the mean arterial pressure: CPP = MAP – ICP

36. Correct answer—C.
The immediate nursing care priority for a patient experiencing seizures should be to observe the seizure activity to help in diagnosis and treatment as well as protect from injury. Protecting from injury does *not* include restraining the patient. This can lead to injuries from the force of muscle contractions. Inserting an artificial airway once seizure activity has begun often is not possible and may actually cause injury to mucous membranes and/or teeth. Anticonvulsant agents are administered only with a physician's order.

37. Correct answer—B.
The most important factor regulating cerebral blood flow is the pCO_2. While pO_2 acidosis and alkalosis all affect cerebral blood flow, the greatest regulator is pCO_2. An increase in pCO_2 causes an increase in cerebral blood flow, whereas a decrease in pCO_2, causes a decrease in cerebral blood flow.

38. Correct answer—D.
The cerebral perfusion pressure should be greater than 50 mm Hg. Cerebral perfusion pressure is calculated by subtracting the intracranial pressure from the mean arterial pressure. An adequate CPP must be maintained to ensure perfusion of the brain.

39. Correct answer—C.
Head circumference on an infant should be measured above the supraorbital ridges to the most distant point over the occipital region. This should provide the largest measurement and serve as a standard for each caregiver to use.

40. Correct answer—A.
Increased intracranial pressure may be a contraindication to performing a lumber puncture because rapid release of the pressure can result in herniation of the brain. A lumber tap may actually be performed to diagnose a central nervous system infection or some intracranial hemorrhages. There is no specific contraindication to lumbar tap following seizure activity.

41. Correct answer—B.
Barbituates may be used to treat intracranial pressure because their primary effect is to decrease metabolic demand of the brain cells. Diuretics such as mannitol and furosemide are used to promote oncotic diuresis. Activity is most effectively reduced by using muscular paralyzing agents such as vecuronium or pancuronium. Relieving pain and reducing anxiety can be best achieved by using morphine sulfate.

42. Correct answer—B.
When morphine sulfate is used to sedate and/or relieve pain in a patient with increased intracranial pressure, the critical care nurse must be particularly alert to the depth and rate of respirations. Morphine sulfate can cause respiratory depression, thus increasing pCO_2 and, in turn, cerebral blood flow and intracranial pressure.

43. Correct answer—B.
For an infant with uncontrolled seizure activity, the pharmacological treatment of choice would be phenobarbital 20 mg/kg as a loading dose. Phenytoin may also be used at the same dosage. Diazepam 0.3 mg/kg may be used if neither phenytoin or phenobarbital are effective. Dextrose should only be given if hypoglycemia is verified.

44. Correct answer—A.
Based on these assessment findings, the critical care nurse recognizes that this infant is most likely also at risk for developing an intraventricular hemorrhage. Factors identified as related to intraventricular hemorrhages include hypernatremia, blood transfusions, shock, acidosis, seizures, and rapid volume expansion.

45. Correct answer—C.
An immediate nursing priority upon admission to the critical care unit would be to begin vasopressive support to improve perfusion, which in turn would help reverse acidosis. The infant has received large amounts of fluid resuscitation, indicating that vasopressive support may be required to improve perfusion. Diuretic therapy would not be indicated until adequate perfusion has been

achieved. There is no evidence suggesting increased intracranial pressure. Sodium bicarbonate may be helpful, but would not correct the underlying metabolic acidosis related to poor perfusion.

46. Correct answer—D.
Hypoxic-ischemic encephalopathy is often accompanied by renal dysfunction, necrotizing enterocolitis and other gastrointestinal disorders, metabolic acidosis, and/or cardiac dysfunction. All these conditions are a result of severe, systemic hypoxia. Hydrocephalus does not result from hypoxia.

47. Correct answer—A.
Common sequelae of hypoxic-ischemic encephalopathy include syndrome of inappropriate antidiuretic hormone (SIADH) secretion, seizures, and general organ systems dysfunction or failure.

48. Correct answer—D.
Elevating the head of the bed can actually help decrease intracranial pressure by promoting cerebral venous return with the help of gravity. Intracranial pressure can be increased in numerous ways. Turning the head to one side may obstruct cerebral venous return by obstructing internal venous jugular flow. Mechanical ventilation, especially with high inspiratory pressures, may also impede venous return, including cerebral venous return, which in turn raises intracranial pressure. A tension pneumothorax may also impede venous return and raise the ICP. Other conditions that increase cerebral blood flow and therefore increase intracranial pressure include hypercarbia, acidosis, anemia, vasodilators, seizures, and hyperthyroidism.

PEDIATRIC-SPECIFIC ANSWERS

49. Correct answer—B.
Cerebral perfusion pressure (CPP) is calculated by subtracting the intracranial pressure (ICP) from the mean arterial pressure (MAP).

$$\text{CPP} = \text{MAP} - \text{ICP}$$

The MAP is calculated from the following formula:

$$\text{MAP} = \frac{\text{systolic pressure} + (2 \times \text{diastolic pressure})}{3}$$

Using this formula, the MAP $= \frac{80 + 2(52)}{3} = \frac{184}{3} = 61$ mm Hg

$$\text{CPP} = \text{MAP} - \text{ICP}$$

$$\text{CPP} = 61 - 20 = 41$$

50. Correct answer—B.

Brudzinski's sign indicates meningeal irritation. As the head and neck are flexed toward the chest, the legs flex at both the hips and the knees in response. Encephalitis, increased intracranial pressure, and intraventricular hemorrhage do not result in meningeal irritation.

51. Correct answer—B.

Based on these findings, the critical care nurse suspects the patient has meningitis. The history of recent illness including fever and chills suggests an infectious process. The assessment finding of Brudzinksi's sign indicates meningeal irritation and supports a diagnosis of meningitis.

52. Correct answer—A.

The nurse would also expect to find on physical examination Kernig's sign, which is pain when the patient attempts to extend the knee with the hip flexed. Like Kernig's sign, this sign indicates meningeal irritation. Cullen's sign is ecchymosis around the umbilicus seen with hemorrhagic pancreatitis. Chvostek's and Trousseau's signs are seen with hypocalcemia.

53. Correct answer—C.

Failure of a child to protest separation from parents or concerning painful procedures needs to be considered abnormal until proven otherwise. The most frequent reasons include compromised neurological or cardiopulmonary function. While a child may be unusually cooperative, separating him from his parents and informing him of a painful procedure should elicit a response. No information about his relationship with his parents should be drawn from this limited interaction.

54. Correct answer—C.

Obtundation is characterized by sleepiness, but when aroused, the patient is oriented. Semicomatose is when a patient responds only to painful stimuli. Lethargy is when a patient sleeps if left undisturbed, but is normally alert when awake. Stuporus is characterized by sleep when left undisturbed, and when awakened the patient is incoherent.

55. Correct answer—B.

Advantages of an intraventricular catheter in monitoring intracranial pressure over other methods include the ability to inject medications directly into the ventricles, to directly sample CSF, and the ability to remove CSF to control intracranial pressure. Placement of an intraventricular catheter is an invasive procedure that can cause trauma to brain tissue. There is an increased rate of infection associated with its use as a result of its invasive nature and direct access to brain tissue.

56. Correct answer—A.

Epdiural bleeding is usually arterial and occurs between the inside of the skull and the peripheral aspect of the dura mater. Venous bleeding is usually associated with subdural bleeding. Bleeding into the brain tissue itself is called intracerebral bleeding. Intraventricular bleeding occurs because of disruption of blood vessels within the ventricles, not surrounding the dura mater.

57. Correct answer—A.
When returning from neurosurgery, the critical care nurse would first assess the airway, breathing, and circulation. These assessments always take priority. Systemic perfusion should be assessed by noting peripheral pulses as well as color, warmth, and capillary refill of extremities. Other assessments such as orientation, presence of reflexes, and pupillary response would follow.

58. Correct answer—D.
Despite the lack or radiographic confirmation of a spinal cord injury, the signs and symptoms exhibited by this patient continue to suggest this injury. A large number of children with spinal cord injuries do *not* exhibit x-ray confirmation of the injury. The critical care nurse should continue to keep the patient's neck and spinal cord immobilized until other tests confirm the injury or the symptoms subside.

59. Correct answer—D.
Following the initiation of antineoplastic therapy, the patient is at no particular risk for intraventricular hemorrhage. However, the critical care nurse observes the patient closely for sepsis related to impairment of the immune system from antineoplastic drugs; increased intracranial pressure from edema, inflammation, or continued tumor growth; and hydrocephalus from impingement of the CSF circulation by tumor growth.

60. Correct answer—B.
When planning the care of a child at risk for spinal cord injury, the critical care nurse should continue with complete neurological assessments every hour even if deficits are not apparent in early assessments. The onset of neurological manifestations of injury are often delayed in children, and the lack of early deficits do not rule out injuries. Diagnostic tests may be helpful in diagnosing a spinal cord injury; however, a large number of children have injuries without radiographic evidence. Neurological assessments for sensation and pain are reliable in children of this age group when performed correctly and any information given by the child should be used in evaluating his condition. Neurological assessments are an excellent indicator of neurological function and injury, but must be used in conjunction with other information and evaluation over time.

NEONATAL-SPECIFIC ANSWERS

61. Correct answer—C.
Preterm infants are prone to intraventricular hemorrhages because they have more vascularization in the ventricular areas. During prenatal life, there is a large and fragile vascular network in the area of the ventricles that receives a

large amount of blood flow. Any event that causes increased blood flow to the brain, such as hypoxia, increases the blood flow and therefore pressure within these fragile vessels, leading to intraventricular hemorrhages. While clotting disorders may be frequently seen in preterm infants as a result of liver dysfunction, metabolic dysfunction, and sepsis, it is not a primary cause of intraventricular hemorrhages. Frequency of head trauma during delivery does not play a major role in intraventricular hemorrhages in preterm infants. Preterm infants only have higher intracranial pressures in the presence of pathology such as hypoxic-ischemic encephalopathy.

62. Correct answer—A.

A preterm infant is at greatest risk for an intraventricular hemorrhage at 1 to 3 days when approximately 90% of the bleeds occur.

63. Correct answer—C.

In preterm infants, the most common source of bleeding in an intraventricular hemorrhage is the germinal matrix. The choroid plexus is the most common site in full term infants. The arachnoid villae are responsible for reabsorption of CSF. The middle meningeal artery is often responsible for epidural bleeds.

64. Correct answer—D.

Neonatal seizures attributed to pyridoxine deficiency are related to a deficiency in vitamin B_6. If seizure activity cannot be attributed to an imbalance of electrolytes, hypoxemia, or hypoglycemia, and is unresponsive to phenobarbital, pyridoxine should be given intravenously at a 50 to 100 mg bolus.

CHAPTER 6

Gastrointestinal Care Problems

Passkeys

GENERAL PRINCIPLES OF GASTROENTEROLOGY

- During fetal life, the placenta performs more nutritional and waste disposal functions than the gastrointestinal (GI) tract.
- The gastrointestinal tract in infants does not reach functional maturity until approximately 2 years of age.
- Assessment of the gastrointestinal system should begin with inspection followed by auscultation, then percussion and palpation. Leaving percussion and palpation for last prevents artificially increasing bowel sounds assessed during auscultation.

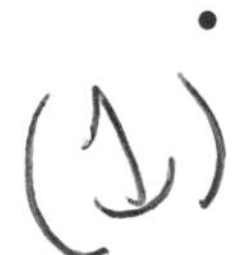

- Gastroeosphageal reflux in infants is a common problem related to the relative functional immaturity of the lower esophageal sphincter (LES). The LES may remain marginally functional until approximately 1 to 6 months of life.
- Adult levels of hydrochloric acid secretion in the GI tract are not reached until approximately 6 months of age.
- The gastrointestinal tract plays an important function in maintaining fluid and electrolyte balance.
- The stomach secretes hydrochloric acid, pepsinogen, and intrinsic factor as digestion is initiated.
- The stomach secretes bicarbonate ions and mucus to protect itself from autodigestion.
- Liquids empty from the stomach more quickly than solids.
- Hypertonic and acidic contents empty from the stomach slowly.
- Children with continuous tube feedings often have residuals of 50% from the previous hour's infusion.
- The splanchnic circulation supplies the stomach and small and large intestines.
- Venous drainage from the stomach, pancreas, and small and large intestines empties into the portal circulation and in turn goes to the liver before emptying into the hepatic vein and inferior vena cava on the way to the heart.

- The small intestine is comprised of the duodenum, jejunum, and ileum. Fats, vitamins, amino acids, and sugars are digested and absorbed primarily in the duodenum and jejunum.
- The cells lining the small intestine turnover rapidly. Failure to feed, malnutrition, ischemia, and other conditions such as infections can seriously affect the small bowel's functional ability.
- The large intestines (colon) are important in reabsorbing water and electrolytes. They store the waste products (feces) for eventual elimination.
- Accessory digestive organs include the pancreas, liver, gallbladder, and salivary glands.
- The pancreas performs important exocrine functions (digestive enzyme and bicarbonate production) and endocrine functions (insulin production).
- Important functions of the liver are found in the following box.
- Caloric requirements are generally highest for the youngest of patients, decreasing with increasing age. Many diseases and illnesses increase caloric needs. See Table 6-1.
- Signs and symptoms of peritonitis associated with gastrointestinal disorders signify a critical emergency. See the accompanying box.

Functions of the Liver

Formation of Clotting Factors	**Storage Site**
clotting factor I	glycogen
clotting factor II	fat-soluable vitamins
clotting factor V	fat
clotting factor VII	**Metabolic Activity**
clotting factor IX	fat
clotting factor X	carbohydrates
clotting factor XI	protein
Synthesis	**Detoxification**
plasma proteins	medications
bile	bilirubin

Table 6-1
Nutritional Requirements for Infants and Children

Age	Calories/kg/24 hr	
Up to 6 mo	120	
6-12 mo	100	
12-36 mo	90-95	
4 yr-10 yr	80	
>10 yr, male	45	
>10 yr, female	38	
Nutrient	**Percent of Total Calories**	
Carbohydrates	40%-45%	Combined 85%-88%
Fat	40%	
Protein	20%	

From Hazinski MF: Nursing care of the critically ill child, ed 2, St Louis, 1992, Mosby.

Signs and Symptoms of Peritonitis

Fever

Abdominal tenderness, especially rebound tenderness

Abdominal rigidity and distension

Diffuse abdominal pain

Nausea and vomiting

Decreased bowel sounds

CONGENITAL GASTROINTESTINAL ABNORMALITIES
Omphalocele

- An omphalocele is the protrusion of abdominal contents including intestines, liver, and/or spleen through the umbilicus. The membranous covering of the contents may have been torn during delivery or ruptured in utero.

- An omphalocele occurs early in gestation, approximately at 10 to 11 weeks.
- Omphaloceles are usually seen in conjunction with other congenital anomalies.
- Neonates with omphaloceles are prone to hypothermia, dehydration, hypoproteinemia, hypoglycemia, shock, and respiratory distress.
- An infant with an omphalocele is not given anything by mouth, and a nasogastric tube is used to decompress the stomach.
- Postoperative care includes antibiotic therapy as well as fluid and electrolyte management. Total parenteral nutrition may be required for long periods postoperatively until the bowel begins to function.

Gastroschisis

- Gastroschisis is the protrusion of abdominal contents through the abdominal wall at a site other than the umbilicus.
- This defect begins earlier than omphaloceles, at about 5 weeks gestation.
- In gastroschisis, there is no thin covering of the protruding contents, which are usually found to the right of the umbilicus.
- This defect may or may not be seen in conjunction with other congenital anomalies.
- Neonates with gastroschisis are prone to hypothermia, dehydration, hypoproteinemia, hypoglycemia, shock, and respiratory distress.
- Before surgical correction, the gastroschisis should be covered with sterile, moist gauze and plastic wrap to avoid fluid loss.
- An infant with gastroschisis is not given anything by mouth, and a nasogastric tube is used to decompress the stomach.
- Postoperative care includes antibiotic therapy as well as fluid and electrolyte management. Total parenteral nutrition may be required for long periods postoperatively until the bowel begins to function.

Volvulus

- A volvulus occurs when the bowel fails to rotate normally at 10 to 12 weeks gestation. Blood circulation to the entire bowel is threatened.
- Most infants with a volvulus do not show symptoms for 3 days to 3 weeks following birth.

Table 6-2
Clinical Problems Associated with Abnormalities of Intestinal Rotation

Stage	Problem
Nonrotation	Midgut volvulus Duodenal obstruction
Incomplete rotation	Midgut volvulus Duodenal obstruction Internal hernia Colonic obstruction (reverse rotation)
Incomplete fixation	Internal hernia Cecal volvulus

From Blumer JL: A practical guide to pediatric intensive care, ed 3, St Louis, 1990, Mosby.

- Symptoms develop rapidly. The abdomen becomes distended, vomiting and pain are significant, and the infant experiences shock often accompanied by bloody stools.

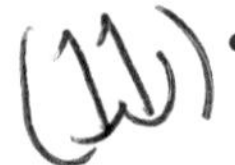

- Hyperkalemia and hypocalcemia often accompany acute symptoms of a volvulus. These may be significant enough to cause cardiac dysrhythmias.
- This condition is a surgical emergency requiring correction within hours of symptom onset to prevent necrosis of affected intestines.
- See Table 6-2 for clinical conditions associated with malrotation of the gut.
- See *Pediatric-Specific Principles* for information about volvulus in older infants and children.

BOWEL INFARCTION/OBSTRUCTION/PERFORATION
Necrotizing Enterocolitis (NEC)

- Necrotizing enterocolitis (NEC) is a disease that most often strikes the ileum and colon, resulting in necrotic ulcerations that may be either diffuse or local.
- NEC most often afflicts low birth weight preterm infants.
- Risk factors for the development of NEC are found in the box on p. 301.
- Ischemia to the intestinal tract often can occur in utero or during the perinatal period.

Risk Factors for the Development of Necrotizing Enterocolitis

Prenatal

Premature rupture of membranes

Perinatal

Low birth weight

Gestation of less than 36 weeks

Asphyxia

Postnatal

Infection

Sepsis

Colonization of *Clostridia*

Polycythemia

Early enteral feeding of premature infant

Hypotension

Shock

Congestive heart failure

Patent ductus arteriosus

Umbilical artery catheterization

Exchange transfusion

- In the ill or severely compromised neonate, blood may be shunted away from the gut to more vital organs such as the brain and heart. During these periods of intestinal ischemia, NEC can begin.
- Once cells in the intestinal tract are compromised by ischemia, they stop secreting protective mucus and the intestinal wall is attacked by digestive (proteolytic) enzymes.
- During NEC, the gut is also ineffective in the synthesis of IgM (immunoglobulin M) so toxins, bacteria, and viruses can more easily gain access to the bloodstream.
- Signs and symptoms of NEC are outlined in the box on p. 302.
- The presence of pneumatosis intestinalis is diagnostic of NEC. This is air seen in the submucosa of the intestines from bacterial invasion. It is often identified by x-ray or during laparotomy.
- Early feeding with breast milk may be an important measure in preventing NEC.
- NEC is treated with prompt cessation of oral feedings, gastric drainage and decompression, discontinuance of umbilical catheters, intravenous antibiotics, intravenous fluids, and parenteral nutrition. Surgical intervention may be required to remove necrotic bowel.
- Indications for surgical intervention include the presence of free air in the abdomen, peritonitis, shock, metabolic acidosis, respiratory failure, and necrotic bowel.

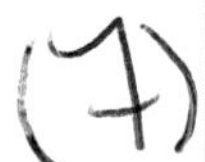

Signs and Symptoms of Necrotizing Enterocolitis	
Abdominal tenderness	Apnea
Abdominal distension	Bradycardia
Gross or occult blood in the stools	Inability to maintain normal body temperature
Decreased bowel sounds	Oliguria secondary to renal dysfuction
Increased residuals if enterally fed	Shock
Vomiting	Hypotension
Lethargy	

- Ileostomies are often necessary because the ends of the resected bowel are inflamed or ischemic.
- Measure abdominal girths and assess all stools for occult blood when caring for the neonate with NEC.
- Do not assess temperatures rectally in the neonate with NEC. Perforation of an inflamed bowel is a serious complication.
- Position the neonate with NEC supine or side-lying to avoid pressure on a distended, often tender, abdomen.
- Oral feedings are usually not begun for at least 7 to 10 days following diagnosis and treatment, but may be delayed for 2 to 3 months or more, depending upon each neonate's clinical course.
- When reintroducing gut feedings following treatment for NEC, usually sterile water or electrolyte solutions are given first, followed by breast milk or predigested formulas.
- Common complications of severe NEC include disseminated intravascular coagulation, sepsis, fistulas, abscesses, and intestinal obstruction.

PEDIATRIC-SPECIFIC PRINCIPLES

CONGENITAL GASTROINTESTINAL ABNORMALITIES

Intussusception

- Intussusception is the invagination, or telescoping, of one part of the intestinal tract into another segment. Invagination leads to intestinal obstruction and impaired circulation.
- Intussusception most commonly occurs in infants under 1 year of age, but may occur from 3 months to 15 years of age and is most commonly found in boys.

- Most common forms include ileocolic (at the ileocecal valve), ileoileal (the ileus into itself), and colocolic (the colon into itself).

- Symptoms include acute abdominal pain (manifested in infants by crying and knee-chest position), vomiting, and red currant jelly stools.

- Physical examination may reveal a sausage-shaped mass in the right upper quadrant while the lower right quadrant feels empty (Dance sign).

- A barium enema, although often not required, is the test of choice in diagnosing intussusception. The barium enema alone may reduce the intussusception.

- Rectal instillation of saline may also be used to reduce the intussusception. This approach to correction is termed hydrostatic reduction because the force or pressure of infusion of the barium or saline alone is responsible for reducing the intussusception. Insufflation of air or oxygen may also be used.

- If perforation or shock are present, surgical correction is preferred.

Malrotation

- Normally during fetal development the bowel undergoes a 270-degree rotation counterclockwise. *Malrotation* is a term used when the bowel fails to rotate, rotates improperly, or is not correctly fixed to the abdominal wall by peritoneal bands.

- Three general types of malrotation include nonrotation, incomplete rotation, or incomplete fixation of the bowel.

- This defect can strike at any age, especially from infancy through adolescence.

- An acute midgut volvulus is a type of nonrotation that causes acute interruption of arterial blood supply. Signs and symptoms include sudden bilious vomiting, abdominal pain, melena, hematochezia, and hematemesis. Hypovolemic shock and sepsis are common. See volvulus under common information mentioned previously.

- Acute or chronic duodenal obstruction may be caused by abnormal peritoneal bands that obstruct or compress on the duodenum rather than anchor the gastrointestinal tract normally. This condition is accompanied by acute abdominal pain, vomiting, electrolyte imbalances, and nutritional deficiencies.

HEPATIC FAILURE/COMA

Portal Hypertension

- Portal hypertension is caused by an obstruction in the portal venous system, and is defined as an increase in pressure above 5 to 10 mm Hg pressure.

- Hypertension in the portal circulation causes venous congestion that leads to clot formation, anemia, and decreased platelet count. Collateral vessels develop

Signs and Symptoms of Portal Hypertension

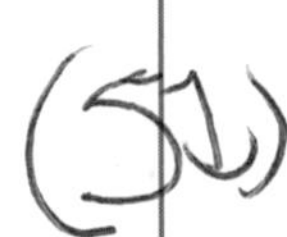

Splenomegaly	Anemia
Hemorrhoids	Thrombocytopenia
Dilated abdominal veins	Leukopenia
Ascites	Upper gastrointestinal bleeding
Hypoalbuminemia	

to the inferior vena cava, which can become enlarged and protrude into the esophagus.

- Extrahepatic obstruction accounts for most cases of portal hypertension in children. This is an obstruction of the portal vein itself or an immediate branch. This commonly occurs from an umbilical venous catheter, a congenital thrombosis, or unknown causes.
- An intrahepatic obstruction is usually associated with primary liver disease such as chronic liver disease, cystic fibrosis, hepatic damage from chemotherapy, or following surgery for biliary atresia.
- Suprahepatic portal hypertension occurs when there is an obstruction of hepatic venous flow into the inferior vena cava.
- Three major complications of portal hypertension are the formation of collateral vessels, impairment of the mesenteric and splenic circulations, and sequestration of blood in the splanchnic circulation.
- Signs and symptoms of portal hypertension are found in the box above.
- Bleeding episodes in portal hypertension may be brought on by an illness accompanied by fever and the use of aspirin which affects platelet function.
- See the box on p. 305 for treatment of hemorrhage associated with portal hypertension.
- Rectal temperatures should not be taken in the child with portal hypertension because of the risk associated with hemorrhage from hemorrhoids.
- Use comfort measures and parents/caretaker to avoid prolonged crying, which can increase the pressure in the esophageal varices. Sedation may be required.
- Monitor bowel elimination patterns for constipation and straining, which can increase or precipitate bleeding episodes. Test all stools for occult or gross blood.

Management of Hemorrhage Associated with Portal Hypertension

I. Resuscitation

Establish intravenous access and appropriate hemodynamic monitoring (arterial line, etc.).

Provide isotonic intravenous fluid (20 mL/kg boluses and repeat as needed) and blood (10 mL/kg as needed). Warm blood products prior to administration in infants and young children.

Evaluate systemic perfusion and hematocrit frequently.

Assess for signs of ongoing hemorrhage (abdominal pain, changes in bowel sounds, hematemesis, or hematochezia).

Monitor fluid and electrolyte balance.

II. Specific Diagnosis

Assess color and location of bleeding.

Monitor for indications that surgical intervention is required (free air observed on abdominal radiograph, severe hemorrhage unresponsive to blood replacement, or continuing hemodynamic instability).

Barium swallow, esophagoscopy, or splenoportography may be performed when the child is stable.

III. Specific Treatment

Sclerotherapy

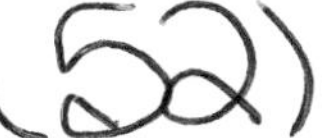

Saline lavage

Vasopressin

Sengstaken-Blakemore tube

From Hazinski MF: Nursing care of the critically ill child, ed 2, St Louis, 1992, Mosby.

- Avoid the Valsalva maneuver or respiratory treatments, which can increase intraabdominal pressure and increase the risk of bleeding.

FULMINANT HEPATITIS

- Acute or fulminant hepatitis results from massive destruction of liver cells and progressive liver function failure.

- The cause of acute hepatic failure may be viral hepatitis, drug-induced or toxin-induced hepatotoxicity, or unknown causes.

- Sulfonamides are among the most common drugs causing fulminant hepatitis. Acetaminophen also is a frequent cause as a result of adolescent suicide attempts. Less common causes include adverse reactions to anesthetic agents and chemotherapy.
- Metabolic causes of fulminant hepatitis include galactosemia and Wilson's disease.
- The pathology and signs and symptoms are related to failure of the liver to perform its functions. (See accompanying box below.)
- Benzodiazepines, narcotics, and barbiturates should not be given because they may contribute to or hasten hepatic coma.
- Dietary protein should be limited to 1g/kg/day.
- Neomycin may be used to destroy bacteria in the gut that contribute to ammonia levels.
- Lactulose also may be given to help facilitate ammonium ion elimination.
- Hemorrhage is treated with packed red cells, platelets, and fresh frozen plasma. Vitamin K therapy is often helpful.
- Prophylactic use of antacids and type II histamine blockers may help decrease the complication of gastrointestinal bleeding.
- The central venous pressure (CVP) needs to be closely monitored. Any increase in CVP can increase the portal pressures.

Signs and Symptoms of Hepatic Failure

Ascites	Lethargy
Dilation of superficial abdominal veins	Irritability
Clubbing of fingernails and toenails	Forgetfulness
Xanthoma formation	Inappropriate moods
Ecchymosis	Slurred speech
Erythema of the palms of the hands	Mild temors
Gynecomastia	Muscle twitching
Spider angiomas	Asterixis
Jaundice	Altered patterns of sleep
Malaise	Coma

BILIARY ATRESIA

- Biliary atresia is a congenital defect characterized by the obstruction or absence of any part or all of the biliary tree. This prevents bile from draining from the liver into the duodenum.

- Surgical correction of biliary atresia must occur before 2 to 3 months of age to prevent hepatic damage that results in cirrhosis and portal hypertension. Even with intervention, these complications often occur.

- Signs and symptoms of biliary atresia include gray-colored stools, dark-colored urine, and pruritus. If the disease progresses, signs and symptoms of liver failure and hepatic encephalopathy also occur.

- Surgical correction includes the resection of the atretic portion of the ducts and connection of the ends to the rest of the biliary tree emptying into the duodenum. In severe cases, liver transplantation may be the only treatment.

LIVER TRANSPLANTATION

- A common and serious complication following liver transplantation is hemorrhage. Bleeding commonly occurs at venous and arterial anastomosis sites.

- Do *not* add heparin routinely to flush solutions of liver transplant patients.

- Hypertension may occur following transplantation. Fluid therapy and all output (urine, drainage, etc.) should be carefully monitored.

- Dopamine therapy at low dose may help improve circulation to the liver.

- Signs of rejection are found in the box on p. 308.

- Rejection commonly occurs between the fourth and tenth days postoperatively.

ACUTE ABDOMINAL TRAUMA

- Most abdominal trauma is blunt trauma.

- In children, the most commonly injured organs are the spleen and liver.

- The liver is commonly injured because the rib cage is more flexible and can be a source of perforation and laceration.

- Liver trauma should be suspected if there are abrasions, bruising, or tenderness over the right upper quadrant of the abdomen or to the rib cage on the right side. A decrease in hemoglobin or hematocrit, right lung injuries, and abdominal distension should also suggest a liver injury.

Signs and Symptoms of Liver Transplantation Rejection

Elevated hepatic enzymes	Fever
Electrolyte imbalances	Right upper quadrant abdominal or flank pain
Hypoglycemia	Jaundice
Coagulopathy	

- Initial treatment of spleen and liver injuries is aimed at medical management through fluid and blood replacement therapies.
- Children breathe with their abdomens. Any abdominal injury can severely affect respiratory excursion and decrease gas exchange.
- Lower left chest wall or upper left quadrant pain, bruising, or injury may suggest injury to the spleen.

NEONATAL-SPECIFIC PRINCIPLES

DUODENAL ATRESIA

- Duodenal atresia is when the duodenum ends abruptly and is not continuous with the rest of the small bowel. It is believed to be caused by an obstruction to blood flow in utero.
- The mother often has polyhydramnios during the pregnancy and the infant is small for gestational age.
- The obstruction may be above the common bile duct, which will make any emesis consist of saliva and undigested oral feedings. If the obstruction is below the common bile duct, the emesis will include bile.
- Signs and symptoms include vomiting; scant, light-colored material from the rectum; and jaundice.
- Early surgical repair is indicated and accomplished by cutting out the atretic portion and reconnecting the bowel segments. Sometimes an ostomy is required.

Questions

GENERAL GASTROINTESTINAL CARE QUESTIONS

1. When performing an abdominal assessment, which order should the nurse follow?
   A. Palpation, percussion, auscultation, inspection
   B. Inspection, palpation, percussion, auscultation
   C. Auscultation, inspection, palpation, percussion
   D. Inspection, auscultation, percussion, and palpation

2. The primary function of the large intestine is to:
   A. Digest carbohydrates
   B. Digest proteins
   C. Reabsorb water
   D. Emulsify fats

3. Which of the following complications would the critical care nurse suspect in the care of a neonate with an omphalocele?
   A. Hypothermia
   B. Fluid overload
   C. Arrhythmias
   D. Cyanosis

4. Which of the following nursing diagnoses would be *most* appropriate for the neonate who has undergone surgical correction for an omphalocele?
   A. High risk for infection
   B. Ineffective airway clearance
   C. Diarrhea
   D. Hypothermia

5. Before surgical correction, nursing care of either an omphalocele or a gastroschisis would include:
   A. A tight abdominal dressing to help reduce the herniation
   B. Leaving the contents open to air to decrease bacterial growth
   C. Covering the sac with moist, saline gauze and plastic
   D. Applying betadine dressings to reduce bacterial colonization

Case Study

During the care of a 2-day-old newborn, the critical care nurse notes that there are decreased bowel sounds and abdominal distension. The baby also appears to be more lethargic. Further examination reveals a gradual decrease in urine output over the last 12 hours, and the neonate's most recent stool tested positive for occult blood. The Apgar scores of this baby were 2 at one minute, and 5 at five minutes. There had been some meconium aspiration that required suctioning and resuscitative efforts in the delivery room. Questions 6 to 9 refer to this case study.

6. Based on the birth history and present signs and symptoms, the nurse suspects:
A. Respiratory distress syndrome
B. Diaphragmatic hernia
C. Hirschsprung's disease
D. Necrotizing enterocolitis

7. Other clinical signs and symptoms of this condition may include:
A. Increased gastric residuals, jaundice, bradycardia
B. Ileus, tachycardia, cyanosis, bright red vomitus
C. Currant jelly stools, dehydration, bowel obstruction
D. Bright red rectal bleeding, jaundice, hypotension

8. After establishing that the baby is maintaining her airway well and her respiratory status is adequate, the *first* priority in caring for this infant would be:
A. Stop oral feedings and begin continuous tube feedings
B. Assess for infection by taking an accurate rectal temperature
C. Stop all feedings and insert an intravenous line for fluids
D. Test any gastric secretions for occult blood

9. Which of the following nursing diagnoses would be of the *highest* priority after surgical repair of gastroschisis?
A. High risk for infection
B. Ineffective breathing pattern
C. Altered nutrition: less than body requirements
D. Colonic constipation

10. Which of the following feedings is preferred for an infant whose bowel function has returned following necrotizing enterocolitis?
A. Full strength soy formula
B. Hyperosmolar feedings to increase caloric intake
C. Low osmotic feedings
D. Full strength milk-based formula

11. A patient with a volvulus should also be assessed for:
    I. Hypocalcemia
    II. Hyperkalemia
    III. Hypermagnesemia
    IV. Hypernatremia
    A. I and II
    B. II and III
    C. III and IV
    D. I and IV

12. Primary functions of the liver include all of the following *except*:
    A. Synthesis of albumin
    B. Production of clotting factors
    C. Storage site for water soluble vitamins
    D. Detoxification of waste products

13. A patient on total parenteral nutrition would *not* be likely to develop which of the following complications?
    A. Infection
    B. Hyperglycemia
    C. Hypoglycemia
    D. Alkalosis

14. For which of the following conditions would intralipids be contraindicated?
    A. Platelet count of 80,000/mm^3
    B. Hematocrit of 28%
    C. Sodium of 150 Meq/L
    D. Negative occult stools

15. The critical care nurse is caring for a patient receiving total parenteral nutrition through a central venous line. When there are 15 cc of solution left in the bottle that is hanging, the nurse discovers that the pharmacy has not yet brought the next bottle to the unit. Which action should the nurse take next?
    A. Slow the infusion rate on the remaining 15 cc
    B. Follow this bottle with normal saline and monitor serum glucoses carefully
    C. Hang a 10% dextrose solution when the first bottle has infused and monitor blood glucoses
    D. Flush the line with heparin when the solution has infused to prevent clotting while the new bottle is prepared

16. Pneumatosis intestinalis is the hallmark of which condition?
    A. Volvulus
    B. Necrotizing enterocolitis
    C. Hirschprung's disease
    D. Tracheoesophageal fistula

17. The critical care nurse identifies all of the following as risk factors associated with the development of necrotizing enterocolitis *except*:
A. Central venous line
B. Umbilical venous line
C. Hypoxia
D. Respiratory distress syndrome

18. The primary cause of hypovolemia in necrotizing enterocolitis is:
A. Blood loss
B. Evaporative loss
C. Decreased oral intake
D. Third spacing of fluids

19. In order to assist in protecting the patient's airway, any infant with gastroschisis should have which of the following placed?
A. Endotracheal tube
B. Oral airway
C. Nasogastric tube
D. Nasopharyngeal airway

20. An important patient outcome associated with caring for a neonate before surgery to repair an omphalocele would include all of the following *except*:
A. A temperature of 37°F
B. Urine output of 1 mL/kg/hr
C. Presence of bowel sounds
D. Serum glucose level greater than 40 mg/dL

21. An elevation in *indirect* bilirubin would *most* likely indicate:
A. Acute hepatic failure
B. Necrotizing enterocolitis
C. Biliary atresia
D. Duodenal atresia

22. To monitor for complications in an infant following surgical repair of gastroschisis, the critical care nurse would look for arterial blood gases that had an elevation in:
A. pO_2
B. pCO_2
C. Base excess
D. pH

23. Hypoglycemia in the infant with an omphalocele is most directly related to:
A. Increased energy needs
B. Increased temperature
C. Altered metabolism
D. Altered intestinal function

24. In planning care for an infant after surgical repair for an omphalocele, the critical care nurse should be aware that:
A. Fluid loss into the bowel continues postoperatively
B. Early feeding is important to promote peristalsis
C. Nasogastric suction will cause metabolic alkalosis
D. A Sengstaken-Balkemore tube will reduce bleeding

25. Infants with gastroesophageal reflux need to be positioned during and after feeding in a/an:
A. Supine position
B. Left lateral position
C. Prone position
D. Upright position

Case Study

A 2-day-old male infant is returned to the critical care unit following surgical repair for gastroschisis. Questions 26 to 28 refer to this case study.

---

26. Upon return to the critical care unit following surgery, the critical care nurse would include which of the following nursing diagnoses in the plan of care? High risk for:
A. Diarrhea related to increased intestinal motility
B. Impaired tissue integrity related to immobility
C. Decreased cardiac output related to decreased venous return
D. Urinary retention secondary to anesthetic agents

27. An appropriate nursing intervention for this high risk infant would be:
A. Use of hyperosmolar feedings to reduce diarrhea
B. Use of skin lotions to prevent skin breakdown
C. Positioning the infant to prevent vena caval compression
D. Administration of cholinergic agents to promote urinary output

28. An appropriate patient outcome for this infant *upon admission* to the critical care unit would include all of the following *except*:
A. Heart rate less than 150 beats per minute
B. Urine output of 1 mL/kg/hr
C. Respiratory rate less than 60 breaths per minute
D. Blood pressure greater than 50/25 mm Hg

29. An infant with gastroschisis has been admitted to the critical care unit from the delivery room. He has a nasogastric tube in place. The tube should be:
A. Attached to gravity drainage
B. Connected to a syringe for frequent aspiration and accurate measurement
C. Secured to suction
D. Wrapped in a towel to collect drainage

30. Upon diagnosis of necrotizing enterocolitis, the nurse should expect administration of antibiotics from which of the following group(s)?
I. Penicillins
II. Aminoglycosides
III. Cephalosporins
IV. Tetracyclines
A. I only
B. I and II
C. III only
D. I and IV

31. Care of the patient receiving total parenteral nutrition (TPN) via a central line should include:
A. Wearing a sterile gown and gloves when changing the dressing
B. Infusing only antibiotics with the TPN when there is no other intravenous site
C. Slowing the infusion when hyperglycemia occurs until the urine tests negative for glucose
D. Clamping extension tubing to prevent retrograde blood flow during bottle changes

32. Which of the following tests would confirm the diagnosis of volvulus?
A. Abdominal x-ray
B. Positive occult stools
C. Barium enema
D. Colonoscopy

Case Study

A 3-day-old female infant is admitted to the critical care unit following acute onset of apparent abdominal pain, distended abdomen, lethargy, hypovolemic shock, and bloody stool. She is diagnosed with a volvulus. Questions 33 to 36 refer to this case study.

---

33. Based on this history and diagnosis, the nurse also would expect all of the following signs and symptoms *except*:
A. Bilious vomiting
B. Hematemesis
C. Shock
D. Hypertension

34. The nurse would expect this patient's initial treatment to be:
A. Management with albumin and blood products to stabilize the blood pressure for 12 hours
B. Administration of antibiotics to prevent sepsis and infection for 48 hours
C. A barium enema to reduce the volvulus immediately
D. Surgical intervention to reestablish blood flow to the gut

35. For which of the following serum electrolyte abnormalities would the critical care nurse be alert?
I. Hyperkalemia
II. Hypomagnesemia
III. Hyponatremia
IV. Hypocalcemia
A. I and III
B. II and III
C. II and IV
D. I and IV

36. For which of the following manifestations of these electrolyte imbalances would the nurse observe?
A. Cardiac dysrhythmias
B. Cullen's sign
C. Edema
D. Poor skin turgor

37. Clay-colored stools may indicate:
A. Necrotizing enterocolitis
B. Liver disease
C. Esophageal atresia
D. Malrotation of the bowel

38. The liver forms all of the following substances *except*:
A. Cholesterol
B. Vitamin K
C. Iron
D. Amino acids

39. Which of the following would be an abnormal finding when inspecting the abdomen during an assessment?
A. Visible peristalsis
B. Visible pulsations
C. Dilated superficial veins
D. Rounded abdomen

40. A patient with gastroschisis usually has:
A. Other associated anomalies
B. An intact membrane covering the defect
C. Minimal fluid losses
D. Thickened, edematous intestines

PEDIATRIC-SPECIFIC QUESTIONS

41. Expected patient outcomes of a barium enema for the infant with intussusception may include:
- **A.** Passage of a meconium stool
- **B.** Reduction of the telescoped bowel
- **C.** Increase in peristalsis
- **D.** Reduction of bleeding

42. For an infant with intussusception, the primary mechanism of intestinal damage is:
- **A.** Bowel ulceration
- **B.** Lack of circulation
- **C.** Abdominal distension
- **D.** Malabsorption

Case Study

A 10-year-old boy is brought to the emergency room with abdominal pain. A review of his history shows he has seen his pediatrician twice in the last 6 months for nonspecific abdominal pain. He reports vomiting with the pain, and serum laboratory studies show low serum protein levels. He is diagnosed with chronic, midgut volvulus. Questions 43 and 44 refer to this case study.

---

43. Which of the following methods is most helpful in diagnosing this condition?
- **A.** Physical examination and Kehr's sign
- **B.** Abdominal x-ray with contrast
- **C.** CT scan of the abdomen
- **D.** Splanchnic angiography

44. The treatment of choice for chronic, midgut volvulus is:
- **A.** Saline enemas to reduce the volvulus
- **B.** Administration of neomycin to sterilize the gut
- **C.** Immediate surgical correction
- **D.** High fiber diet and high oral intake of fluids

Case Study

A 4-month-old male infant is brought to the emergency room with acute abdominal pain manifested by screaming and drawing the knees to the abdomen. His history was negative for any chronic illnesses or other significant health problems. His growth and development appear normal. He had another episode of pain on the way to the emergency room. His latest pain occurred shortly after reaching the emergency room and being put in an examination room. This time he passed a red, currant jelly-like stool. Questions 45 to 47 refer to this case study.

---

45. Based on this data, the nurse suspects:
A. Necrotizing enterocolitis
B. Appendicitis
C. Acute volvulus
D. Intussusception

46. Another expected finding upon physical examination would be:
A. Dance sign
B. Kehr's sign
C. Kernig's sign
D. Cullen's sign

47. Indications for surgical correction include all of the following *except*:
A. Signs of perforation
B. Bloody stools
C. Previous episodes of intussusception
D. Abdominal symptoms for more than 48 hours

Case Study

A 15-year-old boy is referred to the emergency room by his pediatrician for suspected hepatitis. For the past 2 weeks he has had a decreased appetite, nausea, and fatigue. He reports he has been sleeping poorly. Upon physical examination, the pediatrician found yellowing of the sclera, multiple and diffuse ecchymotic areas and ascites. He has been admitted to the intensive care unit. Below are some of his admitting data.

Blood pressure: 84/52 mm Hg
Pulse: 112 beats per minute
Respiratory rate: 31 per minute
Temperature: 36.8°C (100.6°F)

Questions 48 to 50 refer to this case study.

---

48. To follow the severity of his liver disease, the critical care nurse would monitor closely all of the following laboratory values *except*:
A. Alanine aminotransferase (ALT)
B. Aspartate aminotransferase (AST)
C. Alkaline phosphatase (ALP)
D. Acid phosphatase (AP)

49. The critical care nurse would question an order for which of the following medications?
A. Diazepam
B. Dobutamine
C. Potassium chloride
D. Amoxicillin

50. Lactulose is ordered for this patient to:
- **A.** Reduce the incidence of esophageal varices
- **B.** Decrease indirect serum bilirubin levels
- **C.** Decrease ammonia levels
- **D.** Reduce bacteria in the small intestine

51. One of the earliest signs and symptoms of portal hypertension is:
- **A.** Splenomegaly
- **B.** Split S_2 heart sound
- **C.** Ascites
- **D.** Melena

52. A 10-year-old patient with known portal hypertension suddenly develops acute onset of bright red vomiting. Her blood pressure drops quickly to 88/56. The critical care nurse would anticipate *immediate* intervention to include isotonic intravenous fluid administration and:
- **A.** Vasopressin
- **B.** Dopamine
- **C.** Dobutamine
- **D.** Hepatic angiography

53. All of the following are contraindicated for a child with portal hypertension *except*:
- **A.** Use of an incentive spirometer
- **B.** Rectal temperatures
- **C.** Constipation
- **D.** Sedation

54. Which of the following would *most* likely be increased in the early clinical course of biliary atresia?
- **A.** Total serum bilirubin levels
- **B.** Conjugated serum bilirubin levels
- **C.** Total protein
- **D.** Acid phosphatase

55. Encephalopathy associated with decreased liver function is primarily related to:
- **A.** Increased intracranial pressure
- **B.** Hyperproteinemia
- **C.** Sepsis
- **D.** Circulating hepatotoxins

56. Which of the following are signs and symptoms of rejection following a liver transplant?

I. Hypoglycemia
II. Right upper quadrant pain
III. Rectal bleeding
IV. Fever

A. I and II
B. II and III
C. I, II, and IV
D. III and IV

57. The most common site of abdominal trauma in children is the:

A. Liver
B. Spleen
C. Kidney
D. Bladder

58. Initial assessment of the child with abdominal injuries should begin with:

A. Inspection of the abdomen
B. Assessment of ventilation
C. Gentle palpation
D. Rectal examination

59. Following a motor vehicle accident, a child complains of right upper quadrant pain. A chest x-rays reveals a right pleural effusion. The critical care nurse also suspects:

A. Pulmonary infarction
B. Liver trauma
C. Splenic rupture
D. Lacerated kidney

60. Rejection of liver transplants commonly occurs:

A. At the first day
B. Between 4 and 10 days
C. At 1 month
D. Between 4 and 8 weeks

NEONATAL-SPECIFIC QUESTIONS

61. An infant suspected of having duodenal atresia is noted to pass a small amount of light-colored stool from his rectum. The nurse knows this:

A. Rules out a diagnosis of duodenal atresia
B. Is not normal meconium and is consistent with duodenal atresia
C. Makes a diagnosis of intussusception more likely
D. Is more consistent with necrotizing enterocolitis

62. All of the following are factors associated with the development of necrotizing enterocolitis in the preterm infant *except*:
A. Breast milk
B. Early feedings
C. Low birth weight
D. Respiratory distress syndrome

63. Dehydration in the neonate with a omphalocele develops *primarily* because of:
A. Third spacing of fluid
B. Large amounts of watery stools
C. Nasogastric suctioning
D. Evaporative losses

64. A perinatal history consistent with a diagnosis of duodenal atresia includes:
A. Meconium staining
B. Polyhydramnios
C. Preterm labor
D. Metabolic acidosis

Answers

1. Correct answer—D.

When performing an abdominal assessment, the nurse should begin with inspection, then auscultation, and finish with percussion and palpation. Percussion and palpation are performed last because they can increase bowel motility, therefore affecting other findings. If percussion and palpation are performed first, the abdomen can appear to be more active during inspection and bowel sounds are likely to be increased during auscultation. Palpation should be performed last in case and the abdomen is tender. If pain is elicited, it would be hard for a child or infant to be quiet and cooperative with further examination.

2. Correct answer—C.

The primary function of the large intestine is reabsorb water and electrolytes, as well as store the fecal material. Digestion occurs primarily in the small intestines.

3. Correct answer—A.

An omphalocele is the herniation of portions of the intestines, liver, or spleen through the umbilicus. Because the highly vascular, herniated contents are only covered by a thin membrane, the potential for heat loss is great. These neonates generally have problems associated with hypothermia, hypovolemia, hypoglycemia, respiratory distress, and shock.

4. Correct answer—A.

Following surgical correction for an omphalocele, and infant is at high risk for developing infection related to the abdominal incision and surgery on the intestinal tract. Airway clearance is not directly affected by the surgery. Most infants are not given oral feedings postoperatively to avoid aspiration and because bowel function may return very slowly. Hypothermia should not be an increased risk factor following surgery because the herniated organs have been returned inside the abdominal cavity, which reduces heat loss.

5. Correct answer—C.

Before surgical correction, nursing care of either an omphalocele or a gastroschisis would include covering the herniated contents with damp, saline gauze and plastic to keep them moist and minimize heat loss. A tight abdominal dressing would risk damaging the herniated organs and impair circulation. Leaving the contents open to air would increase heat loss, increase bacterial contamination, and damage the delicate mucosa. Applying betaine dressing would be contraindicated because the betaine could be absorbed systemically and prove to be toxic.

6. Correct answer—D.

Based on the birth history and present signs and symptoms, the nurse suspects necrotizing enterocolitis (NEC). The hypoxic episode at birth together with the abdominal distension and blood in the stool are highly suspicious of NEC. Neither respiratory distress syndrome nor a diaphragmatic hernia would cause occult blood in the stool. Hirschsprung's disease is a failure of the gastrointestinal tract to properly develop nervous innervation. This condition is associated with failure to pass meconium and interrupted peristalsis, not blood in the stool.

7. **Correct answer—A.**
Other clinical signs and symptoms of NEC may include increased gastric residuals, jaundice, bradycardia, apnea, lethargy, ileus, vomiting of bile, and shock. Bright red vomitus would be characteristic of upper gastrointestinal bleeding. Currant jelly stools are seen in intussusception. Bright red rectal bleeding is characteristic of Hirschsprung's disease.

8. **Correct answer—C.**
After establishing that the baby is maintaining her airway well and her respiratory status is adequate, the first priority in caring for this infant would be to stop all feedings and insert an intravenous line for fluids to maintain adequate hydration and circulating volume. No oral or tube feedings would be allowed to ensure that the gut is fully rested. Rectal temperatures should never be taken in an infant suspected of having NEC because of the risk of perforation. While gastric secretions should be tested for occult blood, this is not an immediate priority.

9. **Correct answer—B.**
The nursing diagnoses that would be of the highest priority after surgical repair of gastroschisis is an ineffective breathing pattern. When the intestinal contents are returned to the abdominal cavity, they can shift the diaphragm up and seriously decrease the ventilatory efforts of the infant by decreasing the lung capacity. Infection and alterations in bowel function and feeding patterns are postoperative problems. However, those problems associated with airway, breathing, and circulation always are of the highest priority.

10. **Correct answer—C.**
For an infant whose bowel function has returned following necrotizing enterocolitis, low osmotic feedings should be initiated first. Hyperosmolar feedings have been associated with the development of NEC.

11. **Correct answer—A.**
A patient with a volvulus should also be assessed for hypocalcemia and hyperkalemia, frequent electrolyte imbalances that accompany this condition.

12. **Correct answer—C.**
Primary functions of the liver include synthesis of albumin; production of clotting factors; storage site for *fat* soluble vitamins, glycogen, and fat; detoxification of waste products; synthesis of plasma proteins; and metabolism of fat, carbohydrates, and protein.

13. Correct answer—D.
Alkalosis is not a probable complication of total parenteral nutrition (TPN). Acidosis may develop from large protein loads and an inability of the kidneys to excrete ammonia, which is formed from amino acid metabolism. Potential complications associated with total parenteral nutrition include infection, hyperglycemia, hypoglycemia, electrolyte imbalances, mineral deficiencies, thromboemboli, air emboli, and hyperlipidemia.

14. Correct answer—A.
Intralipids are contraindicated in thrombocytopenia because they interfere with platelet function. Intralipids are also contraindicated in patients with liver disease or jaundice because they interfere with the binding of bilirubin to albumin.

15. Correct answer—C.
When another bottle of TPN solution is not immediately available, the critical care nurse should hang a 10% dextrose solution and monitor blood glucoses carefully while waiting for the next bottle of TPN to be prepared. The infusion rate should never be increased or decreased unless titrating or tapering because it can result in severe imbalances of serum glucose. Normal saline solution and flushing the line with a heparinized solution would not provide a source of glucose and could also result in severe hypoglycemia.

16. Correct answer—B.
Pneumatosis intestinalis is the hallmark of necrotizing enterocolitis. Seen on x-ray, it is the presence of trapped pockets of gas in the bowel wall. This condition is unique to NEC.

17. Correct answer—A.
A central venous line does not obstruct splanchnic circulation, and therefore has not been associated with the development of NEC. Risk factors have been found to include umbilical arterial lines, respiratory distress syndrome, shock, hypothermia, early feedings in premature infants, periods of hypoxia, thrombocytopenia, and anemia.

18. Correct answer—D.
The primary cause of hypovolemia in necrotizing enterocolitis is third spacing of fluids in the intestinal tract. Loss of fluids through third spacing may be significant enough to cause shock and oliguria.

19. Correct answer—C.
In order to protect the patient's airway, any infant with gastroschisis should have a nasogastric tube placed to decompress the abdomen and prevent vomiting, which could lead to aspiration. Oral airways are contraindicated in alert patients because they can precipitate the gag reflex and vomiting. A nasopharyngeal airway or endotracheal intubation would be indicated only if the infant were unable to maintain a patent airway or had respiratory insufficiency.

20. Correct answer—C.

Bowel sounds would most likely be absent before surgical repair of an omphalocele. Desired patient outcomes would include a temperature of 37°F, urine output of 1 mL/kg/hr, serum glucose level greater than 40 mg/dL, normal white blood cell count, and signs of adequate peripheral circulation.

21. Correct answer—A.

An elevation in indirect bilirubin would most likely indicate acute hepatic failure. Indirect (unconjugated) levels rise when the liver is unable to conjugate bilirubin. Direct levels rise in biliary atresia, biliary tract obstruction, and conditions that prevent the secretion of conjugated bilirubin into the gastrointestinal tract for excretion.

22. Correct answer—B.

Arterial blood gases in an infant following surgical repair of gastroschisis may have an elevation in pCO_2. When the protruding organs are returned to the abdominal cavity, they may impede movement of the diaphragm and decrease ventilatory movements. A decrease in the excursion of the diaphragm can lead to retained pCO_2. A fall in pO_2, a fall in the pH, and a decrease in the base excess would accompany this deterioration in respiratory function.

23. Correct answer—A.

Hypoglycemia in the infant with an omphalocele is most directly related to increased energy needs from stress, illness, and hypothermia. Infants with an omphalocele generally have decreased temperature from heat loss associated with the protruding abdominal organs.

24. Correct answer—A.

In planning care for an infant after surgical repair for an omphalocele, the critical care nurse should be aware that fluid loss into the bowel continues postoperatively. Because fluid loss continues, these infants need to be closely monitored for hypovolemia and electrolyte imbalances. Urine output may be decreased if there is insufficient intravascular volume. Early feeding is discouraged until the gut has healed and peristalsis returns. Nasogastric suction is necessary until gut motility returns to prevent vomiting and aspiration. A Sengstaken-Blakemore tube is used to treat bleeding associated with esophageal varices.

25. Correct answer—D.

Infants with gastroesophageal reflux need to be positioned during and after feeding in an upright position. Positioning the infant with the head elevated 30 degrees helps reduce the amount of reflux from the stomach into the esophagus.

26. Correct answer—C.

Following surgical repair for gastroschisis, the critical care nurse would include the nursing diagnosis of high risk for decreased cardiac output related to decreased venous return in the plan of care. Because a large amount of visceral organs are being returned to an often small abdominal cavity, there is a risk of compression of the vena cava that in turn reduces venous return to the heart. By decreasing the preload, the cardiac output can fall. Generally following surgery, there is no peristalsis for days to weeks. Impaired tissue integrity related to immobility should not occur if proper positioning and use of pressure reducing aids are employed. Urinary retention is not an expected problem following surgical repair of gastroschisis.

27. Correct answer—C.
An appropriate nursing intervention for this high risk would be positioning the infant to prevent vena caval compression. Side-lying positions may be helpful. The prone position should be avoided to prevent trauma to the suture line and further pressure on the abdomen.

28. Correct answer—A.
Appropriate patient outcomes for this infant upon admission to the critical care unit would include all of the following except a heart rate less than 150 beats per minute. The normal heart rate for a newborn is approximately 100 to 180 beats per minute when awake. The heart rate would be expected to be elevated as a response to stress, blood loss during surgery, any pain, and to increased cardiac output related to metabolic demands. A urine output of 1 mL/kg/hr, respiratory rate less than 60 breaths per minute, and blood pressure greater than 50/25 mm Hg are all normal findings in this age infant.

29. Correct answer—C.
The tube should be attached to suction for drainage to ensure that the stomach is decompressed, bile is drained, and the risk of aspiration from vomiting is minimized. Gravity drainage or using a syringe with frequent aspiration is acceptable only if suction is not available, such as during transport. Wrapping the tubing in a towel would not facilitate accurate measurement of drainage to calculate replacement needs.

30. Correct answer—B.
A penicillin such as ampicillin and an aminoglycoside such as gentamicin are the most common treatments for NEC. Both ampicillin and gentamicin are broad spectrum antibiotics that are bactericidal. This combination of drugs is generally the first-line treatment of NEC.

31. Correct answer—D.
Care of the patient receiving total parenteral nutrition (TPN) via a central line should include clamping extension tubing to prevent retrograde blood flow into the tubing during bottle changes. If the interior of the catheter becomes contaminated with blood, the risk of clot formation increases. Wearing a sterile gown and gloves when changing the dressing is required, but not sufficient without the use of a mask as well. Nothing should ever be infused or piggybacked into the same infusion line with TPN. Only a multilumen catheter would allow infusion of other solutions into

the same catheter, but not the same infusion port. Slowing the infusion when hyperglycemia occurs would risk hypoglycemia or other imbalances of glucose metabolism and should not be done without collaboration with the physician.

32. Correct answer—C.
A barium enema would be used to confirm the diagnosis of volvulus. The barium instilled rectally would allow the visualization of the twisted and enlarged bowel. An abdominal x-ray may or may not show findings to confirm the volvulus. Positive occult stools are found in a variety of gastrointestinal abnormalities. A colonoscopy would not be likely to visualize the affected area and would run the risk of perforation of inflamed bowel.

33. Correct answer—D.
Hypertension would be an unlikely finding because these infants lose a large amount of fluid into the gut and become hypovolemic, which leads to hypotension and shock. An infant with an acute volvulus would be expected to also have bilious vomiting, hematemesis, and shock.

34. Correct answer—D.
The nurse would expect the initial treatment of a patient with a volvulus to be surgical intervention to reestablish blood flow to the gut by untwisting the affected bowel and securing it. Management with albumin and blood products to stabilize the blood pressure would be insufficient treatment because this would not reestablish blood flow to the ischemic bowel. Failure to intervene promptly with surgery risks infarcting the affected bowel. Administration of antibiotics to prevent sepsis and infection would be helpful, but would not reestablish blood flow to the ischemic area. A barium enema may be used to diagnose and reduce intussusception.

35. Correct answer—D.
An infant with a volvulus is at risk for hyperkalemia and hypocalcemia. These may be significantly and seriously altered, causing systemic symptoms.

36. Correct answer—A.
Hyperkalemia and hypocalcemia seen with volvulus can be serious enough to cause cardiac dysrhythmias. Cullen's sign is a bruising around the umbilicus seen with hemorrhagic pancreatitis. Edema would be seen with hyponatremia and hypervolemia. Poor skin turgor would be observed with hypernatremia and dehydration.

37. Correct answer—B.
Clay-colored stools indicate liver or biliary tract disease. The light, clay color comes from an absence of bile in the stool. Bilirubin is a major pigment in bile giving it its characteristic dark color. When the liver cannot conjugate bilirubin, any bile that may be produced is light in color. In biliary tract disease, bile is not eliminated into the stool also resulting in light-colored stools.

38. Correct answer—C.
Iron is stored in the liver, but is not synthesized there. The liver forms cholesterol, Vitamin K, amino acids, albumin, globulins, and clotting factors.

39. Correct answer—C.
An abnormal finding when inspecting the abdomen would be dilated superficial veins, which can indicate liver disease. Peristalsis and arterial pulsations may be normally visible in infants, children, and thin adults. The abdomen is usually rounded as late as puberty.

40. Correct answer—D.
Large fluid losses are associated with gastroschisis because there is no protective saclike covering to prevent evaporative losses. A patient with gastroschisis usually has no other associated anomalies, and has thickened, edematous intestines protruding from the defect.

PEDIATRIC-SPECIFIC ANSWERS

41. Correct answer—B.
Expected patient outcomes of a barium enema for the infant with intussusception include reduction of the telescoped bowel. The pressure of the barium infusion rectally may actually correct the condition. A barium enema would not be expected to increase peristaltic action or reduce bleeding associated with this condition. Passage of a meconium stool has occurred previously because most cases of intussusception peak at 5 to 9 months of age.

42. Correct answer—B.
For an infant with intussusception, the primary mechanism of intestinal damage is lack of circulation. As one segment of the bowel slips, or telescopes, into another segment, the circulation becomes compromised resulting in widespread ischemia or infarction and obstruction at the site. Ulcerations are seen in Meckel's diverticulum and are more focal in nature. Abdominal distension may be a symptom, but is not a cause of intestinal damage. Malabsorption plays no role in intussusception.

43. Correct answer—B.
An abdominal x-ray with contrast will generally visualize this malrotation of the bowel. Physical examination often reveals nonspecific findings. Kehr's sign is seen with injuries to the spleen. A CT scan of the abdomen without contrast would not be as likely to reveal this condition. Angiography is generally reserved for vascular disease.

44. Correct answer—C.
The treatment of choice for chronic, midgut volvulus is immediate surgical correction. No medical management is effective in reducing the malrotation. Failure to correct it surgically can result in severe compromise of blood supply leading to infarction and bowel obstruction.

45. Correct answer—D.
Based on this data, the nurse suspects intussusception. Red, currant jellylike stools are characteristic of this condition. Necrotizing enterocolitis is almost exclusively a disease of premature or newborn infants. Appendicitis and acute volvulus would not give these characteristic stools.

46. Correct answer—A.
Another expected finding upon physical examination of the infant with intussusception would be the Dance sign. This is a sausage-shaped mass felt in the upper right quadrant with a lower right quadrant that feels empty. Kehr's sign is seen with splenic injury. Kernig's sign is seen with meningitis. Cullen's sign is seen with hemorrhagic pancreatitis.

47. Correct answer—B.
The presence of bloody stools alone is not an indication for surgery. Reduction of the intussusception by barium enema or rectal saline solutions should be attempted if there are no clear indications for surgery. Indications for surgical correction include signs of perforation, bloody stools, previous episodes of intussusception, and abdominal symptoms for more than 48 hours.

48. Correct answer—D.
Acid phosphatase (AP) is a laboratory test used primarily to diagnose, stage, and monitor prostatic cancer. To follow the severity of liver disease, the critical care nurse would monitor closely alanine aminotransferase (ALT), aspartate aminotransferase (AST), alkaline phosphatase (ALP), aldolase, prealbumin concentrations, coagulation studies, serum ammonia levels, and serum bilirubin levels (total, direct, and indirect).

49. Correct answer—A.
The critical care nurse would question an order for diazepam (Valium) because benzodiazepines as well as narcotics and barbiturates may promote the development of an hepatic coma. Drugs that are metabolized by the liver should be avoided, or if needed, given at reduced doses with serum levels monitored closely.

50. Correct answer—C.
Lactulose is ordered to decrease serum ammonia levels. Bacteria in the colon break down lactulose into small organic acids, which then combine with NH_3 to form NH_4, reducing the amount of ammonia that enters the blood stream. Bacteria in the colon is reduced by administering neomycin and is another method used to reduce serum ammonia levels. Esophageal varices are formed as a result of portal hypertension. Indirect serum bilirubin levels rise as the liver function fails and bilirubin is not conjugated by the liver for elimination by the gastrointestinal tract.

51. Correct answer—A.

One of the earliest signs and symptoms of portal hypertension is splenomegaly. Because increased pressure occurs in the splanchnic circulation, blood is trapped and results in an increase in the size of the spleen. Ascites, dilated superficial abdominal veins, melena, hypoalbuminemia, anemia, thrombocytopenia, and leukopenia are generally later signs. A split S_2 heart sound is usually associated with pulmonary hypertension or congestive heart failure as well as atrioventricular valvular disease.

52. Correct answer—A.

The critical care nurse would anticipate immediate intervention to include vasopressin. Vasopressin is a powerful vasoconstricting agent that helps stop bleeding by decreasing blood flow to the splanchnic circulation. Administration of vasopressin will help increase the blood pressure by constricting arterioles and increasing water resorption in the kidneys. Dopamine would not be indicated because it would not assist in stopping the bleeding and is not indicated in hypovolemic shock. Dobutamine is not indicated in hypovolemic shock. Hepatic angiography would offer little information for a patient with known portal hypertension and no therapeutic benefits during this emergency.

53. Correct answer—D.

Sedation may be required despite liver metabolism of many of these drugs to calm infants or children who are particularly agitated. Prolonged crying may precipitate or worsen variceal bleeding by increasing portal pressures. The use of an incentive spirometer and straining from constipation would be similarly contraindicated because they increase portal pressure. Rectal temperatures would be contraindicated because rectal hemorrhoids are common manifestations of portal hypertension and the risk of bleeding would be high.

54. Correct answer—B.

The conjugated serum bilirubin level would most likely be increased in biliary atresia because the liver is able to conjugate bilirubin early in the disease process, but is unable to eliminate the conjugated levels as a result of absence of a proper biliary tree. Total serum bilirubin levels are generally normal, or may be only slightly increased. Total protein and albumin levels are also generally normal early in the disease. Alkaline phosphatase levels may be increased, but acid phosphatase is specific to prostate disease.

55. Correct answer—A.

Encephalopathy associated with decreased liver function is primarily related to increased intracranial pressure. Hypoproteinemia generally characterizes impaired hepatic function because the liver is unable to synthesize proteins. Sepsis is a frequent complication of hepatic dysfunction, but is not a cause of encephalopathy.

56. Correct answer—C.

Signs and symptoms of rejection following a liver transplant include hypoglycemia, right upper quadrant pain, flank pain, fever, coagulopathies, and elevation of hepatic enzymes. Rectal bleeding is a sign of portal hypertension.

57. Correct answer—B.

The most common site of abdominal trauma in children is the spleen. The liver is the next most commonly injured intraabdominal organ. Splenic trauma should be suspected in any child with femur and rib fractures, and left-sided abdominal or shoulder pain/bruising.

58. Correct answer—B.

Initial assessment of the child with abdominal injuries should always begin with assessment of the airway, breathing, and circulation. Inspection would follow after these functions have been established as adequate. Palpation would be last because a child with pain, especially elicited during an examination, is generally unable to cooperate with any further examination. Rectal examination of a child with abdominal trauma is generally not performed by the critical care nurse.

59. Correct answer—B.

Because of its location, complaints of right upper quadrant pain associated with trauma are suggestive of liver injury. Pulmonary infarction will cause chest pain and respiratory distress. Splenic injury is associated with left-sided pain, whereas renal damage is associated with flank pain.

60. Correct answer—B.

Rejection of liver transplants commonly occurs between 4 and 10 days, though it can occur any time following transplantation. Rejection as early as the first day is termed *hyperacute* and is rare.

NEONATAL-SPECIFIC ANSWERS

61. Correct answer—B.

A small amount of light-colored stool from the rectum of an infant suspected of having duodenal atresia is not normal meconium and is consistent with the diagnosis. The scant amount does not signify that any oral intake has indeed reached the lower bowel, and the light color indicates that the atretic portion probably is below the entrance of the common bile duct so it does not contain bile. Intussusception is characterized by currant jelly stools, not a scant amount of light-colored material. Necrotizing enterocolitis is characterized by adequate amounts of occult positive stools that may appear dark or red.

62. Correct answer—A.

Incidence of NEC in infants fed with breast milk is lower than those fed with formulas. One possible reason may be the protective effects of immunoglobulins in breast milk against bacterial and viral infections. Factors associated with the development of necrotizing enterocolitis in the preterm infant include early feedings, low birth weight, respiratory distress syndrome, anemia, perinatal asphyxia, exchange transfusions, hyperosmolar feedings, polycythemia, umbilical artery catheterization, shock, hypothermia, and thrombocytopenia.

63. Correct answer—A.

Dehydration in the neonate with an omphalocele develops primarily because of third spacing of fluids into the bowel. There are no large amounts of watery stool, and fluid losses associated with nasogastric suctioning are easily calculated and replaced with intravenous therapy. Evaporative losses are more characteristic of gastroschisis, which has no protective membranous covering over the herniated bowel.

64. Correct answer—B.

A perinatal history consistent with a diagnosis of duodenal atresia includes polyhydramnios, increased oral secretions, bilious vomiting, early abdominal distension, and failure to stool within 48 hours of birth. Excess amniotic fluid develops because of intestinal blockage associated with duodenal atresia. Failure to swallow and clear amniotic fluid as a result of obstruction leads to polyhydramnios.

CHAPTER 7

Renal Care Problems

Passkeys

GENERAL PRINCIPLES OF NEPHROLOGY

- The kidneys are located behind the peritoneum (retroperitoneal). The left kidney is slightly higher than the right kidney. See Fig. 7-1 for an illustration of the renal system. See Fig. 7-2 for an illustration of the gross anatomy of the kidney.

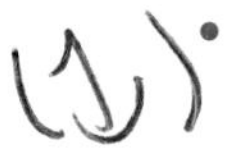

- The nephron is the functional unit of the kidney. There are approximately 1 million nephrons in each kidney. They contain all the essential vascular and urine collecting structures. See Fig. 7-3 for the anatomy of the nephron.

- Juxtamedullary nephrons have a longer loop of Henle that extends deeply into the middle of the kidneys giving them increased ability to concentrate urine.

- The juxtaglomerular apparatus is critical in blood pressure control. It secretes renin that in turn forms angiotensin I, where it is then converted to angiotensin

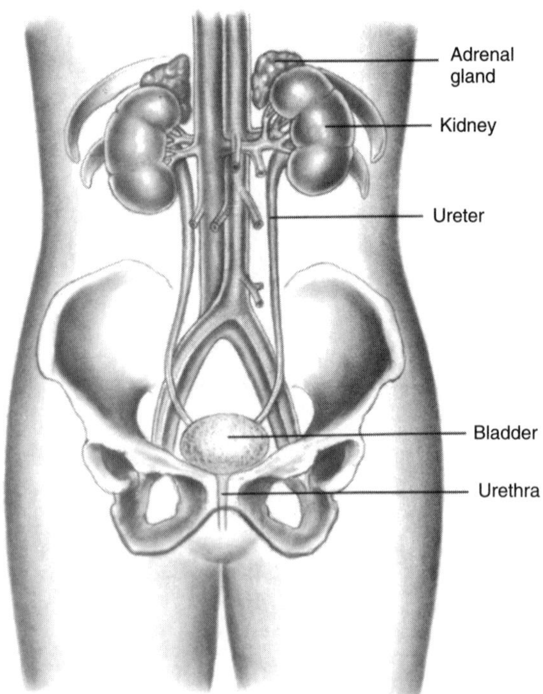

Fig. 7-1 Components of the urinary system. (From Thompson et al: Mosby's clinical nursing, ed 3, St Louis, 1993, Mosby.)

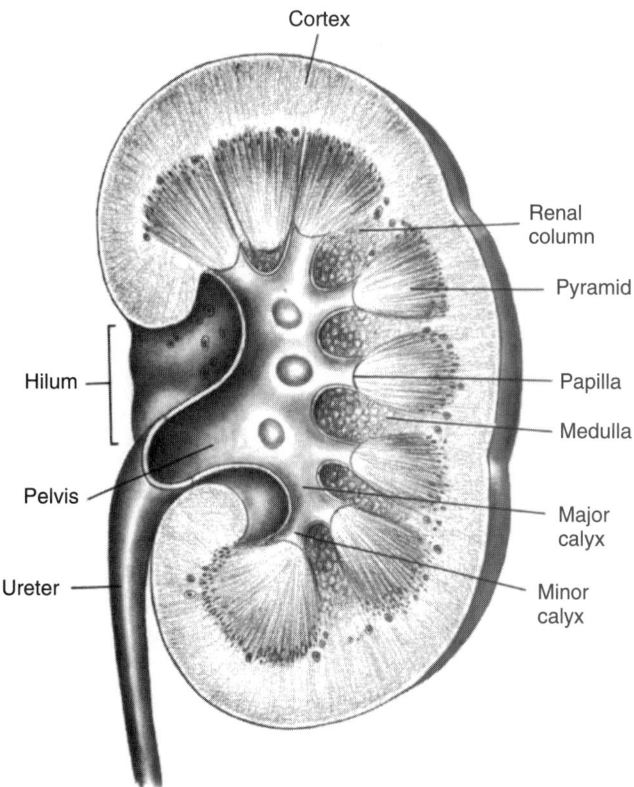

Fig. 7-2 Cross section of kidney. (From Thompson et al: Mosby's clinical nursing, ed 3, St Louis, 1993, Mosby.)

II in the lungs. Angiotensin II is a powerful peripheral vasoconstricting agent. Angiotensin II also causes an increase in aldosterone secretion leading to sodium and water retention that helps increase circulating volume and systemic pressure.

- Glomerular filtration occurs as blood passes through the glomerulus (a capillary bed) and plasma is filtered through the capillary walls into Bowman's capsule. See the box on p. 336 for factors influencing glomerular filtration.
- The glomerular filtration rate is the amount of filtrate (early urine) formed from the glomerulus, expressed as mL/min. The normal glomerular filtration rate is 125 mL/min/1.73 m^2.
- The kidneys in the neonate do not concentrate urine or conserve sodium well.
- Neonates are prone to acidosis as a result of the decreased ability of the renal tubules to reabsorb bicarbonate ions.

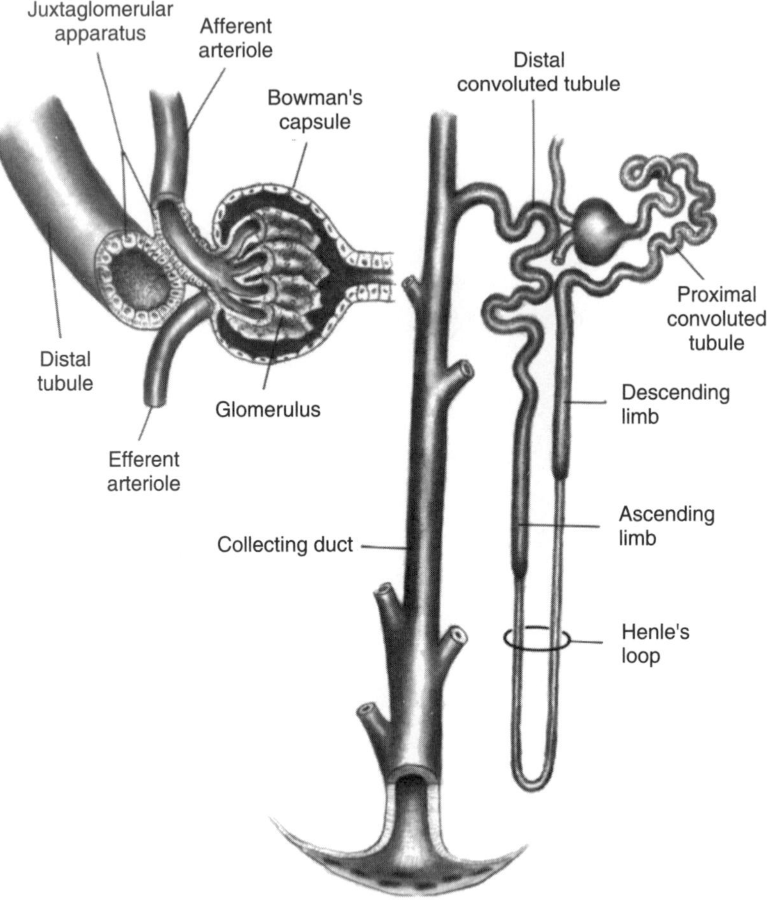

Fig. 7-3 Components of nephron. (From Thompson et al: Mosby's clinical nursing, ed 3, St Louis, 1993, Mosby.)

Factors Influencing Glomerular Filtration

- Systemic arterial pressure
- Rate of renal blood flow
- Glomerular capillary permeability
- Hydrostatic pressure within Bowman's capsule
- Hydrostatic pressure within the glomeruli
- Changes in afferent or efferent arteriolar vasoconstriction
- Obstruction to urinary flow
- Dehydration
- Hypoproteinemia
- Interstitial edema in the kidneys

- The glomerular filtration rate in the newborn is only 30 to 40 mL/min/1.73 m^2. It gradually rises from 55 to 65 mL/min/1.73 at 2 weeks of age to adult levels by 1 to 2 years of age.
- Serum creatinine levels should be about 0.4 mg/dL in term infants by the first week of life.
- Oliguria is defined as urine output less than 1 mL/kg/hr, except in the first 2 days of life. During the first 48 hours of life, oral intake may be low, so the kidneys are appropriately conserving fluid by decreasing urinary output.
- Cephalosporin antibiotics can affect laboratory determinations of the serum creatinine level. Serum creatinine levels should be drawn during the time of lowest serum cephalosporin levels.
- Antidiuretic hormone works on the distal convoluted tubules and collecting ducts allowing water to be reabsorbed into the bloodstream and decreasing urine output.
- Serum uric acid is elevated in the newborn as a result of increased production. It can appear red in color when passed through the urinary tract and mistaken for blood.
- Trace quantities of glucose can be normal in a term infant.
- Proteinuria is common in term infants and is related to gestational age. Proteinuria is highest at birth and should fall rapidly.
- The bladder is innervated by the parasympathetic branch of the autonomic nervous system.

Acid-Base Balance

- Acid-base balance is maintained by the bicarbonate-carbonic acid buffering system, plasma buffers, renal hydrogen ion excretion and bicarbonate reabsorption, and respiratory buffering action.
- The sodium bicarbonate dose to treat metabolic acidosis can be calculated by: mEq $NAHCO_3$ = base deficit × kg body weight × 0.3.
- See Table 7-1 for the mechanisms of the major buffering systems.

Pharmacological Principles

- Thiazide is preferred over furosemide in neonates requiring diuretic therapy. Furosemide causes losses of potassium as well as calcium. Urine calcium losses with furosemide have been responsible for renal calcifications. Furosemide use may also increase the incidence of patent ductus arteriosus as a result of its effect on prostaglandin synthesis.

Table 7-1

Buffering Systems

The bicarbonate-carbonic acid buffering system

$$CO_2 + H_2O \rightarrow H_2CO_3 \rightarrow HCO_3^-$$

Excessive amounts of carbon dioxide produced by cellular metabolism combine with water to form carbonic acid which quickly dissociates to hydrogen ions and bicarbonate ions. Excessive amounts of hydrogen ions can be eliminated by the kidney, or bicarbonate ions can be saved by the kidney to maintain normal acid base balance.

The renal hydrogen ion excretion and bicarbonate reabsorption buffering system

$$H^+ + HCO_3^- \rightarrow H_2CO_3 \rightarrow CO_2 + H_2O$$

Hydrogen ions can also combine with bicarbonate ions to form carbonic acid which dissociates to water and carbon dioxide, normally eliminated by the lungs.

The plasma buffering system

Hemglobin binds with H^+.

Hemoglobin transports CO_2 to the lungs for elimination

Respiratory buffering system

Hyperventilation helps eliminate CO_2 which in turn decreases hydrogen ions formed when CO_2 combines with water. This can help compensate for metabolic acidosis, or can be the cause of respiratory alkalosis.

Hypoventilation helps retain CO_2 which in turn increases hydrogen ions formed when CO_2 combines with water. This can help compensate for metabolic alkalosis, or be the cause of respiratory acidosis.

- Aminoglycosides must be closely monitored when used in neonates as a result of the variability of renal excretion.
- Indomethacin can cause or worsen renal failure in neonates by decreasing renal blood flow.
- Hypokalemia can decrease the effectiveness of diuretics.
- Hypokalemia can precipitate digitalis toxicity.
- Low dose dopamine at 1 to 4 mcg/kg/min is indicated for oliguric patients with poor cardiac output. It improves renal perfusion by dilating renal arteries and increasing the glomerular filtration rate. Dobutamine or isoproterenol also may be used.

GENERAL PRINCIPLES OF FLUID AND ELECTROLYTE BALANCE

- In the full term neonate, approximately 70% of body weight is water. This gradually decreases to 65% in young adult males and 52% in young adult females.

- Infants and children will develop a decrease in cardiac output and systemic perfusion if fluids totalling 7% to 10% of body weight are lost. In adolescents, only 5% to 7% of body weight need to be lost in fluids.

- Signs and symptoms of dehydration can be found in Table 7-2.

- Normal urine output is:
  Infants: ≥ 2 to 3 mL/hr
  Children (infant to preschooler): ≥ 2 mL/hr
  Children (school age): ≥ 1 to 2 mL/hr
  Adolescent: 0.5 to 1.0 mL/hr

Table 7-2

Assessment of Degree of Dehydration in Isotonic Fluid Losses*

Clinical Parameters	Mild	Moderate	Severe
Body weight loss			
Infant	5% (50 mL/kg)	10% (100 mL/kg)	15% (150 mL/kg)
Adult	3% (30 mL/kg)	6% (60 mL/kg)	9% (90 mL/kg)
Skin turgor	Slightly ↓	↓↓	↓↓↓
Fontanelle	May be flat or depressed	Depressed	Significantly depressed
Mucous membranes	Dry	Very dry	Parched
Skin perfusion	Warm, normal color	Extremities cool Pale color	Extremities cold Mottled or grey color
Heart rate	Mild tachycardia	Moderate tachycardia	Extreme tachycardia
Peripheral pulses	Normal	Diminished	Absent
Blood pressure	Normal	Normal	Reduced
Sensorium	Normal or irritable	Irritable or lethargic	Unresponsive
Urine output	Slightly ↓	Mild oliguria	Marked oliguria or anuria
Azotemia	Absent	Present	Present and severe

*The interpretation of the assessments must be appropriately modified for age and for *type* of dehydration (hypotonic or hypertonic dehydration).

From Hazinski MF: Nursing care of the critically ill child, ed 2, St Louis, 1992, Mosby.

- Normal fluid requirements:
  0 to 10 kg: 100 mL/kg/day
  11 to 20 kg: 1000 mL for the first 10 kg + 50 mL/kg/day
  More than 20 kg: 1500 mL for the first 10 kg + 25 mL/kg/day

- Normal insensible fluid losses:
  Infants: 35 mL/kg/day
  Children greater than 10 kg: 15 to 20 mL/kg/day + urine loss

- Electrolyte requirements:
  Sodium: 3 to 8 mEq/kg/day
  Potassium: 2 to 4 mEq/kg/day

- Aldosterone is secreted by the adrenal cortex in response to adrenal corticotropic hormone (ACTH) released by the pituitary gland. Aldosterone causes sodium to be retained and potassium to be excreted. A drop in systemic pressure, increased serum potassium, and decreased right atrial distension result in increased levels of aldosterone.

- Antidiuretic hormone (ADH) is produced in the hypothalmus and secreted by the pituitary in response to an increase in intracellular and serum osmolality, a decrease in blood volume, an increase in serum sodium levels, a decrease in systemic arterial pressure, and fear, exercise, or pain. ADH causes an increase in water resorption in the tubules.

- Dehydration is graded by percent of body weight lost:
  Mild: 5% of body weight lost
  Moderate: 10% of body weight lost
  Severe: 15% of body weight lost

LIFE-THREATENING ELECTROLYTE IMBALANCES

Potassium

- Normal serum potassium is 3.5 to 5.0 mEq/L.

- Potassium is the most abundant ion *inside the cells.*

- Potassium plays an important role in acid-base balance, cardiac depolarization, and neuromuscular function.

- See the following boxes on p. 341 for causes of potassium imbalances and signs and symptoms of potassium imbalances.

Hyperkalemia

- Hyperkalemia causes characteristic tall, tented T-waves on the electrocardiogram tracing.

Causes of Potassium Imbalances

Hyperkalemia	Hypokalemia
Extreme prematurity	Bicarbonate therapy
Hypoperfusion	Alkalosis
Renal failure	Inadequate dietary intake
Crushing injuries	Nasogastric suctioning
Hemorrhage, bruising	Diuretic therapy
Acidosis	Diarrhea
Rhabdomyolysis	Prolonged vomiting
Iatrogenic administration of excessive potassium chloride	Renal tubular acidosis
Hypoaldosteronism	Hyperaldosteronism
Transfusion of blood greater than 3 days old	

Signs and Symptoms of Potassium Imbalances

Hyperkalemia	Hypokalemia
Muscle weakness	Muscle weakness
Ventricular tachycardia	Constipation
Ventricular fibrillation	Rapid, weak, irregular pulse
Peaked T-waves	Abdominal distension
Wide QRS complexes	Vomiting
Abdominal cramping	ST segment depression
Diarrhea	Flat T-waves
Decreased or absent urine output	Presence of a U-wave

- Hyperkalemia is associated with acidosis. As the excess positively charged potassium ions move into the cells, positively charged hydrogen ions are forced out into the blood.

- Hyperkalemia may be treated with glucose and insulin or bicarbonate to drive the potassium into the cells and lower serum levels. This is only a temporary solution because no potassium is actually removed from the body. Be alert to recurring hyperkalemia.

- Calcium chloride or calcium gluconate may also be used in hyperkalemia to stimulate cardiac contractility, which is often depressed with hyperkalemia. *This treatment is contraindicated in patients on digoxin.*

- Kayexalate and sorbital are used to treat hyperkalemia and actually remove potassium, rather than shift it into cells. Kayexalate works as an ion exchange resin trading a sodium ion for a potassium ion. Sorbitol is a sugar that causes diarrhea and helps eliminate excess potassium by the gastrointestinal system.

Hypokalemia

- Intravenous (IV) potassium supplements must always be given very slowly and never given as a bolus! High concentrations of potassium supplements given rapidly IV can cause tissue and vessel necrosis as well as ventricular fibrillation.

- Flattened T-waves characterize the electrocardiogram tracing in a patient with hypokalemia.

Sodium

- Normal serum sodium is 135 to 145 mEq/L.

- Sodium is the most common ion *outside the cells.*

- Sodium plays an important part in determining the osmotic pressure of extravascular fluids, cardiac depolarization, and neuromuscular function.

- See the following boxes on p. 343 for causes of sodium imbalances and for signs and symptoms of sodium imbalances.

- Neonates have a decreased ability to excrete excessive sodium.

- Usually hypernatremia is more likely to reflect a water loss resulting in concentration of sodium rather than a true excess of total body sodium.

- True sodium excess with water losses should be treated with intravenous solutions, which contain little sodium. Dextrose 5% in water or 1/2 normal saline solutions would be indicated.

Causes of Sodium Imbalances

Hypernatremia

Inadequate water intake

Dehydration

Diabetes insipidus

Hypercalcemia

Excessive water loss

Mineralocorticoids

Increased adrenocortical secretion of aldosterone

Hyponatremia

Excessive water intake

Syndrome of inappropriate antidiuretic hormone

Diuretic therapy

Diarrhea

Nasogastric suctioning

Hyperglycemia

Congestive heart failure

Hepatic cirrhosis

Prematurity

Medications:

- indomethacin
- furosemide
- methylxanthines

Signs and Symptoms of Sodium Imbalances

Hypernatremia

Sunken fontanelle

Dry mucous membranes

Cool, pale skin

Tachycardia

Diminished or absent peripheral pulses

Normal or reduced systemic arterial pressure

Irritability, lethargy, unresponsiveness

Decreased urine output

Fever

In infants: high-pitched cry, apnea, seizures, coma

Hyponatremia

Weakness

Apathy

Headaches

If dilutional: dyspnea, edema

If dehydration: thirst

In infants: apnea, irritability, seizures

Table 7-3
Normal Values of Phosphorus, Calcium, and Magnesium

Electrolyte	Normal Value
Phosphorus	Newborn: 4.3-9.3 mg/dL Child: 4.5-6.5 mg/dL
Calcium (total)	Newborn: 9.0-10.6 mg/dL Child: 8.8-10.8 mg/dL
Magnesium	Newborn: 1.8-2.4 mg/dL Child: 1.8-2.4 mg/dL

- Rapid lowering of high serum sodium levels can cause cerebral edema or intraventricular hemorrhage in infants.
- Hyponatremia is treated by ensuring adequate oral intake or supplementation by IV sodium containing solutions.

Phosphorus, Calcium, and Magnesium

- See Table 7-3 for normal serum values of phosphorus, calcium, and magnesium.
- Phosphorous, calcium, and magnesium levels are closely related. Magnesium and calcium tend to rise and fall together. Phosphorous levels rise and fall inversely to magnesium and calcium.
- See Table 7-4 for causes of phosphorous, calcium, and magnesium imbalances and Table 7-5 for signs and symptoms of imbalances.
- Hypocalcemia may resolve without calcium supplements. If treatment is required, boluses or continuous infusions of calcium gluconate are preferred. If boluses are given, they must be given slowly over 20 to 30 minutes by infusion pump under constant ECG monitoring to prevent bradycardia or asystole.
- Calcitonin infusions or furosemide may be used to treat hypercalcemia.
- Calcium gluconate or furosemide may be used to treat hypermagnesemia.
- Hypomagnesemia may be treated by correcting hypocalcemia or magnesium sulfate infusions.

Table 7-4

Etiology of Phosphorous, Calcium, and Magnesium Imbalances

Electrolyte	Etiology of Imbalance
Phosphorous	*Increased levels:* hypoparathyroidism, renal failure, liver disease, hypocalcemia *Decreased levels:* poor dietary instake, hyperparathyroidism, hypercalcemia, rickets
Calcium (total)	*Increased levels:* hyperparathyroidism, Addison's disease, Paget's disease of bone *Decreased levels:* hypoparathyroidism, renal failure, malabsorption, pancreatitis
Magnesium	*Increased levels:* renal failure, Addison's disease *Decreased levels:* prolonged vomiting or diarrhea, renal failure

Table 7-5

Signs and Symptoms of Phosphorous, Calcium, and Magnesium Imbalances

Electrolyte	Signs and Symptoms of Imbalance
Phosphorous	*Increased levels:* paraesthesia, twitching, dysrhythmias, hypotension, laryngospasm *Decreased levels:* lethargy, bone pain, decreased muscle tone, nausea, vomiting, anorexia, constipation, flank pain, headache, thirst, increased urinary output
Calcium (total)	*Increased levels:* lethargy, bone pain, decreased muscle tone, nausea, vomiting, anorexia, constipation, flank pain, headache, thirst, increased urinary output *Decreased levels:* bone pain, lethargy, constipation, nausea, vomiting, cramps, shallow breathing, bronchospasm, dysrhythmias, decreased urinary output, increased abdominal girth, tetany, Chvostek's sign, Trousseau's sign
Magnesium	*Increased levels:* lethargy, hypotension, flushing, diaphoresis, nausea, vomiting, diminished reflexes, drowsiness, muscle weakness, hypoventilation *Decreased levels:* tremors, convulsions, hyperactive reflexes, leg and foot cramps, cardiac dysrhythmias, muscle weakness, tetany

Multisystem Effects of Acute Renal Failure

Cardiovascular

Congestive heart failure

Dysrhythmias

Hypertension

Pericarditis

Pulmonary

Pulmonary edema

Pneumonia

Pleural effusions

Neurological

Altered level of consciousness

Cerebral edema

Hematological/Immunological

Anemia

Abnormal platelet function

Diminished white blood cell function

Infection

Hemorrhage

Gastrointestinal

Anorexia

Nausea

Vomiting

Gastrointestinal hemorrhage

Disorders of Electrolyte and Acid-Base Balance

Metabolic Disturbances

ACUTE RENAL FAILURE

- Acute renal failure (ARF) can be divided into three major etiologies: prerenal, intrarenal, and postrenal failure
- Renal failure causes multisystem problems. See the box above for expected systemic complications associated with ARF.
- Congenital renal anomalies should be suspected in any infant with ARF who has not voided and has bladder distension, malpositioned ears, ambiguous genitalia, abnormal abdominal muscles, epispadias, hypospadias, or a single umbilical artery.

PRERENAL FAILURE

- Prerenal failure occurs when there is an inadequate circulatory supply to the kidneys so that adequate filtration of the blood cannot occur. The result is a failure of the kidneys to maintain normal fluid and biochemical homeostasis. Causes of acute renal failure can be found in the box on p. 347.

Causes of Acute Renal Failure

Prerenal Failure

Hypotension

Hemorrhage

Sepsis

Dehydration

Congestive heart failure

Renal artery thrombosis/stenosis

Hypoxia

Respiratory distress syndrome

Intrarenal Failure

Hemolytic uremic syndrome

Glomerulonephritis

Pyelonephritis

Polycystic kidney disease

Crush injuries

Acute tubular necrosis

Potter's syndrome

Postrenal Failure

Posterior urethral valves

Ureterocele

Neurogenic bladder

Stenosis/obstruction of urinary drainage system

- Acute renal failure is usually defined as a blood urea nitrogen (BUN) level greater than 80 mg/dL and a serum creatinine greater than 1.5 mg/dL.

- Oliguria is an expected, but not required, finding in ARF. Anuria, or the absence of urinary output, is expected only in obstructive disorders of the urinary tract.

- Prerenal failure can be distinguished from intra-renal and postrenal failure by a low urinary sodium level, a urine osmolality in excess of the serum osmolality, and a BUN:serum creatinine ratio greater than 20:1.

INTRARENAL FAILURE

- Intrarenal failure occurs when the kidneys themselves are damaged or abnormal. It may be the primary cause of renal failure, or result from prerenal or postrenal causes that have not been corrected and progressed to renal parenchymal damage.

PEDIATRIC-SPECIFIC PRINCIPLES

RENAL TRAUMA

- Many children with renal trauma do *not* have hematuria.

- Laceration of the kidney should be suspected if there is a lower rib fracture or spinal fracture.
- Despite renal vascular damage, nonoperative intervention such as complete bed rest may successfully avoid surgical intervention.
- Injuries to the ureters are not common.
- Bladder trauma or rupture should be suspected in any child with pelvic fractures.
- Signs of urethral trauma include blood at the urinary meatus, perineal edema, and distended bladder with inability to void.

NEONATAL-SPECIFIC PRINCIPLES

- In the preterm infant, as much as 80% to 85% of body weight is water.
- Preterm infants have a very low glomerular filtration rate and immature nephrons. Renal function is best judged by ensuring the neonate's serum creatinine is no higher than the maternal level or below 1.5 mg/dL.
- Glomerular filtration rate in preterm infants less than 34 weeks gestation may be only 0.5 mL/min.
- Trace quantities of glucose in the urine are normal in preterm infants.
- In ARF, the neonate may be limited to a rise in BUN of only 5 mg/dL/day because of low urea production and high total body fluids.

POLYCYSTIC KIDNEYS

- Perinatal history of an infant with polycystic kidney disease includes oligohydramnios, oliguria, abdominal distension, hypertension, congestive heart failure, and dyspnea.
- Care is supportive and directed at clinical manifestations.
- Some infants will die in the neonatal period, whereas others may survive many years before ultimately developing chronic end-state renal disease.

EXTROPHY OF THE BLADDER

- In exstrophy of the bladder, the bladder is exposed externally and the condition is often associated with epispadias. However, the upper urinary tract and kidneys are usually normal.

- The anus is often displaced, associated inguinal hernias are common, and frequently there are abnormalities of the pelvic bone structure.
- The bladder is protected preoperatively by a clear, sterile, plastic dressing until surgical correction takes place usually within 48 hours after birth.

POTTER'S SYNDROME

- Potter's syndrome is associated with severe failure of the renal and genitourinary systems to develop during fetal life.
- These infants have distinct facial characteristics including low set ears, broad nasal bridge, widely spaced eyes, and receding chin.
- The prognosis is 100% mortality, generally in the first 1 to 2 days of life.

Questions

GENERAL RENAL CARE QUESTIONS

1. The basic functional unit of the kidney is the:
   A. Nephron
   B. Collecting tubules
   C. Calyces
   D. Glomerulus

2. Many medications that are secreted by the kidneys need to be adjusted in dosage when given to infants because:
   A. They are nephrotoxic to infants
   B. They can cause hepatorenal syndrome
   C. The glomerular filtration rate is decreased
   D. They may cause acid-base imbalances

3. The kidneys conserve or eliminate water in the body primarily in response to levels of:
   A. Potassium (K^+)
   B. Antidiuretic hormone (ADH)
   C. Aldosterone
   D. Angiotensin II

4. Normal urinary output for infants should be greater than or equal to:
   A. 0.5 to 1.0 mL/kg/hr
   B. 1.0 to 3.0 mL/kg/hr
   C. 2.0 to 3.0 mL/kg/hr
   D. 3.0 to 4.0 mL/kg/hr

5. Which of the following patients is most likely to have an increased need for maintenance fluid requirements? A patient:
   A. On the first day following open-heart surgery
   B. With hepatic encephalopathy
   C. With acute tubular necrosis
   D. On mechanical ventilation

Case Study

A 3.3 kg infant is admitted to the critical care unit and diagnosed with severe dehydration associated with diarrhea. She is irritable, with very dry mucous membranes and no tears with crying. Questions 6 to 9 refer to this case study.

---

6. The *most* important priority in the first minutes of intervention for this patient is:
A. Establishment of a vascular access
B. Calculation of mean arterial pressure
C. Determination of life-threatening electrolyte imbalances
D. Intubation with assisted ventilation

7. This infant would be expected to have a fluid loss that is what percentage of her body weight?
A. 1%
B. 5%
C. 10%
D. 15%

8. She would also be expected to have which of the following clinical signs and symptoms?
A. Decreased urine specific gravity, cool and pale skin, decreased serum pH, and tachycardia
B. Decreased urine specific gravity, cool and mottled skin, decreased serum pH, and hypotension
C. Increased urine specific gravity, cool and pale skin, increased serum pH, and hypertension
D. Increased urine specific gravity, cool and mottled skin, decreased serum pH, and tachycardia

9. Immediate fluid resuscitation for this infant most likely would include:
A. 10 mL bolus of a crystalloid solution given over 3 minutes
B. 35 mL bolus of a crystalloid solution given over 5 minutes
C. 65 mL bolus of a crystalloid solution given over 15 minutes
D. 100 mL bolus of a crystalloid solution given over 1 hour

10. The kidneys help regulate acid-base balance by all of the following mechanisms *except*:
A. Reabsorption of bicarbonate ions
B. Secretion of hydrogen ions
C. Increased filtration of ions
D. Production of buffers

11. An example of a cause of prerenal failure would be:
A. Potter's syndrome
B. Hypovolemic shock
C. Neurogenic bladder
D. Glomerulonephritis

12. Normal sodium balance is primarily regulated by:
A. Aldosterone
B. Antidiuretic hormone
C. Parathyroid hormone
D. Glomerular filtration rate

13. An oliguric patient with rising blood urea nitrogen (BUN) and serum creatinine levels has a urine specific gravity of 1.010. His serum and urine osmolalities are both 285 mOsm/L. This patient most likely has:
A. Prerenal failure
B. Postrenal failure
C. Intrarenal failure
D. Hepatorenal failure

14. For a patient on furosemide therapy, which of the following is *not* an expected or desired patient outcome?
A. Urine output of 1 mL/kg/hr or greater
B. No adventitious breath sounds
C. Absence of S_3 heart sounds
D. Resolution of pleural effusion

15. Interventions for acute renal failure may include the following *except*:
A. Kayexelate
B. Sodium bicarbonate
C. Increased protein intake
D. Increased intravenous fluids

16. Neonates have decreased renal function in the early weeks of life because:
A. The glomerular filtration rate is decreased
B. Sodium is poorly excreted
C. Their glomeruli are excessively permeable
D. They have fewer nephrons

17. During acidosis, the kidneys compensate by:
A. Increasing bicarbonate excretion
B. Forming ammonia
C. Decreasing hydrogen ion excretion
D. Decreasing urine pH

Case Study

A female infant was admitted to the critical care unit for perinatal asphyxia and 4 days later developed acute renal failure. She had a prolonged episode of hypotension during her delivery and an immediate resuscitation period. Her urine output has fallen to 0.35 mL/kg for the last 24 hours. Questions 18 to 20 refer to this case study.

---

18. For which of the following electrolyte imbalances is this infant most at risk?
A. Hyperkalemia
B. Hypernatremia
C. Hypercalcemia
D. Hypophosphatemia

19. To prevent complications, initial treatment of this infant focusing on her history should include:
A. Fluid bolus of 20 mL/kg of Ringer's lactate
B. 10 mL/kg of red packed cells
C. Dopamine 2 to 5 mcg/kg/min
D. Calcium gluconate

20. Which of the following medications would be *least* likely to require an adjustment in dosage for this infant?
A. Gentamicin
B. Digoxin
C. Pancuronium bromide
D. Dobutamine

21. Which of the following causes of renal failure will most likely result in prerenal failure?
A. Neurogenic bladder
B. Cardiogenic shock
C. Polycystic kidney disease
D. Glomerulonephritis

22. Care of the patient in oliguric acute renal failure should include which of the following?
A. Weigh every other day
B. Protein-restricted diet
C. Monitor for signs of dehydration
D. Observe for Turner's sign

Case Study

A 4.0 kg 5-day-old patient is admitted to the critical care unit in congestive heart failure. Over 8 hours his urinary output has averaged 0.3 cc/kg/hr. His laboratory studies are as follows:
Na+: 128 mEq/L
K+: 5.8
BUN: 41 mg/dL
Creatinine: 0.6 mg/dL
Serum osmolality: 265 mOsm/L
Serum phosphates: 2.6 mEq/L
Serum calcium: 9.1 mg/dL

Questions 23 and 24 refer to this case study.

---

23. Which of the following orders is *contraindicated* in this patient?
A. 30 to 50 mcg/kg digoxin for digitalizing dose
B. 400 mL/day of isotonic solutions
C. Furosemide 1 mg/kg IV
D. Dopamine infusion of 3 mcg/kg/min

24. This patient's sodium level is most likely related to:
A. Hypervolemia
B. Hypovolemia
C. Sodium wasting
D. Sodium retention

25. When taking a blood pressure using an automatic blood pressure monitor, the critical care nurse notices that the patient has a carpopedal spasm. This is most likely because of:
A. Hypophosphatemia
B. Hypermagnesemia
C. Hypokalemia
D. Hypocalcemia

26. A critically ill patient with hypocalcemia is at risk for all of the following *except*:
A. Bleeding abnormalities
B. Respiratory arrest
C. Alkalosis
D. Cardiac arrest

27. In planning nursing interventions for the patient with hyperkalemia, the most critical action would be to:
A. Administer calcium chloride for patients on digoxin therapy
B. Administer racemic epinephrine to prevent bronchospasm
C. Administer sodium bicarbonate to correct alkalosis
D. Administer glucose and insulin to shift potassium into cells

28. For the nursing diagnosis of altered renal tissue perfusion related to hypovolemia, the patient outcomes within 4 hours of admission would include all of the following *except*:
A. Age appropriate normal sinus rate and rhythm
B. Moist mucous membranes and warm extremities
C. Urinary output greater than 1.0 mL/kg
D. Infusion of 20 mL/kg bolus of crystalloids

29. Acute renal failure can result in hyperkalemia specifically related to:
A. Decreased aldosterone production
B. Increased secretion of ADH
C. Decreased urinary output
D. Increased sodium retention

30. An acutely ill, postoperative patient begins to have a decrease in urinary output over a 2-hour period. The blood pressure is within normal limits. Which of the following therapies is most appropriate to initiate *first*?
A. Fluid bolus of 20 mL/kg of crystalloids
B. Dobutamine at 15 mcg/kg/min
C. Dopamine at 12 mcg/kg/min
D. Furosemide bolus 1 mg/mL IV

31. A patient with rotovirus is admitted to the critical care unit in hypovolemic shock. After fluid infusion and establishment of adequate circulating volume, the patient continues to be lethargic with shallow respirations; rapid, weak, irregular pulse; abdominal distension; and the ECG shows ST segment depression, flat T waves, and the presence of a U wave. The nurse suspects:
A. Hyperkalemia
B. Hypokalemia
C. Hypercalcemia
D. Hypocalcemia

32. Which of the following would *most likely* confirm the diagnosis of *pre*renal acute renal failure in a patient?
A. Urinary output less than 1.0 mL/kg/hr
B. Serum creatinine greater than 1.0
C. BUN:creatinine ratio of 20:1
D. Renal ultrasound

33. In planning nursing interventions for the patient with hypocalcemia, the critical care nurse should be aware that:
A. Bolus doses are preferred over continuous infusions
B. Peripheral infiltrations of calcium should be treated with phentolamine mesylate (Regitine)
C. Bolus doses should be given quickly to get the maximum serum level
D. Liver necrosis can occur with calcium infused through umbilical catheters

34. Infants and children with hypocalcemia need continuous cardiac monitoring because this electrolyte imbalance causes:
A. Prolonged QT intervals
B. Prolonged PR internals
C. Third-degree heart block
D. Supraventricular tachycardia

35. A patient in acute renal failure is found to have flaccid muscle tone, lethargy, and deep, rapid respirations. His blood gases reveal a pH of 7.25 and serum electrolytes are deranged, including a potassium of 6.8 mEq/L. His electrocardiogram shows multiple ventricular ectopic beats and tall, tented T waves. The critical care nurse anticipates immediate administration of:
A. Kayexelate
B. Glucose and insulin
C. Normal saline fluid bolus
D. Magnesium sulfate

36. A patient in the critical care unit develops acute renal failure following a prolonged hypotensive episode. Her most recent arterial blood gases are:
pH: 7.26
pCO_2: 28 mm Hg
pO_2: 94 mm Hg
HCO_3^-: 16 mEq/L
% arterial saturation: 98%
Base deficit: -3
The most likely physiological cause of this patient's abnormal blood gas results is:
A. Retention of bicarbonate ions
B. Retention of hydrogen ions
C. Hypoventilation
D. Hyperventilation

37. In identifying potential risk factors, the critical care nurse recognizes that hypocalcemia is generally found with:
A. Hypophosphatemia
B. Hypokalemia
C. Hypomagnesemia
D. Hyponatremia

38. Neonates at risk for hypermagnesemia include those with a maternal history of:
A. Toxemia of pregnancy
B. Diabetes mellitus
C. Hyperthyroidism
D. Hypocalcemia

39. The critical care nurse recognizes compensation for metabolic acidosis by which of the following changes?
A. Decrease in pCO_2
B. Increase in pCO_2
C. Decrease in HCO_3^-
D. Increase in HCO_3^-

40. When administering sodium bicarbonate to a neonate, the critical care nurse should be aware that the:
A. Correct dose is 2 to 4 mEq/kg
B. Concentration should not exceed 0.5 mEq/mL
C. Bolus infusion rate should not be more than 2 mEq/kg/min
D. Route of administration may be IV or IM

PEDIATRIC-SPECIFIC QUESTIONS

Case Study

A 4-year-old girl is admitted to the critical care unit with hypovolemic shock and a serum potassium of 2.8 mEq/L related to diarrhea. Questions 41 to 43 refer to this case study.

---

41. Which of the following signs and symptoms related to hypokalemia would the critical care nurse expect to find during an assessment?
A. Weakness, bradycardia, prolonged PR interval
B. Nausea, tented T waves, fatigue
C. Fatigue, weakness, flattened T wave
D. Muscle pain, nausea, wide QRS

(hyper)

42. Which of the following pharmacological treatments is indicated for treating this patient?
A. Kayexalate given as an enema or orally
B. Potassium infusion of 15 to 20 mEq/L/hr
C. Potassium replacement by bolus
D. Digoxin for cardiac dysrhythmias

43. This patient is also at risk for developing which acid-base imbalance?
A. Metabolic alkalosis
B. Metabolic acidosis
C. Respiratory alkalosis
D. Respiratory acidosis

44. The critical care nurse would recognize all of the following as risk factors for renal trauma *except* injury to the:
A. Lumbar spine
B. Lower right ribs
C. Lower left ribs
D. Pelvis

45. Which of the following signs would be important in identifying renal trauma?
A. Turner's sign
B. Cushing's triad
C. Cullen's sign
D. Trousseau's sign

46. A 10-year-old child was admitted to the critical care unit after being hit by a car. She complains of needing to void, but she appears unable. Physical examination reveals an easily palpable and full bladder. The next action the critical care nurse should take is to:
A. Immediately catheterize the patient to minimize bladder damage
B. Inspect the urinary meatus for blood before catheterization
C. Delay catheterization until a renal ultrasound can be completed
D. Gently crede the bladder to assist in voiding

Case Study

A 16-year-old patient is admitted to the critical care unit following a basketball injury where he sustained a blow to the right flank. He was noted in the emergency room to have bruising over the area of hematuria. He was admitted to the intensive care unit because of severe pain, hypotension, and further stabilization. Questions 47 and 48 refer to this case study.

---

47. Which of the following interventions would *not* be indicated in the initial treatment of this patient?
A. Obtain a blood sample
B. Administer intravenous fluids
C. Initiate antimicrobial therapy
D. Administer narcotic analgesics

48. How long should this patient remain on bedrest? Until his:
A. Flank pain is controlled without medication
B. Hemoglobin and hematocrit return to normal
C. Renal ultrasound demonstrates no perirenal hematoma
D. Hematuria resolves

49. In a trauma patient with genitourinary (GU) injuries, which of the following is most likely to be an *abnormal* finding?
A. Palpable bladder
B. Palpable right kidney
C. Palpable left kidney
D. Palpable symphysis pubis

50. Which of the following statements is *not* true about GU trauma?
A. Most GU trauma is a result of motor vehicle accidents
B. The use of seat belts has increased the incidence of GU trauma
C. GU trauma is usually accompanied by trauma to other organ systems
D. A full bladder increases the risk of GU trauma in motor vehicle crashes

NEONATAL-SPECIFIC QUESTIONS

Case Study

A 24-hour-old 4 kg neonate is admitted to the critical care unit with a diagnosis of infantile polycystic disease. Questions 51 to 53 refer to this case study.

---

51. Assessment of this neonate is likely to reveal all of the following *except*:
A. Polyuria
B. Flank masses
C. Respiratory distress
D. Hematuria

52. Infantile polycystic kidney disease is characterized by which of the following laboratory tests?
A. Hyperkalemia, hypocalcemia, hyperphosphatemia, and acidosis
B. Hypokalemia, hypocalcemia, hyperphosphatemia, and acidosis
C. Hyperkalemia, hypercalcemia, hypophosphatemia, and alkalosis
D. Hypokalemia, hypercalcemia, hypophosphatemia, and alkalosis

53. Positive patient outcomes in the treatment of this neonate would *not* include:
A. Blood pressure of 60 to 80/20 to 55 mm Hg
B. Absence of adventitious breath sounds
C. Palpable liver border 3 cm below the costal margin
D. Urinary output of 50 cc/24 hours

54. Which of the following statements about extrophy of the bladder is *not* true?
A. It is often associated with epispadias
B. There are often other associated renal anomalies
C. This condition is more common in boys
D. An umbilical hernia is often found in association

55. In counseling the family of a neonate with extrophy of the bladder, the most appropriate statement for the critical nurse to share would be:

A. "Most of the infants have a great deal of trouble with bed-wetting and bladder control as they get older."

B. "These children can achieve normal bladder control with surgery that involves six stages."

C. "Most infants can achieve good bladder control with surgery and medical therapy."

D. "Your infant will probably have surgery to correct this condition within the first week of life."

56. The critical care nurse's care of the neonate with extrophy of the bladder would include:

A. Covering the exposed bladder with petroleum gauze

B. Use of a sterile cord clamp on the umbilical cord

C. Insertion of an indwelling urinary catheter

D. Using a clear, occlusive dressing to cover the bladder

Case Study

A neonate is admitted to the critical care unit directly from the delivery room in respiratory distress. He is small for his gestational age. Physical examination reveals low set ears, widely spaced eyes, large hands, and bowed legs. The labor and delivery room nurse reports a perinatal history of oligohydramnios. Questions 57 to 59 refer to this case study.

---

57. The most likely cause of these findings is:

A. Polycystic kidney disease

B. Turner's syndrome

C. Potter's syndrome

D. Hydronephrosis

58. The most likely cause of this neonate's respiratory distress is:

A. Bronchiolitis

B. Pneumothorax

C. Aspiration

D. Tracheoesophageal fistula

59. Interventions for this infant would most likely be planned to:

A. Increase urinary output

B. Decrease metabolic acidosis

C. Provide comfort measures

D. Maximize nutritional status

Answers

GENERAL RENAL CARE ANSWERS

1. **Correct answer—A.**
The basic functional unit of the kidney is the nephron because it contains all essential elements for the formation of urine. Within the nephron are both capillaries, which permit the filtration of blood, and a urine collecting system. Essential circulatory components include the afferent arteriole, glomerulus, efferent arteriole, and peritubular capillaries. The critical elements of the urine collecting system include Bowman's capsule, the proximal convoluted tubule, loop of Henle, distal convoluted tubule, and tubular collecting system.

2. **Correct answer—C.**
Many medications that are secreted by the kidneys need to be adjusted in dosage when given to infants because the glomerular filtration rate takes as long as 2 years to reach adult levels. Because the glomerular filtration rate is lower in infants under 2 years of age, medications may be poorly excreted by the kidneys, thus requiring lower doses or close monitoring of serum levels.

3. **Correct answer—B.**
The kidneys conserve or eliminate water in the body primarily in response to levels of antidiuretic hormone (ADH). ADH acts directly on the renal tubular cells and makes it easier for water to move from the urine collecting ducts back into the circulatory system. Potassium is lost when urinary output increases, but it doesn't *cause* an increase in output. Aldosterone regulates sodium balance. Angiotensin II is produced in the lungs in response to renin secretion in the kidneys, but it causes arterial and venous vasoconstriction and plays no direct role in the excretion or conservation of water.

4. **Correct answer—B.**
Normal urinary output for infants should be greater than 1.0 to 3.0 mL/kg/hr. Children should have urinary output greater than or equal to 1.0 to 2.0 mL/kg/hr.

5. **Correct answer—D.**
All of the following patients have a decreased need for maintenance fluid requirements *except* a patient on mechanical ventilation. Mechanical ventilation is generally associated with increased insensible water losses, which increase a patient's daily fluid need. On the first day following open-heart surgery, a patient's fluid needs are generally less than the full maintenance amount because of the stress response to surgery that results in fluid retention. Most neurological conditions, such as encephalopathy, also demand conservative fluid therapy to avoid increasing intracranial pressure. Acute tubular necrosis (ATN) also would decrease a patient's fluid requirements because of the oliguria that accompanies ATN.

6. **Correct answer—A.**
The most important priority in the first minutes of intervention for this patient is establishment of a vascular access. Resuscitation always begins with ensuring a patent airway and adequate breathing. Nothing in this patient's history demonstrates an increased risk immediately. Following airway and breathing, circulation is the next priority in resuscitation. This infant, because of her diagnosis of severe dehydration, has inadequate circulation making establishment of a vascular access for fluid resuscitation the highest priority. Determining the mean arterial pressure and assessing for life-threatening electrolyte imbalances are important, but follow the priority of improving circulation.

7. **Correct answer—D.**
This infant would be expected to have a fluid loss that is 15% or more of her body weight. Mild dehydration is associated with only 5% body weight loss and moderate dehydration is associated with 10% loss.

8. **Correct answer—D.**
An infant with severe dehydration would be expected to have increased urine specific gravity, cool and mottled skin, decreased serum pH, and tachycardia. In addition, findings would include oliguria, hypotension, hypernatremia, and sunken fontanelles. Urine specific gravity is increased because of the body's effort to conserve water and decrease urine output. Skin is cool and mottled from shock and severely compromised cardiac output and peripheral perfusion. Serum pH falls as peripheral tissues, which are poorly perfused, produce lactic acids. Tachycardia and hypotension result from the heart's efforts to attain an adequate cardiac output with an inadequate circulatory volume.

9. **Correct answer—C.**
Immediate fluid resuscitation for this infant most likely would include a 65 mL bolus of a crystalloid solution given over 15 minutes. Fluid resuscitation for a patient with severe dehydration or loss of circulating volume is generally given at 20 mL/kg bolus of crystalloids or 10 mL/kg bolus of blood/colloid over 10 to 15 minutes.

10. **Correct answer—C.**
Filtration occurs in the glomerulus and does not increase or decrease to excrete bicarbonate or hydrogen ions. The kidneys help regulate acid-base balance by reabsorption of bicarbonate ions, secretion of hydrogen ions, and production of buffers.

11. **Correct answer—B.**
An example of a cause of prerenal failure would be hypovolemic shock. Prerenal failure occurs when there is inadequate perfusion to the kidneys so that the kidneys are unable to adequately filter the blood and maintain normal homeostasis. Other examples of prerenal failure include hemorrhagic and septic shock, dehydration, congestive heart failure, cardiac tamponade, pulmonary embolism, or

renal artery occlusion. Potter's syndrome and glomerulonephritis are examples of intrarenal failure as a result of renal parenchymal damage. A neurogenic bladder is an example of postrenal failure where the function of the kidneys is impaired because of obstruction to the urinary drainage system.

12. Correct answer—A.
Normal sodium balance is primarily regulated by aldosterone. Aldosterone is responsible for retaining or eliminating sodium in the urine based on physiological need. Antidiuretic hormone regulates water balance. Parathyroid hormone regulates calcium and phosphorous balance. The glomerular filtration rate is responsible for adequate initial filtration of the blood, but is not specifically responsible for fluid or electrolyte balance by regulating resorption or excretion.

13. Correct answer—C.
A rising blood urea nitrogen (BUN) and serum creatinine levels along with relatively equal serum and urine osmolalities are characteristic of intrarenal failure. Prerenal failure is characterized by very concentrated urine with a high specific gravity and urine osmolality as the body tries to conserve fluid. The kidneys' ability to concentrate or dilute urine is not affected in prerenal failure unless the condition persists and damage to the renal tissue itself occurs. Postrenal failure is characterized by anuria as a result of obstruction of urinary flow.

14. Correct answer—D.
Furosemide is a loop diuretic that increases urinary output and therefore decreases excess body water. Pleural effusions are an accumulation of excess fluid in the pleural space, but are not generally responsive to diuretic therapy. For a patient on furosemide therapy, expected or desired patient outcomes would include urine output of 1 mL/kg/hr or greater, absence of adventitious (abnormal) breath sounds, and absence of S_3 heart sounds (gallop rhythm).

15. Correct answer—C.
Interventions for acute renal failure would not include increasing the protein intake. Increased protein intake would increase the blood urea nitrogen level and worsen azotemia. Kayexelate may be used to decrease hyperkalemia and sodium bicarbonate may be required to treat acidosis often associated with ARF. Increased intravenous fluids may be indicated in treating prerenal failure, which was caused by an inadequate circulating volume.

16. Correct answer—A.
Neonates have decreased renal function in the early weeks of life because the glomerular filtration rate is decreased. Sodium is actually lost or wasted in the neonate because the tubules are initially poorly capable of selective and active resorption. Neonates' glomeruli are small, but are not more permeable than older infants, children, or adults. Increased permeability of the glomerulus is *always* abnormal and can result in hematuria and proteinuria. Although nephrons are immature at birth, there is no increase in number over the life span.

17. Correct answer—B.

During acidosis, the kidneys compensate by forming ammonia, which helps to eliminate excess hydrogen ions. Bicarbonate ion excretion is decreased, whereas hydrogen ion excretion is increased. The urine pH ideally decreases as hydrogen ions are excreted in larger numbers and bicarbonate ions are excreted less.

18. Correct answer—A.

This infant is most at risk for hyperkalemia related to her diminished urinary output. When urine output falls below minimal levels, potassium cannot be removed and life-threatening hyperkalemia can result. Hyponatremia is another common complication related to the dilutional effects of increased fluid retention. Hyperphosphatemia occurs because the kidneys are unable to effectively remove phosphorous, which in turn causes a reciprocal hypercalcemia.

19. Correct answer—C.

To prevent complications, initial treatment of this infant, focusing on her history, should include low dose dopamine therapy at 2 to 5 mcg/kg/min. Dopamine at this dosage would help support systemic arterial pressure, but more importantly improve renal perfusion by selectively dilating renal arteries. A fluid bolus or infusion of packed cells would be more appropriate for a neonate with a hypovolemic or hemorrhagic volume depletion. Calcium gluconate may increase cardiac output and blood pressure temporarily, but does not effectively improve renal perfusion.

20. Correct answer—D.

Dobutamine would be least likely to require an adjustment in dosage for a patient with acute renal failure. This medication is rapidly metabolized in the liver. Gentamicin, digoxin, and pancuronium bromide are all dependent upon renal function for excretion.

21. Correct answer—B.

Cardiogenic shock results in prerenal failure by failing to provide enough perfusion to the kidneys for an adequate glomerular filtration rate and urine formation. Neurogenic bladders may result in *post*renal failure by blocking the flow of urine. Both glomerulonephritis and polycystic disease are examples of *intra*renal failure, which is related to damage to the kidneys themselves.

22. Correct answer—B.

Care of the patient in oliguric acute renal failure should include a protein-restricted diet to reduce azotemia. Adequate protein intake must be maintained, but should be restricted to essential amino acids. The patient should be weighed at least daily, infants as often as three times a day. A patient in oliguric renal failure should most often be monitored for sign of hypervolemia, not dehydration. Turner's sign is usually seen in association with renal trauma and is a bruising over the flank area.

23. Correct answer—B.

An order for 100 mL/kg/day (400 mL) of isotonic solutions would be contraindicated in this patient because it is an order based on normal fluid requirements. Because this infant is oliguric, fluid therapy needs to be restricted to insensible losses (35 mL/kg/day) plus urine or other measurable fluid losses. Digoxin may be given at 30 to 50 mcg/kg for a digitalizing dose, but should be divided over 24 hours. Furosemide 1 mg/kg IV may be used to promote urinary output, but if unsuccessful, should not be continued because it is nephrotoxic. Dopamine infusion of 3 mcg/kg/min may be helpful in increasing renal artery blood flow and thus improve urinary output.

24. Correct answer—A.

This patient's low sodium level is most likely related to hypervolemia. Because urinary output has fallen, this patient has an excess of fluid diluting his serum sodium level. Hypovolemia would raise the serum sodium level. Sodium wasting would support a low serum sodium such as this patient's, but is not likely to be occurring because the urine output is low. Sodium retention would raise the serum sodium *above* normal levels.

25. Correct answer—D.

A carpopedal spasm during blood pressure measurement is most likely because of hypocalcemia. Hypocalcemia is also seen in conjunction with hyperphosphatemia and hypomagnesemia. Alterations in potassium levels do not result in carpopedal spasms. A carpopedal spasm is an involuntary contraction of the affected hand and arm.

26. Correct answer—C.

A critically ill patient with hypocalcemia is at risk for bleeding abnormalities, respiratory arrest, cardiac arrest, renal calculi, tetany, and seizures. Alkalosis is associated with hypercalcemia.

27. Correct answer—D.

In planning nursing interventions for the patient with hyperkalemia, the most critical action would be to administer glucose and insulin to ship potassium into cells to reduce serum levels. Calcium chloride is used to treat hyperkalemia, but is contraindicated in patients on digoxin therapy. Bronchospasm is a risk associated with hypocalcemia, not potassium imbalances. Sodium bicarbonate is used to correct *acidosis*, not alkalosis.

28. Correct answer—D.

Infusion of 20 mL/kg bolus of crystalloids is not a patient outcome, but rather an accomplishment of therapy or intervention. Carrying out a therapy or intervention does not guarantee a positive patient outcome. For the nursing diagnosis of altered renal tissue perfusion related to hypovolemia, the patient outcomes within 4 hours of admission would include age appropriate normal sinus rate and rhythm, moist mucous membranes, warm extremities, and urinary output greater than 1.0 mL/kg.

29. Correct answer—C.

Acute renal failure can result in hyperkalemia specifically related to decreased urinary output. Without adequate urinary output, potassium cannot be excreted. Aldosterone production is not decreased in renal failure. Secretion of antidiuretic hormone influences water balance, and an increase in ADH does not generally occur during renal failure. Increased sodium retention generally leads to increased renal excretion because of aldosterone's role in regulation of these electrolytes.

30. Correct answer—A.

The therapy which is most appropriate to initiate first would be a fluid bolus of 20 mL/kg of crystalloid fluids. Postoperatively, this patient is at risk for hypovolemia as a result of blood loss and third-spacing of fluid. A fluid challenge should be given first, which may increase urinary output by increasing renal perfusion. Dobutamine and dopamine should be used only when adequate circulatory volume is established, and in lower doses than these for optimal renal perfusion. A furosemide bolus of 1 mg/mL IV also is most indicated *after* adequate circulatory volume has been established.

31. Correct answer—B.

The history of diarrhea and hypovolemic shock makes this patient at risk for hypokalemia as a result of potassium losses from the gut. The signs and symptoms are consistent with hypokalemia. Hyperkalemia would cause tall, tented T waves. This patient is not at a significant risk of calcium imbalance.

32. Correct answer—C.

A BUN:creatinine ratio of 20:1 or greater would most likely confirm the diagnosis of *pre*renal acute renal failure. In prerenal failure, because of decreased renal blood flow, the BUN is reabsorbed and rises quickly. The serum creatinine rises more slowly. Urinary output less than 1 mL/kg/hr may simply signify dehydration or hypovolemia. A drop in urine output is also not diagnostic of *pre*renal failure, but may be seen in any type of renal failure. A fluid bolus would be given to establish that the kidneys intrinsically are unable to increase urinary output. A serum creatinine greater than 1.0 would indicate renal failure, but not specifically *pre*renal failure. A renal ultrasound can help visualize the anatomy of the kidneys, but would be of little value in diagnosing function.

33. Correct answer—D.

In planning nursing interventions for the patient with hypocalcemia, the critical care nurse should be aware that liver and intestinal necrosis can occur with calcium infused through umbilical catheters. Continuous infusions are preferred over bolus doses because bolus doses given too rapidly can cause bradycardia and cardiac arrest. Peripheral infiltrations of calcium should be treated with hyaluronidase. Phentolamine meslate (Regitine) is given for dopamine infiltration.

34. Correct answer—A.
Infants and children with hypocalcemia need continuous cardiac monitoring because this electrolyte imbalance causes prolonged ST and QT intervals, which predispose them to cardiac arrest. Prolonged PR intervals are associated with first-degree heart block and cardiac glycoside toxicity.

35. Correct answer—B.
This patient is exhibiting serious signs and symptoms of hyperkalemia as manifested by ventricular dysrhythmias and acidosis. Administration of glucose and insulin are indicated to *immediately* move excess serum potassium inside cells and quickly reduce serum K+ levels. Kayexelate will permanently remove potassium from the body, but takes longer to act and would be indicated *after* glucose and insulin work without delay. Normal saline fluid bolus would not be effective in treating hyperkalemia. Magnesium sulfate is indicated in treating hypomagnesemia.

36. Correct answer—B.
The most likely physiological cause of this patient's abnormal blood gas results in metabolic acidosis related to retention of hydrogen ions from the kidneys' inability to perform their normal role in acid-base balance. Bicarbonate ions are wasted, not retained in renal failure. Although the body is hyperventilating to eliminate excess carbon dioxide and raise the pH, it is not the primary cause of these abnormal blood gases, but rather is a compensatory mechanism for metabolic acidosis. Hypoventilation would result in an increase in pCO_2.

37. Correct answer—C.
In identifying potential risk factors, the critical care nurse recognizes that hypocalcemia is generally found with hypomagnesemia and hyperphosphatemia. Calcium levels do not directly rise and fall in relation to potassium or sodium.

38. Correct answer—A.
Neonates at risk for hypermagnesemia include those with a maternal history of toxemia of pregnancy. These mothers may have received magnesium sulfate therapy during labor causing maternal hypermagnesemia, which crosses the placenta to the fetus.

39. Correct answer—A.
The critical care nurse recognizes compensation for metabolic acidosis by a decrease in pCO_2 on the arterial blood gases. The lungs compensate for acidosis by eliminating a respiratory acid, pCO_2. An increase in pCO_2 would only worsen acidosis by increasing the respiratory acid component. Changes in HCO_3^- are part of a metabolic compensatory mechanism that would not be effective if the acidosis were respiratory in origin.

40. Correct answer—B.

When administering sodium bicarbonate to a neonate, the critical care nurse should be aware that the concentration should not exceed 0.5 mEq/mL or severe side effects may result. The correct dosage is 1 to 2 mEq/kg and should be administered at not more than 1 mEq/kg/min intravenously or through an umbilical or central catheter only.

PEDIATRIC-SPECIFIC ANSWERS

41. Correct answer—C.

Signs and symptoms related to hypokalemia include lethargy, flattened T wave, malaise, shallow respirations, nausea, fatigue, and a weak, irregular heart rate. Hyperkalemia is characterized by weakness, bradycardia, prolonged PR interval, tented T wave, and a wide QRS complex.

42. Correct answer—B.

A potassium infusion of 15 to 20 mEq/L/hr is indicated for treating this patient's hypokalemia. Kayexalate is given to treat *hyper*kalemia. Potassium replacement by bolus is never indicated because it can lead to tissue necrosis and lethal ventricular dysrhythmias. Digoxin for cardiac dysrhythmias is *not* indicated for patients with hypokalemia because toxicity is enhanced in the presence of low potassium levels.

43. Correct answer—A.

This patient is also at risk for developing metabolic alkalosis. As positively charged potassium ions (K+) leave the cells to raise the serum potassium level, positively charged hydrogen ions (H+) must enter the cells to balance the spaces electrically. As hydrogen ions enter the cells, a general deficit occurs in the blood leading to metabolic alkalosis. Metabolic acidosis is associated with hyperkalemia. Respiratory acidosis and alkalosis are associated primarily with respiratory disease or dysfunction.

44. Correct answer—D.

Pelvis injuries would more likely result in bladder and urethral injuries than renal trauma. The kidneys are located higher and outside the pelvic cavity. Risk factors for renal trauma would include injuries to the lumbar spine and lower right and left ribs.

45. Correct answer—A.

Turner's sign is bruising over the flank and lower back and is associated with a retroperitoneal bleed. The kidneys are located in the retroperitoneal space. Cushing's triad is an ominous change in vital signs associated with increasing intracranial pressure. Cullen's sign is seen in hemorrhagic pancreatitis. Trousseau's sign is associated with hypocalcemia.

46. Correct answer—B.

The urinary meatus should be inspected before attempting to catheterize a trauma patient who is having difficulty voiding. Passing a catheter in the presence of urethral trauma could worsen any damage. A renal ultrasound is not likely to reveal information on urethral or bladder trauma. Manual pressure to the bladder to assist in voiding would be contraindicated because it might worsen bladder or urethral damage.

47. Correct answer—D.
Narcotic analgesics would not be indicated until other abdominal and pelvic injuries were ruled out. Administering pain medication might mask other injuries and worsen his blood pressure before it is stabilized. Obtaining a blood sample would be important in evaluating blood loss. Administering intravenous fluids would be important in treating his blood loss and stabilizing his blood pressure. Antimicrobial therapy is indicated in renal trauma to prevent renal and urinary tract infections.

48. Correct answer—D.
This patient should remain on bedrest until his hematuria resolves. Flank pain is not a reliable indicator of healing of the actual contusion, laceration, or other renal trauma. The hemoglobin and hematocrit will usually not return to normal until after the trauma has healed. Perirenal hematoma is only one indicator of renal trauma, and would not be indicative of a renal contusion, which also would require bedrest.

49. Correct answer—C.
In a trauma patient with genitourinary injuries, a palpable left kidney is most likely to be an *abnormal* finding. The right kidney is lower than the left and may be normally palpable. A palpable bladder may indicate urethral trauma resulting in an inability to void, but may also be palpable simply if the patient hasn't had the opportunity to void. The symphysis pubis is part of the pelvic bone structure and is normally palpable in all but the extremely obese.

50. Correct answer—B.
The use of seat belts has *decreased* the incidence of GU trauma by offering better protection against steering wheel injuries to the pelvic region, and decreased incidence of injuries from femur compression into the pelvis. Most GU trauma is a result of motor vehicle accidents. A full bladder increases the risk of GU trauma in motor vehicle crashes resulting in bladder ruptures, usually at the dome. GU trauma is usually accompanied by trauma to other organ systems, seldom occurring in isolation.

NEONATAL-SPECIFIC ANSWERS

51. Correct answer—A.
Assessment of the neonate with polycystic kidney disease would reveal a *decreased* urinary output, bilateral flank masses from enlarged kidneys, respiratory distress related to fluid overload, and hematuria from renal parenchymal disease.

52. Correct answer—A.

Infantile polycystic kidney disease is characterized by hyperkalemia, hypocalcemia, hyperphosphatemia, and acidosis. Because polycystic disease leads to acute renal insufficiency and failure, the signs and symptoms of renal failure are found. Hyperkalemia, hyperphosphatemia, and acidosis result from an inability of the kidneys to clear potassium, phosphorous, and hydrogen ions as well as an inability to retain bicarbonate ions. Hypocalcemia results from its reciprocal relationship to serum phosphate levels. As serum phosphate levels rise, serum calcium levels fall.

53. Correct answer—C.

Positive patient outcomes in the treatment of this neonate would not include a palpable liver border 3 cm below the costal margin. This finding would indicate hepatomegaly and be suggestive of either hepatic or congestive heart failure. A blood pressure of 60 to 80/20 to 55 mm Hg is within normal limits for a neonate of this age. Absence of adventitious breath sounds would indicate clear lung fields and a desirable fluid balance. Urinary output of 50 cc/24 hours would also be within normal limits because it represents approximately 0.5 cc/kg/hr.

54. Correct answer—B.

Renal and upper urinary tract anomalies are not commonly associated with extrophy of the bladder. It is, however, often associated with epispadias, which is a lower urinary tract anomaly. This condition is more common in boys than girls and is often accompanied by an umbilical hernia as well as anterior displacement of the anus and undescended testes.

55. Correct answer—C.

In counseling the family of a neonate with extrophy of the bladder, the most appropriate statement for the critical nurse to share would be "most infants can achieve good bladder control with surgery and medical therapy." These infants do not generally have significantly more trouble with bed-wetting and bladder control as they get older. The surgery is usually accomplished by closing the bladder within the abdominal cavity within the first 48 hours of life, followed by correction of the epispadias at 1½ to 2 years of age, and completed by reimplantation of the ureters at 2 to 3 years of age.

56. Correct answer—D.

The critical care nurse's care of the neonate with extrophy of the bladder would include using a clear, occlusive dressing to cover the bladder. Petroleum gauze is not recommended because it may leave material on the exposed membranes. A cord tie, rather than a clamp, should be used because the clamp may rub or lay against the exposed and delicate tissues. Insertion of an indwelling urinary catheter would not be routinely indicated and would increase the risk of urinary tract infection.

57. Correct answer—C.

The most likely cause of these findings is Potter's syndrome. In addition to these findings, other signs and symptoms include dry skin, a bell-shaped chest, and a skin fold beneath the eyes. Polycystic kidney disease, Turner's syndrome, and hydronephrosis would not be characterized by these facial and hand deformities.

58. Correct answer—B.

The most likely cause of this neonate's respiratory distress is a pneumothorax, which is a complication associated with Potter's syndrome. Hypervolemia related to oliguria or anuria might also result in congestive heart failure and pulmonary edema. Bronchiolitis, tracheoesophageal fistula, and aspiration are not increased occurrences in these infants.

59. Correct answer—C.

Interventions for this infant would most likely be planned to provide comfort measures. Most of these infants do not survive beyond the second day of life because of the absence of kidneys and multiple anomalies.

CHAPTER 8

Multisystem Care Problems

Passkeys

GENERAL PRINCIPLES OF MULTISYSTEM PATIENT CARE PROBLEMS

Septic or Distributive Shock

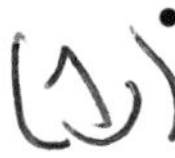

- All types of shock—septic, hypovolemic, and cardiogenic—are defined as a dysfunction of the cardiovascular system resulting in inadequate perfusion to meet the needs of tissues.

- Septic shock occurs when endotoxins are released from microorganisms resulting in myocardial dysfunction, massive vasodilation, vascular endothelial dysfunction leading to capillary leakage, and an abnormal distribution of blood in the circulatory system. Blood vessels vasodilate resulting in venous pooling and an inadequate amount of blood for the arterial/systemic circuit. (See Fig. 8-1.)

- Gram negative bacteremia is one cause of sepsis and septic shock. This often occurs from translocation (migration) of bacteria across the wall of the gastrointestinal tract into the circulatory system.

- Nosocomial infections are a frequent cause of sepsis and septic shock. The most common sources of infection include bacteremia, lower respiratory tract infections, and skin infections.

- Signs and symptoms of compensated and uncompensated septic shock can be found in Table 8-1.

- The treatment goal of septic shock focuses on maximizing oxygen delivery and minimizing oxygen demands. This involves support of heart rate, circulation, airway, ventilation, intravascular volume, acid-base balance, and electrolyte imbalances.

- Treatment of septic shock includes fluid resuscitation, antibiotic therapy, beta-receptor stimulants, vasopressors, and supportive therapy. If shock is not treated quickly and effectively, cell functions will be interrupted, resulting in acidosis, cell death, and ultimately the patient's death.

- Persistent pulmonary hypertension of the neonate is often seen in newborns with septic shock.

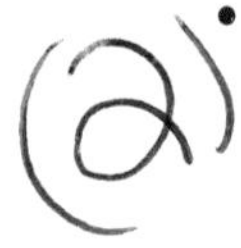

- Distinguishing factors of septic shock from other factors include positive cultures, edema, sclerema, proteinuria, and sometimes a normal blood pressure with clinically evident hypoperfusion (cold, mottled skin, weak pulses, oliguria, sluggish capillary refill).

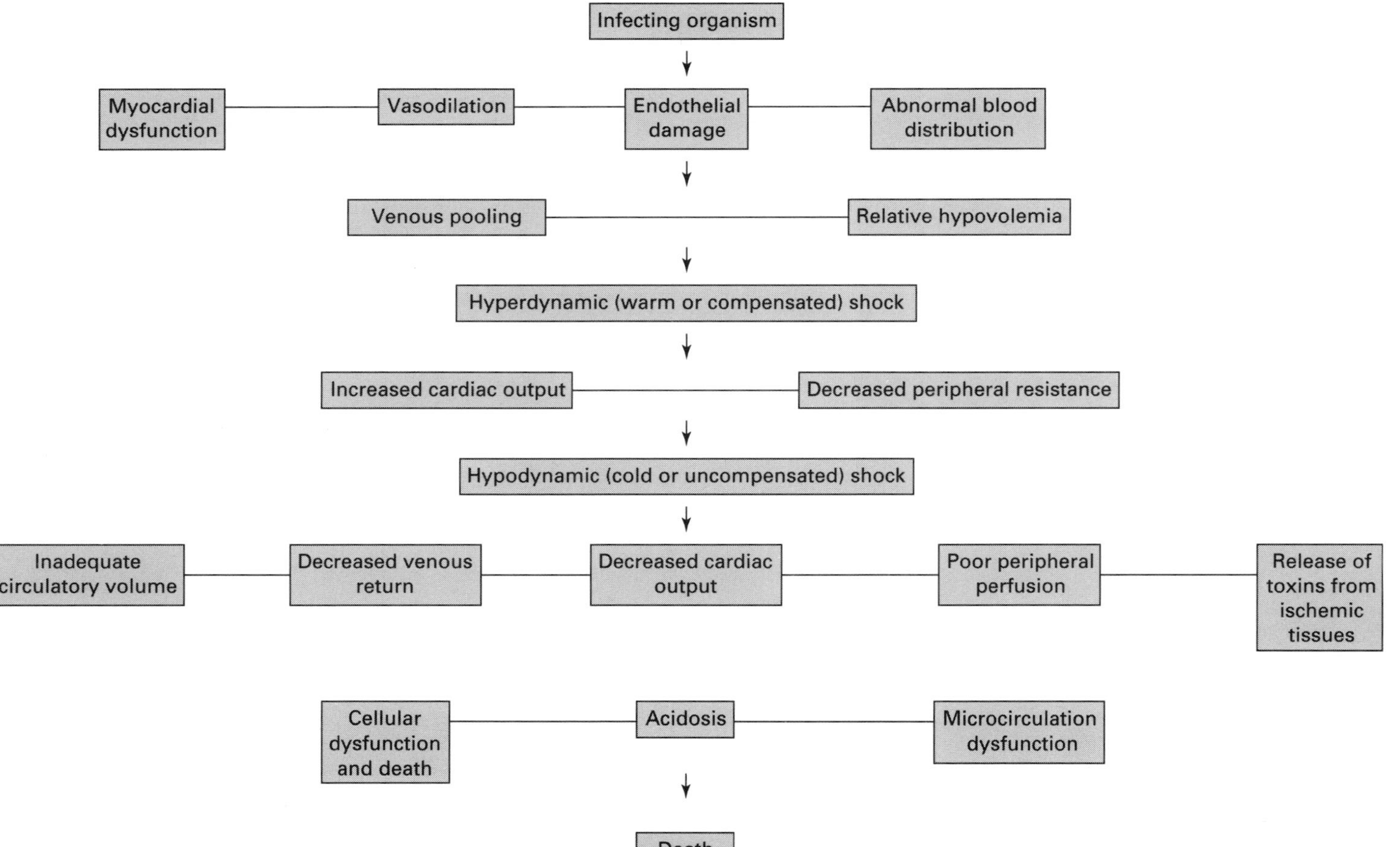

Fig. 8-1 Progression of septic shock.

Table 8-1
Signs and Symptoms of Compensated and Uncompensated Septic Shock

Compensated	Uncompensated
Rapid capillary refill	Sluggish capillary refill
Warm, pink to flushed skin	Cold, mottled skin
Hyperthermia	Hypothermia
Normal blood pressure progressing to a decrease in diastolic pressure	Hypotension with falls in systolic and mean arterial pressures after diastolic pressure falls
Bounding peripheral pulses	Decreased peripheral pulses
Decreased systemic vascular resistance	Increased systemic vascular resistance
Increased cardiac output	Decreased cardiac output
Increase in serum glucose levels from sympathetic stimulation	Decrease in serum glucose from hepatic hypoperfusion and dysfunction
Early increase in urine output progressing to a decrease	Decreased urine output
Changes in level of consciousness, restlessness, irritability	Decreased level of consciousness
Respiratory alkalosis followed by metabolic acidosis	Severe metabolic and respiratory acidosis
Thrombocytopenia	Disseminated intravascular coagulation

Hypovolemic Shock

- Hypovolemic shock occurs as a result of inadequate circulating volume leading to progressive circulatory dysfunction. Intravascular volume is inadequate relative to vascular space.

- Avoid administration of hypotonic fluids. They will be distributed throughout total body water and less than 8% will remain in the vascular space.

Cardiogenic Shock

- Cardiogenic shock occurs when abnormal cardiac function results in inadequate perfusion. Depressed cardiac output is most commonly the result of decreased myocardial contractility or systolic failure.

- Heart rate abnormalities in cardiogenic shock may include supraventricular tachycardias, ventricular dysrhythmias, and bradycardia.

- Treatment goals in the management of cardiogenic shock are to minimize myocardial oxygen demands and maximize myocardial performance.

PEDIATRIC-SPECIFIC PRINCIPLES

TOXIC INGESTIONS

- Toxic ingestion should be suspected in any previously healthy infant or child with unexplained drowsiness, seizures, coma, or other unusual symptoms.

- Initial treatment and stabilization of toxic ingestions should focus on the ABC's—airway, breathing, and circulation.

- Monitoring of vital signs and level of consciousness should be continuous.

- Emesis and aspiration are a threat from both the ingested toxin itself and treatments for the toxin. Precautions to guard against aspiration should be continuous.

- A change in level of consciousness and respiratory depression are clear indications for intubation in the suspected poisoning victim.

- When inducing emesis is verified, ipecac syrup is the treatment of choice. It should not be used in any patient who has a poor gag reflex, decreased level of consciousness, seizures, or has ingested a hydrocarbon (kerosene, pine oil cleaners, lighter fluid, turpentine), corrosive agent (bleach), or organophosphates (insecticide).

- The potential number of toxic agents in suspected poisonings is almost limitless. To aid in diagnosis and treatment, toxidromes (groups or classes of toxins) can help identify the specific class of compounds or syndrome based on symptoms. See Table 8-2 for specific toxidromes.

- Activated charcoal works by preventing the absorption of ingested toxins from the gastrointestinal tract into the circulatory system *and* enhancing elimination of toxins already absorbed into the bloodstream. It should be administered to almost all toxin ingestion victims, especially those requiring admission to an intensive care unit. Activated charcoal is also sometimes mixed with sorbital to increase the rate of excretion through the gastrointestinal tract by temporarily causing diarrhea.

- Children under 5 years of age are at risk for hypoglycemia following ethanol poisoning. Common sources of ethanol poisoning in this age group include mouthwashes, cough medicines, cold medicines, and colognes.

Table 8-2
Selected Toxidromes

Toxin	Treatment	Symptoms
Narcotics/opiates	Naloxone	Pinpoint pupils, bradycardia, hypoventilation, hypotension, euphoria or coma, possible seizures
Organophosphates (insecticides)	Atropine for muscarinic symptoms; pralidoxime for nicotinic symptoms	Cholinergic symptoms: *Muscarinic:* salivation, lacrimation, urination, diarrhea, bronchoconstriction, wheezing, bradycardia, diaphoresis, nausea, vomiting, increase in pulmonary secretions, constriction of pupils *Nicotinic:* muscle fatigue, twitching, fasiculations, paralysis, hypoventilation, tachycardia, hypertension, hyperglycemia, pallor *Central nervous system:* headache, anxiety, restlessness, confusion, slurred speech, hypotension, ataxia, emotional lability, central cardiovascular and pulmonary depression, coma
Tricyclics	Sodium bicarbonate	Prolonged QRS interval, ventricular dysrhythmias, seizures, tachycardia, hypotension or hypertension, hyperthermia, dilated pupils, agitation or coma
Sedatives/ hypnotics	Gastric lavage or ipecac syrup (if fully conscious and not at risk for aspiration) followed by activated charcoal; supportive treatment of symptoms; hemodialysis	Hypoventilation, hypothermia, hypotension, nystagmus, slurred speech (age appropriate), barbiturates may produce excitability in children, hyporeflexia, coma, no response to naloxone
Hydrocarbons (kerosene, pine oil cleaners, lighter fluid, turpentine, etc.)	Intubation and mechanical ventilation with respiratory symptoms; gastric lavage	Coughing, choking, grunting, emesis, lethargy, coma, respiratory arrest

- Ethanol poisoning in older children and adolescents is most often associated with alcoholic beverages. The possibility of chronic abuse and nutritional deficiencies should be considered.

- Peak serum ethanol levels usually occur 30 to 60 minutes after ingestion. They may take as long as 6 hours to peak if gastric emptying is delayed.

- Management of ethanol poisoning includes intravenous administration of dextrose solutions, gastric lavage, and intubation and mechanical ventilation if central nervous system depression is present. Activated charcoal is not effective. In extreme cases (blood alcohol levels greater than 350 mg/dL), hemodialysis may be required.

NEAR-DROWNING

- *Near-drowning* is defined as survival past 24 hours following a submersion event that is serious enough to require emergency medical treatment.

- The morbidity and mortality associated with near-drowning is directly related to the degree of hypoxia suffered.

- Pulmonary complications seen in near-drowning victims include noncardiogenic pulmonary edema, infection, aspiration of gastric contents, aspiration of foreign material found in the submersion fluid, and dysfunction of surfactant in the lungs.

- The clinical differences between freshwater and saltwater drownings are insignificant. Fluid shifts, hemolysis, and electrolyte derangements are unusual in all near-drowning victims.

- Hypothermia and cold fluid submersion are important, usually positive, predictors of morbidity and mortality.

- Although hypothermia decreases damage to the central nervous system, it complicates resuscitation because it increases susceptibility to ventricular fibrillation and asystole. It also impairs the effectiveness of resuscitation drugs, glucose metabolism, and oxygen delivery. At least some of the injury to any organ occurs during reperfusion rather than during ischemia. Limited blood flow may provide oxygen and substrate, but toxic products are generated that cannot be cleared.

- Approximately ⅓ of all near-drowning victims that are admitted to a pediatric intensive care unit in a coma and flaccid do have a successful neurological outcome and survival.

- Treatment focuses on correcting hypothermia, improving respiratory and cardiac dysfunction, and minimizing central nervous system damage. These patients need to be normothermic and have an adequate glucose source, cardiac output, and peripheral perfusion. Seizures should be treated aggressively. Positive end expiratory pressure, surfactant, and appropriate FiO_2 are important respiratory and ventilatory tools in treating the near-drowning victim.

- Prevention is important. Secure pools and hot tubs with fences at least 5 feet tall. Latches should be at least 4½ feet high.

BURNS

- Important normal functions of the skin include temperature regulation, excretion, sensory, protection, and barrier to infection.
- The degree of injury is related to the temperature and length of contact with the thermal source.
- Table 8-3 describes two classification systems for burn injuries.
- The magnitude of the burn injury may be determined using several methods. The Rule of Nines, although commonly used in adults, is less reliable in infants and children. The palmar method uses the victim's own hand to represent 1% of body

Table 8-3
Methods of Classifying Burn Injuries

Zone of Tissue Damage	Depth of Injury
Zone of Coagulation The most severely damaged area of the burn injury The tissue is coagulated and necrotic	*First-Degree Burn* Superficial injury Damage to the top of the epidermis layer only
Zone of Stasis An area that has suffered milder injury With improper management or further ischemia, the damage to this area can increase	*Second-Degree Burn* Partial thickness injury Damage to the epidermis and part of the dermis
Zone of Hyperemia The most peripheral area of a burn injury Injury to this area is usually minimal	*Third-Degree Burn* Deep tissue injury Damage to the entire epidermis and dermal layers
	Fourth-Degree Burn Deepest tissue injury Damage beyond epidermal and dermal layers to muscle and bone

surface area and estimates the size of the burn from this reference. The Lund and Browder method is probably the most accurate method for use in infants and children. Fig. 8-2 illustrates a method based on age for use in pediatric patients.

- Thermal injuries affect every body system. See Table 8-4 for a listing of the effects of thermal injuries on various body systems.

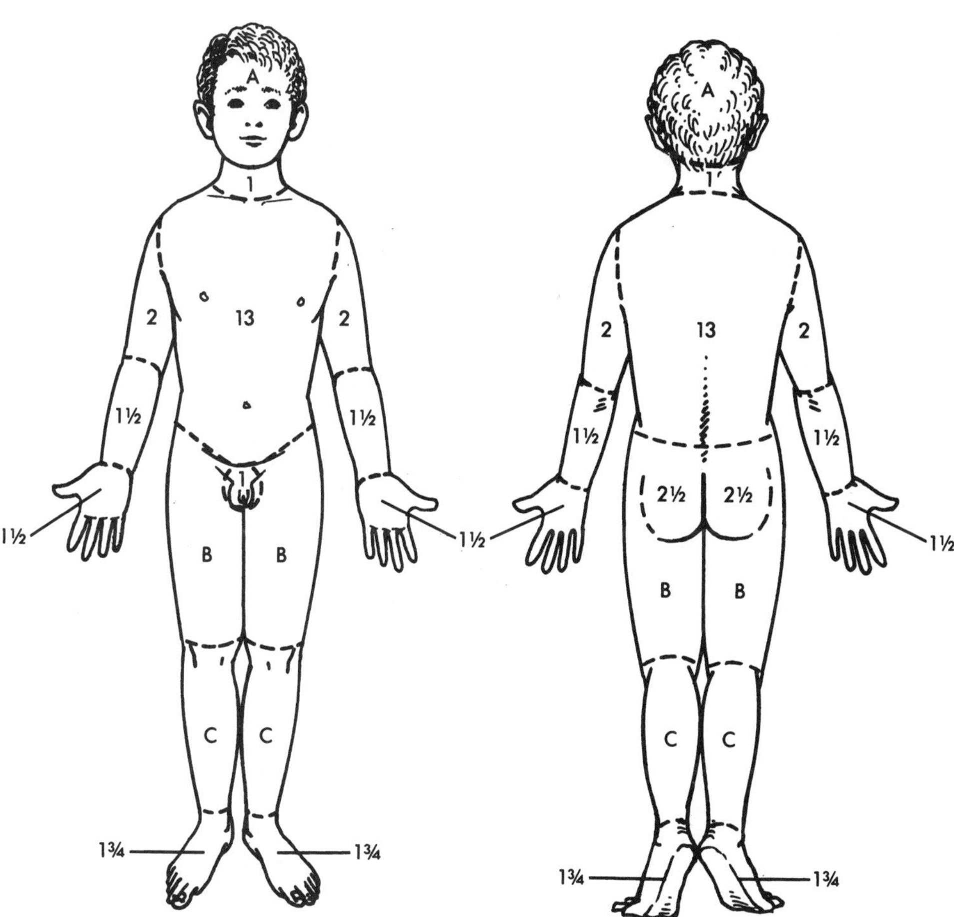

Fig. 8-2 Percentage of surface area of head and legs at various ages.

Area in diagram	*0*	*1*	*5*	*10*	*15 (years)*
A ½ of head	9½	8½	6½	5½	4½
B ½ of one thigh	2¾	3¼	4	4¼	4½
C ½ of one lower leg	2½	2½	2¾	3	3¼

This chart of body areas, together with the table showing the percentage of surface area of the head and legs at various ages, can be used to estimate the surface area burned in a child. (From Blumer JL: A practical guide to pediatric intensive care, ed 3, St Louis, 1990, Mosby.)

Table 8-4
Effects of Thermal Injuries on Body Systems

Body System	Effect of Thermal Injury
Cardiovascular and hematological systems	Increased capillary permeability Decreased circulating volume Decreased cardiac output Increase in systemic and pulmonary vascular resistance Hypoalbuminemia
Pulmonary	Direct damage from inhaled smoke, toxins, superheated air Loss of airway patency as a result of airway edema Pulmonary edema Intrapulmonary shunting Hypoxemia Decreased compliance of lung tissues Respiratory distress syndrome
Neurological	Most neurological problems occur secondary to dysfunction of other organ systems Decreased and absent peripheral sensation in third- and fourth-degree burns
Gastrointestinal	Decreased splanchnic flow Intestinal ischemia Translocation of intestinal bacteria Curling's ulcer Hypermetabolic state Hepatic dysfunction Alterations in glucose, fat, and protein metabolism
Renal	Decreased urine output with fall in circulating volume and cardiac output Renal failure related to myoglobinuria and acute tubular necrosis Increased secretion of antidiuretic hormone
Immunological	Initial decreased lymphocyte response Dysfunction of phagocytic processes Decreased levels of complement Infection Sepsis

- Fluid losses and hypovolemia in burn victims result from actual fluid loss through the thermal injury as well as capillary leakage and third-spacing of fluid.

- When the thermal injury is greater than 15% of body surface area (BSA), fluids must be replaced intravenously. Boluses of 20 cc/kg administered over 5 to 15 minutes are repeated until peripheral perfusion and urine output are adequate.

- A modified Parkland formula for children helps guide fluid resuscitation in pediatric patients:
  - 4 cc/kg/%BSA of crystalloid fluids + maintenance fluid requirements (1500 ml/m^2 BSA)
  - Half of calculated fluids are given in the first 8 hours, the other half administered over the following 16 hours.

- Table 8-5 reviews advantages and disadvantages of various resuscitation fluids.

HEMOLYTIC UREMIC SYNDROME (HUS)

- HUS is characterized by hemolytic anemia, decreased platelet levels, and renal failure. Widespread involvement of many organ systems exists.

- The most common form of HUS follows a gastrointestinal illness in children 1 to 3 years of age. Other forms may follow other infections or in association with some medications.

Table 8-5

Advantages and Disadvantages of Resuscitation Fluids in Treating Thermal Injuries

Resuscitation Fluid	Advantages	Disadvantages
Crystalloids	Inexpensive Easily available	Rapidly shifts into extravascular space Requires large amounts of fluids May worsen peripheral edema
Colloids	Increases intravascular oncotic pressures Requires less volume than crystalloids Hinders third spacing of fluids if capillary membranes are not leaking	May worsen systemic edema if capillary leakage occurs More expensive

Table 8-6
Potential Multisystem Effects of Hemolytic Uremic Syndrome (HUS)

Body System	Effect of HUS
Cardiovascular and hematological	Anemia Thrombocytopenia Leukocytosis Elevated reticulocyte count Hypertension Congestive heart failure
Pulmonary	Pulmonary edema
Neurological	Seizures Coma
Gastrointestinal	Hepatomegaly Splenomegaly Bowel necrosis
Renal	Decreased urine output Renal failure related to cortical necrosis and tubular damage Renal intravascular coagulation
Immunological	No detectable antibodies responsible for HUS Generally normal studies

- Anemia and thrombocytopenia may be severe, with a hemoglobin of only 4 to 6 g/L and platelet count of 20,000 to 50,000/mm^3.

- Systemic manifestations of HUS are summarized in Table 8-6.

- Therapy is generally supportive and aimed at fluid and electrolyte balance, as well as stabilization of the hemoglobin, hematocrit, and platelet count.

- Dialysis may be required in anuric patients or those with abnormal fluid and electrolyte balance.

NEONATAL-SPECIFIC PRINCIPLES

FETAL EXPOSURE TO DRUGS AND ALCOHOL

- Most mothers who use drugs are using more than one drug. Toxicology screens should be employed in neonates suspected of fetal drug exposure. For example, samples of urine, feces, meconium, or hair may be obtained from infants to reveal maternal use of cocaine.

- Most abused drugs cause any of the following: intrauterine growth retardation, intrauterine deaths, malformations, prematurity, asphyxia, and central nervous system abnormalities.

- Maternal substance abuse has a strong relationship to infection with the human immunodeficiency virus (HIV).

- Decrease sensory input and environmental stimuli for most drug-exposed infants. Actively assess and prepare for seizure activity.

- Tight swaddling and rocking in a vertical position may be effective in reducing irritability.

- Breast-feeding is contraindicated in mothers using cocaine, methamphetamines, heroin, marijuana, and in those who are HIV positive.

Cocaine

- Cocaine causes vasoconstriction, hypertension, and tachycardia in both the fetus and the mother.

- Placental abruptio and fetal cerebral infarcts are common complications associated with maternal cocaine use.

- The cocaine metabolite may persist in maternal circulation for up to 1 week.

- Cocaine provides an adrenergic-like response resulting in a stimulant effect. Euphoria is followed by dysphoria.

- Cocaine causes vasoconstriction in the placenta, seriously compromising blood flow to the fetus resulting in fetal hypoxia.

- The fetus/neonate of a mother using cocaine is often malnourished because cocaine causes anorexia in the mother.

- Infants of mothers using cocaine are often growth retarded and microcephalic.

- Use during the first trimester injures placental vessels even if cocaine use is stopped. Use during later trimesters can cause fetal tachycardia and induce uterine contractions. Spontaneous abortions and premature labor are common.

- Neonates of cocaine mothers have many problems. See the box on p. 386 for common effects.

Fetal and Neonatal Effects of Maternal Cocaine Use

- Hypoxia
- Spontaneous abortions
- Premature labor
- Intrauterine growth retardation
- Renal anomalies
- Genitourinary anomalies
- Limb defects
- Cardiac anomalies
- Cranial defects
- Tremors
- Irritability
- Hypertension
- Poor feeding
- High-pitched cry
- Tachypnea
- Hyperreflexia
- Fever
- Poor interaction with people and environment
- Exaggerated startle reflex
- Difficult to comfort
- Bowel infarctions

Methamphetamines

- Symptoms at birth may be less severe than those associated with other abused drugs.
- Long-term effects on infants include tremors, hypotonia, abnormal eye movements, and hemiparesis. These may not be evident until school age.

Heroin and Methadone

- Heroin causes withdrawal in neonates, but is not believed to be responsible for congenital abnormalities.
- Reduction in placental blood flow with opiate use frequently results in fetal distress and death.
- Other common perinatal problems are listed in the box on p. 387.

Alcohol

- Alcohol most likely adversely affects the fetus by causing hypoxia, impairing protein synthesis, and by producing teratogenic effects.
- Alcohol results in congenital anomalies by interfering with normal cell differentiation and growth.

Fetal and Neonatal Effects of Maternal Heroin and Methadone Use

Fetal	Neonatal
Infections	Hypoxia
Malnutrition	Meconium aspiration
Growth retardation	Infections
Anemia	Sudden infant death syndrome
Meconium staining	
Prematurity	

- Amount, frequency, and duration of alcohol exposure in utero are important factors in determining the severity of fetal anomalies.
- Spontaneous abortion, abruptio placentae, growth retardation, and neural tube defects are common fetal problems associated with maternal alcohol use.
- A diagnosis of fetal alcohol syndrome (FAS) must include growth retardation, facial dysmorphology, and abnormalities of the central nervous system.
- See Table 8-7 for physical assessment findings of infants with FAS.

Cigarettes

- Smoking adversely affects the fetus by causing hypoxia, vasoconstriction, and increased carbon monoxide levels.
- Abruptio placentae, premature rupture of membranes, placentae previa, and placental dysfunction are commonly associated with maternal smoking.
- Newborns frequently exhibit low weight and decreased length at birth.

Perinatal Asphyxia

- See the box on p. 389 for risk factors for perinatal asphyxia.
- In utero asphyxia is characterized by tachycardia, prolonged bradycardia, loss of baseline variability, fetal respiratory movements, and alterations in fetal heart rate patterns, especially late decelerations.

Table 8-7
Physical Assessment Findings in Fetal Alcohol Syndrome

Growth Abnormalities	Facial Dysmorphology	Central Nervous System Abnormalities	General Abnormalities
Decreased weight Decreased length Microcephaly	Face: small and underdeveloped chin, bulging forehead Eyes: strabismus ptosis, epicanthal folds Mouth: cleft lip, cleft palate, small teeth, poor sucking, upper lip is long and straight, poorly developed groove of upper lip	Hyperactivity Feeding problems Abnormal sleep patterns Hypotonia Hyporeflexia Mental retardation Developmental delays	Congenital cardiac defects: ventricular or atrial septal defects, patent ductus arteriosis, and tetralogy of Fallot Renal defects: hydronephrosis, renal hypoplasia Nonspecific neoplasms Slowed bone growth Abnormal creases in the palms of the hands Irregular hair patterns

- In utero asphyxia often results in the passage of meconium into amniotic fluid and potential meconium aspiration.

HYPOXIC-ISCHEMIC ENCEPHALOPATHY (HIE) (BRAIN INJURY)

- See the box on p. 390 for signs and symptoms of hypoxic-ischemic encephalopathy (HIE).
- Multiorgan dysfunction is common, with the kidneys, central nervous system, and cardiorespiratory systems most commonly affected.
- If muscle tone returns within 1 to 2 hours after birth, the prognosis for recovery and normal function is encouraging.
- The return of muscle tone within 24 hours, which is hypertonic, often prognosticates survival but with significant neurological damage.
- Cranial ultrasound is most helpful in evaluating preterm infants whereas a computed tomographic scan is more useful in evaluating full term infants.

Risk Factors for Perinatal Asphyxia

Maternal Medical History

toxemia
diabetes
pyelonephritis
chronic renal disease
anemia
drug abuse
placenta previa
abruptio placentae
hypertension
hypotension
lupus anticoagulant
cholestasis
older maternal age
polyhydramnios
low urinary estriol levels
sedative and analgesics just prior to delivery

History of Previous Pregnancies

stillbirth
neonatal death
perinatal asphyxia

Perinatal History

low birth weight
intrauterine growth retardation
decreased fetal movement
premature delivery
postmature delivery
cord prolapse
cord compression
prolonged labor
prolonged rupture of membranes
meconium-stained amniotic fluid
breech presentation
fetal heart rate decelerations
cesarean section
multiple gestation

Neonatal Medical History

congenital heart disease
lung disease
recurring apnea
significantly large patent ductus arteriosus
sepsis with hemodynamic instability
fetal malformations

LOW BIRTH WEIGHT/PREMATURITY

Gestational Age

- Variations of gestational age are categorized as prematurity and postmaturity. *Prematurity* is defined as a neonate who has completed less than 38 weeks gestation. *Postmaturity* is defined as a neonate who has completed more than 42 weeks

Signs and Symptoms of Hypoxic-Ischemic Encephalopathy

Mild

Poor sucking

Irritability

Hyperalertness

Overactivity of the sympathetic system

Uninhibited reflexes

Moderate

Hypotonia

Poor reflexes

Stupor

Lethargy

Seizures

Severe

Flaccid muscle tone

Coma

Poor brainstem function

Seizures

Increased intracranial pressure

Multiorgan dysfunction

gestation. Therefore, a term infant is a neonate who has completed more than 38 weeks but less than 42 weeks gestation.

- Physical features vary with gestational age. Assessment of the following can help determine neonatal maturity:

  skin: The preterm infant has thin, opaque, ruddy skin with blood vessels that are easy to see. The term infant has thicker, pinker skin with fewer visible blood vessels. The postterm infant has thick skin that peels, cracks, and is almost leathery in appearance with few visible blood vessels.

  lanugo: Soft, downy hair appears over the entire body from 21 to 33 weeks gestation. It is absent from the face by about 34 weeks gestation, and may be present only on the shoulders by 38 weeks gestation. Lanugo is very rare in postterm infants.

  plantar creases:
  34 to 35 weeks: only 1 to 2 creases on the anterior sole
  36 to 38 weeks: creases cover anterior ⅔ of sole
  38 to 42 weeks: creases are found over sole and heel
  >42 weeks: deeper and more numerous creases over entire sole of foot

  breast size:
  34 weeks: areola beings to appear
  36 weeks: breast bud of 1 to 2 mm can be seen
  38 to 42 weeks: breast bud grows to 12 mm

ear form:
<28 weeks: little cartilage, flat, shapeless
28 weeks: external part of ear (pinna) beings to turn in
36 weeks: good cartilage formation leading to firm ear that recoils. Upper ⅔ of pinna are folded
38 to 42 weeks: clear curving in of pinna
>42 weeks: definite curving of ear; ears stand away from the head

genitalia:
Male:
<28 weeks: testes are undescended, scrotum is high and close to body
28 to 36 weeks: rugae appear, testes are in inguinal canal
36 to 40 weeks: testes are in upper scrotum, rugae on anterior scrotum
>42 weeks: deep rugae, pendulous scrotum
Female:
30 to 36 weeks: prominent clitoris, labia majora are small and separated
36 to 40 weeks: labia majora are larger, nearly covering clitoris
>40 weeks: labia majora cover both labia minora and clitoris

- The Dubowitz method of determining gestational age uses ten physical and eleven neurological criteria.

- The Ballard scoring system uses six neurological and six physical criteria. The Ballard scoring system can be used on ill or fragile babies.

- Besides being classified by gestational age, neonates are also classified by birth weight for gestational age. Small for gestational age (SGA) is an infant whose birth weight falls in the bottom 10th percentile for the gestational age. Large for gestational age (LGA) is an infant whose birth weight is above the 90th percentile for gestational age.

Small for gestational age (SGA)
- SGA results from intrauterine growth retardation (IUGR). The causes and comorbidities are diverse and summarized in the box on p. 392.

Large for gestational age (LGA)
- The leading cause of LGA is maternal diabetes.

- Common complications include risk of premature labor, high incidence of unexplained death, birth injuries, and other commonly associated conditions. (See the box on p. 393.)

LIFE-THREATENING MATERNAL-FETAL COMPLICATIONS
Abruptio Placentae

- Abruptio placentae is a separation of the placenta from the uterine wall that is sudden, pathological, and results in severe maternal bleeding and fetal hypoxia/anoxia.

Causes of Intrauterine Growth Retardation (IUGR) and Comorbidities for SGA

Intrauterine Growth Retardation

Fetal and Placental Abnormalities

- Infarction
- Umbilical vascular abnormalities
  - Single umbilical artery
  - Umbilical vascular thrombosis
- Premature placental separation
  - Placenta previa
  - Placenta abruptio
- Hemangiomas
- Aberrant cord insertion
- Placental membrane abnormalities
- Poor placental blood flow
  - Multiple pregnancy
  - Substance abuse
  - Pregnancy induced hypertension
  - Chronic hypertension
  - Renal disease
  - Infection (TORCH)
  - Vascular tumors
- Monozygotic twins

Maternal Conditions

- Toxemia
- Cardiac disease
- Renal disease
- Chronic systemic hypertension
- Smoking
- Malnutrition
- Substance abuse
  - Heroin
  - Cocaine
  - Methadone
  - Alcohol
- Short interpregnancy interval
- History of SGA for the mother herself
- Use of anticonvulsants

Comorbidities for SGA Neonates

Perinatal Conditions

- Asphyxia
- Meconium aspiration
- Respiratory distress
- Pulmonary air trapping
- Pneumothorax
- Pulmonary hypertension
- Cerebral hypoxia
- Polycythemia
- Poor microcirculatory perfusion
- Altered carbohydrate metabolism

Long-term Conditions

- Impaired growth
- Immunologic deficiency
- Speech and language development impairments
- Hyperactivity
- Hyperreflexia
- Poor coordination
- Learning problems
- Delayed intellectual development
- Delayed neurological development

Conditions Commonly Associated with Large for Gestational Age Neonates

Birth Injuries

Fractures
- Skull
- Clavicular

Head injuries
- Cephalhematoma
- Intracranial bleeding

Nerve damage
- Facial nerve
- Phrenic nerve
- Brachial plexus palsy

Commonly Associated Conditions

Congenital anomalies
- Beckwith-Weidemann syndrome
- Transposition of the Great Vessels

Other conditions
- Rh isoimmunization
- Erythroblastosis fetalis
- Polycythemia
- Hypoglycemia
- Hypocalcemia
- Increased bilirubin production

Perinatal complications
- Umbilical cord prolapse
- Risk of premature labor
- Respiratory distress
  - meconium aspiration
  - intrauterine asphyxiation

- Abruptio placentae is a common cause of bleeding in the last half of pregnancy and during labor.
- Risk factors for abruptio placentae are listed in the box on p. 394.
- Maternal signs and symptoms of abruption include increasing uterine size from accumulation of blood, frank hemorrhage (although blood may be trapped between the placenta and uterine wall and not escape through the vagina), tender abdomen, rigid abdomen, sharp abdominal pain, rust to red colored amniotic fluid.
- Fetal signs and symptoms of abruption include tachycardia, late decelerations, decreased fetal heart rate variability, weak fetal heart tones, and absent fetal heart tones.
- Maternal complications associated with abruptio placentae include anemia, disseminated intravascular coagulation, shock, renal failure, Couvelaire uterus, and death.
- Fetal complications associated with abruptio placentae include anemia, hypoxia, asphyxia, and death.

Risk Factors for Abruptio Placenta

Maternal	Placental-uterine
Cigarette smoking	Short umbilical cord
Poor weight gain	Uterine leiomyomas
Cocaine use	Uterine anomalies
High multiparity	Polyhydramnios
Abdominal trauma	
Multiple pregnancy	
Supine hypotension	
History of previous abruption	

- If bleeding is severe or the fetus is distressed, an emergency cesarean section will be performed.
- If bleeding does not result in a serious health threat to the fetus or mother, the mother is placed on bed rest and monitored closely for abdominal rigidity, shock, fetal distress, and amount of vaginal bleeding.
- Ultrasound is the test of choice for evaluating the degree of placental separation.

PREGNANCY-INDUCED HYPERTENSION (PIH)

- Risk factors for pregnancy-induced hypertension (PIH) are listed in the box on p. 395.
- Potential maternal and placental-fetal complications are listed in the box on p. 395.
- HELLP syndrome (hemolysis, elevated liver function tests, low platelet count) is a maternal complication of PIH.

Preeclampsia

- Place on bed rest and in a left lateral position.
- Institute seizure precautions.

Risk Factors for Development of Pregnancy-Induced Hypertension (PIH)

- Malnutrition
- Maternal diabetes
- Hydatidiform mole
- Primigravidas
- Older maternal age
- Younger maternal age
- Multiple gestation
- Family history of PIH
- Poor weight gain in pregnancy
- History of use of barrier contraceptives
- Multigravidas with different paternity for varying pregnancies

Potential Fetal and Maternal Complications Related to Pregnancy-Induced Hypertension

Maternal Complications

Cardiopulmonary

- Cardiopulmonary failure
- Cardiomyopathy
- Cardiopulmonary arrest

Neurological

- Grand mal seizures
- Cerebrovascular accident
- Retinal detachment

Renal

- Renal cortical necrosis
- Renal failure

Hematologic

- Disseminated intravascular coagulation
- Low platelet count
- Hemolysis

Hepatic

- Elevated liver enzymes

Placental-Fetal Complications

Placental

- Abruptio placentae
- Premature placental aging
- Infarction
- Oligohydramnios

Fetal

- Intrauterine growth retardation
- Fetal distress
- Preterm delivery

- A high protein (1.5 g/kg/day) with low to moderate sodium diet is indicated.
- Placental-fetal tests are done to ensure viability and health of fetus.
- Magnesium sulfate is used prophylactically as a CNS depressant to prevent seizures.
- Sedation may be achieved with phenobarbital. This may make the nonstress test nonreactive because of fetal effects.
- Fetus is closely observed for short-term variability.
- Hydralazine may be used to lower maternal blood pressure. Sudden changes in maternal pressure, however, can result in fetal distress such as bradycardia, tachycardia, late decelerations.

ECLAMPSIA

- Management of a seizure is like any emergency—it begins with airway, breathing, and circulation.
- Magnesium sulfate and hydralazine are commonly used to treat eclampsia.
- The fetus is closely monitored for bradycardia or distress.
- Cesarean section or induction of labor is indicated when the mother and fetus recover from the seizure event.

NEONATAL COMPLICATIONS

- Intrauterine growth retardation and prematurity are commonly associated with PIH.
- Hypoxia, hypomagnesemia, and acidosis are common metabolic complications associated with PIH.

MATERNAL DRUG EFFECTS ON NEONATE

- Diazepam can cause hypothermia in the neonate.
- Hydralazine given to the mother for PIH can cause thrombocytopenia in the infant.
- Infants of mothers treated with phenobarbital have reduced neurological functioning as manifested by poor sucking, respiratory depression, and lethargy.
- Hypermagnesemia from maternal magnesium sulfate administration can cause a variety of symptoms listed in the box on p. 397.

Neonatal Complications Associated with Maternal Magnesium Sulfate Administration

Neuromuscular

Lethargy

Hypotonia

Weakness

Flaccidity

Cardiopulmonary

Respiratory depression

Hypotension

Dysrhythmias

Gastrointestinal

Decreased gut motility

Genitourinary

Urinary retention

Risk Factors for Umbilical Cord Prolapse

Malposition

Breech

Transverse lie

Small Fetal Size

Small for gestational age

Prematurity

Other Factors

Cephalopelvic disproportion

Multiple pregnancy

Polyhydramnios

Long cord

UMBILICAL CORD PROLAPSE

- The umbilical cord prolapses when it falls through the pelvic inlet well because the presenting part of the fetus does not close the inlet sufficiently. This occurs most often when the membranes rupture.
- Risk factors for umbilical cord prolapse are listed in the box above.
- Umbilical cord prolapse can occur even when cord is not visible or palpable on vaginal examination. Occult prolapse occurs when the cord is compressed between the presenting part and either the cervix or the pelvis.

- Clinical signs and symptoms of prolapse include fetal tachycardia (accelerations to 180 to 200 beats per minute) followed by bradycardia if compression of cord is not relieved.

- Fetal complications include fetal hypoxia, anoxia, neurological injury, neonatal infection, and perinatal mortality of approximately 35%.

- Maternal complications are related to rapid forceps or cesarean delivery.

- If prolapse occurs, interventions include administration of oxygen to the mother, continuous monitoring of fetal heart rate, and positioning mother in a knee-chest or Trendelenburg position with hips higher than the head. The examiner should keep the examining hand within the vagina to push the presenting part up and relieve pressure on the cord. Palpation of the cord for pulsation is desirable.

Questions

GENERAL MULTISYSTEM CARE QUESTIONS

1. Shock is best defined as:
   A. Decreased cardiac output
   B. Insufficient circulating volume
   C. Inadequate tissue perfusion
   D. Decreased systemic vascular resistance

2. Which of the following is a distinguishing characteristic of *septic* shock?
   A. Hypotension
   B. Cardiac dysrhythmias
   C. Proteinuria
   D. Weak pulses

3. Simulation of the sympathetic nervous system to improve blood pressure in distributive shock is best accomplished by which pharmacologic agents?
   A. Beta-adrenergic blocking agents
   B. Beta-adrenergic agonists
   C. Alpha-adrenergic blocking agents
   D. Calcium channel blockers

Case Study

A normotensive neonate is admitted to the critical care unit with an increase in serum glucose levels, decreased urinary output after 24 hours of increased output, and respiratory alkalosis. The critical care nurse closely monitors this infant in compensated shock for signs and symptoms of decompensation. Questions 4 to 6 refer to this case study.

---

4. This infant in compensated shock will likely exhibit all of the following signs and symptoms *except*:
   A. Bounding upper and lower extremity pulses
   B. Increased cardiac output and index
   C. Increased serum glucose levels
   D. Compensated metabolic acidosis

5. The critical care nurse knows this neonate with septic shock is most directly at risk for developing which of the following additional conditions?
   A. Persistent pulmonary hypertension
   B. Aspiration pneumonia
   C. Intraventricular bleeding
   D. Generalized seizures

6. Symptoms of decompensation for which the critical care nurse would be alert in this newborn include all of the following *except*:
A. Decreased level of consciousness
B. Metabolic alkalosis
C. Prerenal failure
D. Disseminated intravascular coagulation

7. Which outcome indicates effective management of an infant in uncompensated septic shock?
A. Urinary output of 1 mL/kg/hr
B. Capillary refill of 2.5 sec
C. Arterial pH of 7.33
D. Cardiac index of 2.3 L/min/m^2

8. The nurse is most likely to find peripheral edema while assessing a patient with:
A. Septic shock
B. Decreased circulating volume
C. Hemorrhagic shock
D. Systemic hypotension

9. The *first* step in the clinical management of distributive shock is to administer:
A. Beta-adrenergic agents to increase the systemic resistance
B. Blood products to raise the systemic blood pressure
C. Clotting factors to treat associated coagulopathies
D. Crystalloid or colloid fluids to increase circulating volume

10. In distributive shock, the nursing diagnostic category of fluid volume deficit is related to all of the following factors *except*:
A. Vascular endothelial dysfunction and leakage
B. Abnormal distribution of intravascular volume
C. Release of endotoxins causing vasodilation
D. Myocardial dysfunction from depressant factors

PEDIATRIC-SPECIFIC QUESTIONS

11. When caring for a child suspected of ingesting a toxic agent, the *first* action that should be taken is:
A. Administer activated charcoal to prevent absorption of toxin
B. Induce vomiting to stop exposure and absorption of the toxic agent
C. Ensure a patent airway and adequate ventilation
D. Identify the toxic agent to determine an antidote and/or treatment

Case Study

A 4-year-old boy is admitted to the critical care unit with a 2-hour history of drowsiness progressing to seizures at which point his parents immediately called emergency medical services and brought him to the emergency room. He had no previous history of seizures or head injury. The parents deny he was sick before this episode. Toxic ingestion was immediately suspected based on his history and presenting symptoms. Questions 12 and 13 refer to this case study.

12. Which of the following common toxidromes is most likely to be responsible for this child's presentation?
A. Salycilates
B. Narcotics
C. Methanol
D. Tricyclic antidepressants

13. Which of the following would be helpful in treating this child?
A. Atropine
B. Sodium bicarbonate
C. Mucomyst
D. Naloxone

14. Common problems associated with ingestion of aliphatic hydrocarbons include all of the following *except*:
A. Cardiac dysrhythmias
B. Chemical pneumonitis
C. Respiratory arrest
D. CNS depression

15. Aspiration of hydrocarbons is most likely to present with which of the following clinical pictures?
A. Cough, sputum, fever, and infiltrates
B. Dyspnea, cough, pulmonary edema, hypoxemia
C. Dyspnea, wheezing, cyanosis, pulmonary edema
D. Fever, wheezing, and cough with sputum

16. Contraindications to the use of syrup of ipecac include all of the following *except*:
A. Poor gag reflex
B. Acidosis
C. Seizures
D. Hydrocarbon ingestion

17. Which statement best describes how activated charcoal works?
   A. Prevents absorption and enhances elimination of toxins
   B. Inactivates toxins within the gastrointestinal tract
   C. Promotes emesis to eliminate toxins from the gut
   D. Neutralizes gastric acid to reduce hazard of aspiration

18. Which symptoms are *not* associated with ingestion of corrosives?
   A. Burning in the mouth, stomach, and throat
   B. Anxiety and apprehension
   C. White and swollen mucous membranes
   D. Increased oral secretions and swallowing

Case Study

A 15-year-old boy is admitted to the critical care unit with a diagnosis of acute alcohol toxicity. He is unconscious and responding only to noxious stimuli. His friends report a 3-hour drinking binge that began 4 hours ago and stopped just 1 hour before admission to the unit. Questions 19 and 20 refer to this case study.

---

19. Serum alcohol levels in this child can be expected to peak:
   A. ½ to 1 hour after ingestion
   B. Up to 12 hours after ingestion (L6)
   C. Up to 8 hours after ingestion
   D. ¼ to ½ hour after ingestion

20. The *immediate* priority in treating this child is to:
   A. Administer charcoal to absorb any remaining alcohol
   B. Induce vomiting to empty the stomach of alcohol
   C. Intubate endotracheally and nasogastrically
   D. Administer naloxone to reverse his alcohol poisoning

21. Proper administration of charcoal for a toxic ingestion is:
   A. Administer charcoal immediately, then induce vomiting
   B. Administer charcoal within 1 hour of poisoning after vomiting is induced
   C. Administer charcoal after emetic to absorb toxin and remaining emetic
   D. Administer charcoal within 1 hour of poisoning before vomiting is induced

22. Which nursing diagnostic category is appropriate for the child with an accidental poisoning that occurred at home?
   A. Impaired gas exchange
   B. Self-care deficit: feeding
   C. Impaired swallowing
   D. High risk for poisoning

Case Study

A 3-year-old girl is admitted to the critical care unit after a near-drowning episode. She is flaccid and comatose. According to the emergency medical technician at the scene, she was severely bradycardic and apneic when they arrived, but the parents were doing rescue breathing. They immediately intubated her, administered atropine, and had a good response. Questions 23 to 25 refer to this case study.

23. The prognosis for this child is most closely related to:
A. The temperature of the water
B. The length of submersion time
C. Saltwater versus freshwater drowning
D. The extent of hypoxia suffered

24. Priorities for treating this child will focus on all of the following *except*:
A. Maintaining mild hypothermia
B. Improving peripheral perfusion
C. Ensuring adequate glucose stores
D. Improving cardiac function

25. The critical care nurse would expect to observe signs and symptoms of increased intracranial pressure after how many hours in this child?
A. 12 to 24 hours
B. 24 to 48 hours
C. 48 to 72 hours
D. 72 to 96 hours

26. Which statement about neurological outcome for a child who was admitted flaccid and comatose following near-drowning is *true*?
A. Approximately ½ of victims have a successful outcome
B. Approximately ⅓ of victims have a successful outcome
C. Approximately ¼ of victims have a successful outcome
D. Approximately ⅕ of victims have a successful outcome

27. When caring for a near-drowning victim, the critical care nurse observes an elevated urine sodium level (>120 mEq/L), a serum sodium level of 122 mEq/L, and a urine specific gravity of 1.044. The nurse suspects this patient is developing:
A. Syndrome of inappropriate antidiuretic hormone secretion
B. Diabetes insipidus
C. Acute respiratory distress syndrome
D. Electrolyte shifts related to saltwater near-drowning

Case Study

A 7-year-old boy is admitted to the critical care unit with thermal injuries covering 40% of his body surface area acquired in a bedroom fire where he was playing with matches and his clothes caught on fire. Questions 28 to 31 refer to this case study.

28. Outcome criteria related to cardiac function within the first 12 hours of injury would include all of the following *except*:
A. Peripheral pulses: 3+
B. Cardiac index of 3.5 to 4.5 L/min/m^2 of body surface area
C. Intracompartmental pressures <30 mm Hg
D. Absence of peripheral paresthesia

29. All of the following nursing diagnosis for cardiac function are appropriate for this patient *except*:
A. Decreased cardiac output related to extravascular fluid shift
B. Decreased cardiac output related to myocardial dysfunction
C. Decreased cardiac output related to insufficient intravascular volume
D. Decreased cardiac output related to low central venous pressure

30. The physician may prescribe vasodilators for this patient. What would be an indication for their use?
A. The systemic vascular resistance is elevated
B. The intravascular volume is elevated
C. Capillary leakage is creating significant third-spacing
D. The fluid remobilization period has begun

31. After restoring adequate intravascular volume, the nurse would expect the physician to prescribe which medication to improve the function of his heart and improve his cardiac output?
A. Nitroprusside
B. Dobutamine
C. Digoxin
D. Dopamine

32. The nurse would anticipate outcome criteria during the first 12 hours for a patient with significant thermal injuries to include:
A. Urinary output of 0.5 cc/kg/hr
B. Resolution of an S_3 heart sound
C. A central venous pressure of 18
D. Normal skin temperature

33. When changing a dressing on a child with a large thermal injury, the nurse notes that the wound area has blisters and the area below where blisters have been removed is pink and sensitive to both touch and temperature. The area is also edematous. Based on this information, the nurse classifies this injury as:
A. First degree
B. Second degree
C. Third degree
D. Fourth degree

34. Which of the following is *not* an accurate method for determining the extent of a thermal injury in children, especially those under 4 years of age?
A. Lund and Browder method
B. Palmar method
C. Rule of Nines
D. Calculation of BSA affected

35. The critical care nurse would be alert to which of the following electrolyte and metabolic derangements associated with severe thermal injuries?
A. Hyperkalemia
B. Hypernatremia
C. Hypercalcemia
D. Hypermagnesemia

36. Which of the following is a *late* sign of inadequate intravascular volume resuscitation in a burn injured patient?
A. Diminished pulses
B. Tachycardia
C. Hypotension
D. Oliguria

Case Study

A 10 kg child is calculated to have a total BSA of 0.47 m^2. This child has a 40% BSA thermal injury. Questions 37 and 38 refer to this case study.

---

37. What would be the approximate fluid resuscitation needs of this child?
A. 865 cc
B. 565 cc
C. 1000 cc
D. 300 cc

38. How should fluid resuscitation for this child be administered?
- **A.** The first ⅓ calculated volume over the first 8 hours, the next ⅔ of the calculated volume over the next 16 hours
- **B.** The first ⅔ calculated volume over the first 12 hours, the next ⅓ of the calculated volume over the next 8 hours
- **C.** The first ½ calculated volume over the first 8 hours, the second ½ of the calculated volume over the next 8 hours
- **D.** The first ½ calculated volume over the first 8 hours, the second ½ of the calculated volume over the next 16 hours

39. Which of the following is *not* an appropriate fluid for volume resuscitation in the first 24 hours following a thermal injury?
- **A.** Albumin
- **B.** 0.45% normal saline
- **C.** Ringer's lactate
- **D.** 1.5% normal saline

40. Outcome criteria for fluid resuscitation in a burn injured patient would include all of the following *except*:
- **A.** Administration of the total calculated volume
- **B.** Return of peripheral pulses
- **C.** Warm, pink extremities
- **D.** Central venous pressure of 5 mm Hg

41. In a child with a smoke inhalation injury, oxygen saturation should be measured by:
- **A.** Pulse oximetry
- **B.** Calculating arterial pH and PaO_2
- **C.** Cooximetry
- **D.** Transcutaneous monitoring

42. Immune dysfunction in children with burn injuries is related to all of the following *except*:
- **A.** Loss of skin integrity
- **B.** Invasive monitoring and therapies
- **C.** Poor lymphocyte function
- **D.** Low immunoglobulin levels

Case Study

An 8-month-old infant is admitted to the critical care unit with a platelet count of 55,000/mm^3, a blood urea nitrogen (BUN) level of 90 mg/dL, a serum creatinine level of 2.2 mg/dL, and a hemoglobin of 6.2 g/L. The parents report that the baby recently had diarrhea and some vomiting several days before admission. She is admitted to the unit with a diagnosis of hemolytic uremic syndrome. Questions 43 to 45 refer to this case study.

---

43. Physical examination of this infant's skin would be expected to reveal:
- **A.** Purpuric lesions with flushed skin
- **B.** Pale skin with bruising
- **C.** Mottled skin with red blotching
- **D.** Ulcerations and bruising

44. Dialysis would be instituted for this child if:
- **A.** Anuria persisted for 24 hours
- **B.** Serum potassium rose to 6.4 mEq/L
- **C.** BUN became greater than 110 mg/dL
- **D.** Urinary output <0.5 mL/kg/hr

45. Which of the following blood products would be preferred to treat anemia in HUS?
- **A.** Irradiated red blood cells
- **B.** Whole blood
- **C.** Fresh, packed red blood cells
- **D.** Platelets

NEONATAL-SPECIFIC QUESTIONS

46. Maternal cocaine use is a high risk factor for all of the following complications *except*:
- **A.** Congenital cardiac defects
- **B.** Hydrocephalus
- **C.** Meconium aspiration
- **D.** Placenta previa

Case Study

A 35-week small for gestational age (SGA) infant is admitted to the NICU. Twelve hours after birth she is tachypneic, has temperature lability, sweating, sneezing, tremors, and a poor cry. She is a poor feeder and has slept little. Questions 47 to 50 refer to this case study.

---

47. These signs and symptoms are most likely to be a result of:
- **A.** Maternal cocaine use
- **B.** Narcotic abstinence syndrome
- **C.** Fetal alcohol syndrome
- **D.** Fetal tobacco syndrome

48. This infant would *least* likely be at risk for which of the following?
A. Respiratory distress syndrome
B. Skin breakdown
C. Malnutrition
D. Seizures

49. In order to reduce irritability in this neonate, the critical care nurse would:
A. Position the infant prone
B. Cover the hands with mittens
C. Reduce eye contact
D. Minimize verbal stimuli

50. The critical care nurse recognizes that this infant is also at risk for:
A. HIV infection
B. Respiratory distress syndrome
C. Hyperglycemia
D. Congenital diaphragmatic hernia

51. Which of the following abused substances is *least* likely to cause congenital anomalies?
A. Alcohol
B. Heroin
C. Cocaine
D. Cigarettes

52. A neonate with a history of abruptio placentae and suspected maternal substance abuse should be screened for which of the following substances?
A. Marijuana
B. Amphetamines
C. Heroin
D. Cocaine

53. An important nursing intervention when caring for the infant of a mother with substance abuse is:
A. Ample eye contact to promote bonding
B. Minimal physical contact to avoid overstimulation
C. Use of a firm mattress to promote sense of security
D. Swaddling and rocking for comfort measures

54. When working with drug dependent mothers, the critical care nurse should:
A. Encourage the mother to consider adoption or foster care
B. Look to a grandparent for a more stable parenting model
C. Be open and honest and avoid judgmental behavior
D. Order testing for HIV for the neonate

Case Study

An infant is admitted to the neonatal intensive care unit following meconium aspiration with a diagnosis of hypoxic-ischemic encephalopathy (HIE). Initial Apgar scores were 4 at one minute and 6 at five minutes. Questions 55 and 56 refer to this case study.

55. The final Apgar score:
A. Represents severe distress
B. Does not predict severity of HIE very well
C. Indicates mild to moderate HIE
D. Suggests clinical recovery

56. Physical examination of an infant with mild hypoxia would be expected to reveal:
A. Flaccid muscle tone, seizures, increased intracranial pressure
B. Poor brainstem function, convulsions, poor muscle tone
C. Lethargy, hypotonia, seizures, stupor
D. Irritability, poor sucking, uninhibited reflexes

57. Which of the following are common complications in other organ systems for the infant with hypoxic-ischemic encephalopathy?
A. Cardiogenic shock
B. Hyperbilirubinemia
C. Urinary retention
D. Pulmonary hypoplasia

58. A positive outcome for cardiac dysfunction related to HIE would include all of the following *except*:
A. Warm, pink extremities
B. Urinary output of 1 mL/kg/hr
C. Bounding peripheral pulses
D. Absence of pulmonary edema

59. The most important initial nursing measure for the infant with HIE would be to:
A. Obtain a computed tomographic scan (CT scan) to evaluate neurologic injury
B. Maintain a patent airway, optimize oxygenation and ventilation
C. Evaluate renal function by monitoring urinary output closely
D. Assess for necrotizing enterocolitis by monitoring for occult blood in stool

60. Which of the following statements is most appropriate for the critical care nurse to share with the parents of an infant with mild HIE?
A. "Generally there are not long-term problems with brain damage."
B. "Between two and four infants out of ten will have long-term brain damage."
C. "Nearly all infants will have permanent brain damage."
D. "Brain damage depends upon how long the baby is artificially ventilated."

61. In assessing an infant with HIE, the critical care nurse recognizes which of the following findings as likely indicating persistent and permanent neurological dysfunction?
A. Seizure activity more than 48 hours following birth
B. Hypotonia 24 hours after birth
C. Dilation of pupils during the first 24 hours
D. Little spontaneous movement during the first 12 hours

Case Study

A 1550 g female infant is born at 38 weeks gestation. She is 46 cm in length and has a head circumference of 32 cm. Questions 62 and 63 refer to this case study.

---

62. This infant is properly classified as:
A. Appropriate for gestational age (AGA)
B. Small for gestational age (SGA)
C. Large for gestational age (LGA)
D. Symmetrically growth retarded

63. For what complication is this infant at greatest risk in the first 8 to 12 hours after birth?
A. Hyperbilirubinemia
B. Apnea
C. Respiratory distress syndrome
D. Hypoglycemia

Case Study

The critical care nurse is caring for an infant of a diabetic mother (IDM) who is large for gestational age (LGA). The cardiac monitor is showing abnormal heart rhythms. Questions 64 to 66 refer to this case study.

---

64. Which of the following electrolyte imbalances that can cause dysrhythmias is most common in an IDM who is LGA?
A. Hypernatremia
B. Hyponatremia
C. Hypercalcemia
D. Hypocalcemia

65. Which of the following orders would the critical care nurse recognize as appropriate for this patient?
A. Monitor serum calcium. Elevated levels usually normalize without treatment
B. Administer calcium gluconate 10% 3 mL/kg for hypocalcemia
C. Restrict fluids and improve ventilation to normalize hyponatremia
D. Restrict sodium in IV fluids, sodium bicarbonate, and other medications

66. Which nursing diagnosis is appropriate for this infant?
A. High risk for altered body temperature
B. Fluid volume deficit
C. Impaired swallowing
D. Altered tissue perfusion

67. A full-term infant weighing 9720 g is admitted to the critical care unit with cyanosis, metabolic acidosis, and hypoxemia. No murmur is auscultated. This patient's pulse oximetry reading at admission is 75% on 100% oxygen after being intubated in the delivery room. Which of the following diagnoses is most likely?
A. Transient tachypnea of the newborn
B. Respiratory distress syndrome
C. Transposition of the great arteries
D. Peripheral pulmonary stenosis

68. What abnormal laboratory results would the critical care nurse anticipate in a LGA infant?
A. Hematocrit: 65%
B. White blood cell count: 26,000/mm^3
C. Hemoglobin: 12.7 g/dL
D. Platelets: 100,000/mm^3

69. Which of the following defines large for gestational age?
A. A postterm infant weighing more than the 75th percentile
B. A preterm infant weighing more than the 10th percentile
C. A term infant weighing more than the 50th percentile for gestational age
D. Any infant weighing more than the 90th percentile for gestational age

70. Small for gestational age infants who are term are at risk for which of the following:
A. Hypoglycemia, meconium aspiration, congenital malformations
B. Apnea, hyperbilirubinemia, hyaline membrane disease
C. Congenital malformations, hyperbilirubinemia, hyperglycemia
D. Meconium aspiration, apnea, hyaline membrane disease

71. In anticipating home discharge needs, the critical care nurse would identify potential need for which of the following for the preterm appropriate for gestational age (AGA) infant?
A. Home apnea monitoring
B. Home enteral nutritional therapy
C. Home oxygen therapy
D. Home shift nursing care

72. An appropriate nursing diagnosis related to the complications discussed above would be:
A. High risk for ineffective breathing pattern
B. Altered nutrition: less than body requirements
C. Impaired gas exchange
D. Caregiver role strain

Case Study

A small infant admitted to the neonatal intensive care unit weighs 1400 g and is 42 cm in length. Physical examination is performed to help determine gestational age.

Questions 73 and 74 refer to this case study.

---

73. Examination of the skin reveals no transparency, no lanugo, and the underlying blood vessels are difficult to visualize. There is no visible wrinkling or desquamation. Based on this information, the critical care nurse estimates the gestational age at:
A. 30 to 32 weeks
B. 33 to 34 weeks
C. 36 to 37 weeks
D. 39 to 41 weeks

74. Which of the following statements is important when the nurse assesses sole creases for estimation of gestational age?
A. Creases first appear on the posterior portion of the foot
B. After 12 hours, sole creases are not a valid indicator
C. Creases first appear on the heel and progress to the toes
D. Sole creases diminish with increasing gestational age

75. An infant with a raised areola but without any nodule of palpable breast tissue is estimated to be what gestational age?
A. 28 weeks
B. 30 weeks
C. 34 weeks
D. 40 weeks

76. An infant is born at 37 weeks gestation and is plotted to be at the 5th percentile for weight and the 50th percentile for length. This neonate is correctly classified as:
A. A symmetrically AGA preterm
B. An asymmetrically SGA preterm
C. A symmetrically SGA preterm
D. An asymmetrically AGA preterm

77. At what gestational age are the testes completely descended into the scrotum?
A. 30 weeks
B. 33 weeks
C. 36 weeks
D. 40 weeks

78. A major reason for accurately determining gestational age and size for gestational age is to:
A. Assess nutritional needs
B. Prevent apnea
C. Determine metabolic needs
D. Predict common complications

79. A neonate is determined to be small for gestational age and 34 weeks gestation. She has been intubated for hypoxia and apnea. She is on an FiO_2 of 0.8, pressure support, and a rate of 30 breaths/min. Her physical examination reveals clear, bilateral breath sounds. At the end of her assessment, however, the critical care nurse notices a sudden drop in the pulse oximeter from 95% to 78%. The most important *immediate* nursing action would be to:
A. Check the patency of the endotracheal tube
B. Increase the FiO_2 to 1.0
C. Suction aggressively for a mucous plug
D. Pull back the endotracheal tube 1.5 cm

80. Which of the following would be *most* helpful in determining the amount of placental separation in a placentae abruptio?
A. Complete blood cell count
B. Ultrasound
C. Amniocentesis
D. Vaginal examination

81. A mother during labor suddenly complains of sharp, continuous pain in her abdomen. The nurse's assessment reveals a rigid and tender abdomen, decreased blood pressure, tachycardia, and diaphoresis. The nurse ensures that the physician is notified immediately and should take what *initial* action?
A. Prep the abdomen
B. Insert a Foley catheter
C. Order a type and cross match
D. Insert a large bore intravenous line

82. A desired outcome in treating a patient with abruptio placentae is:
A. Liver palpable <2 to 3 cm below the costal margin
B. Evidence of a Couvelaire uterus
C. Urinary output of ≥30 cc/hr
D. Absence of seizure activity

83. A nurse is caring for a mother who just experienced abruptio placentae. After ensuring her airway, breathing, and circulation were stable, attention turned to assessing fetal well-being. The best assessment of fetal well-being would be which of the following?
A. Fetal movement count
B. Evaluation of fetal heart rate
C. Vaginal examination
D. Ultrasound of the abdomen

84. Which of the interventions listed below would be the *highest* priority when preparing a patient for an emergency cesarean section following a placentae abruptio?
A. Sending a urine for toxicology screen when catheterizing
B. Omitting surgical consent because of the urgency of surgery
C. Obtaining liver function studies with other blood work
D. Notifying the primary pediatrician

85. When caring for a neonate born by emergency cesarean section for abruptio placentae, for which of the following signs and symptoms of expected complications would the nurse be most alert?
I. Urine output <0.5 cc/kg/hr, periorbital edema
II. Platelet count 110,000/mm^3, oozing from venipuncture sites
III. Liver palpable 4 cm below costal margin, total bilirubin 21.5 µmol/L
IV. Hypotonia, seizures, arterial pH 7.10, pO_2 192 torr, pCO_2 16 torr
A. I and II
B. II, III, and IV
C. III and IV
D. I, II, and IV

86. The critical care nurse would review cardiac tests such as the echocardiogram and electrocardiogram for which of the following conditions when caring for an infant born by emergency cesarean section for prolapsed cord?
A. Right ventricular dilatation
B. Left ventricular hypertrophy
C. Coronary artery insufficiency
D. Junctional nodal rhythms

87. Which of the following signs and symptoms of electrolyte disturbance would the critical care nurse anticipate in caring for an infant born of a mother treated for eclampsia?
A. Weakness, lethargy, hypotonia, poor suck, apnea, and hypotension
B. Muscle weakness, peaked T waves on electrocardiogram, widened QRS complex
C. Apnea, irritability, twitching, seizures
D. Listlessness, irritability, apnea, seizures, coma

88. The critical care nurse would follow the complete blood count carefully in a neonate born of a mother with pregnancy induced hypertension for which of the following complications?
A. Neutrophilia
B. Thrombocytopenia
C. Eosinophilia
D. Leukopenia

Answers

GENERAL MULTISYSTEM CARE ANSWERS

1. **Correct answer—C.**
All types of shock are defined as a dysfunction of the cardiovascular system that *results in inadequate perfusion to meet the needs of tissues.*

2. **Correct answer—C.**
Proteinuria is a distinguishing characteristic of septic shock. Additional distinguishing characteristics include positive cultures, edema, sclerema, and occasionally a normal blood pressure accompanied by clinical evidence of poor peripheral perfusion. Hypotension and poor peripheral pulses may accompany any form of shock. Cardiac dysrhythmias may also accompany any form of shock, especially if myocardial oxygen demands are not being met.

3. **Correct answer—B.**
Stimulation of the sympathetic nervous system to improve blood pressure in distributive shock is best accomplished by beta-adrenergic agonists. An agonist is an agent that mimics or produces a specific response. Beta-adrenergic agonists result in vasoconstriction to improve systemic vascular resistance and systemic blood pressure. In forms of distributive shock, such as septic shock, one of the major causes of hypotension and poor perfusion is vasodilation. Beta-adrenergic blocking agents would only worsen the vasodilatory effects of distributive shock by facilitating more vasodilation. Alpha-adrenergic blocking agents and calcium channel blockers also would worsen peripheral vasodilation.

4. **Correct answer—D.**
Compensated shock does not include symptoms of compensated or uncompensated metabolic acidosis. Metabolic acidosis occurs when shock is *not* adequately compensated for by increased output leading to poor peripheral perfusion and metabolic acidosis. Bounding upper and lower extremity pulses occur in compensated shock because cardiac output and index are increased to try to maintain peripheral tissue perfusion and oxygen demand. An increase in serum glucose levels also often occurs as a result of sympathetic nervous system stimulation. Other signs and symptoms of compensated shock include hyperthermia, rapid capillary refill, flushed skin, thrombocytopenia, and mild changes in the level of consciousness.

5. **Correct answer—A.**
The neonate with septic shock is most directly at risk for developing persistent pulmonary hypertension of the newborn. Alveolar hypoxia and hypoxemia are powerful pulmonary vasoconstrictors. Poor perfusion and capillary leak, which accompany septic shock, inhibit the normal transition from fetal circulation

resulting in persistent pulmonary hypertension. Aspiration pneumonia, intraventricular bleeding, and generalized seizures are not directly related to septic shock, but may accompany any severe illness.

6. Correct answer—B.

Metabolic alkalosis would not be present in distributive forms of shock. Because shock results in inadequate tissue perfusion, metabolic *acidosis* would occur as cells switch to anaerobic metabolism and acids accumulate. Symptoms of decompensation for which the critical care nurse would be alert include decreased level of consciousness from poor cerebral perfusion, prerenal failure from poor renal perfusion, disseminated intravascular coagulation probably related to hepatic hypoperfusion and dysfunction, decreased cardiac output and index, respiratory acidosis, sluggish capillary refill, hypothermia, pale or mottled skin, and hypotension with the diastolic pressure effected first.

7. Correct answer—A.

Urinary output of 1 mL/kg/hr is an outcome that indicates effective management of an infant in uncompensated septic shock. Capillary refill of 2.5 seconds represents a delayed refill and therefore still inadequate peripheral perfusion. Normal arterial pH is 7.35 to 7.45; a pH of 7.33 indicates acidosis and continued inadequate peripheral tissue perfusion. A cardiac index of 2.3 L/min/m^2 is below the lower limits of normal, which is 2.5 L/min/m^2 and shows a cardiac output that is still inadequate.

8. Correct answer—A.

The nurse is most likely to find peripheral edema while assessing a patient with septic shock because of the capillary leak associated with the inflammatory response of sepsis. Decreased circulating volume, hemorrhagic shock, and systemic hypotension are not associated with capillary leakage and edema.

9. Correct answer—D.

The first step in the clinical management of distributive shock is to administer crystalloid or colloid fluids to increase circulating volume. Beta-adrenergic agents are used later to increase the systemic vascular resistance only after an adequate circulating volume has been established. Pharmacologically inducing systemic vasoconstriction without adequate intravascular volume would only worsen peripheral perfusion. Blood products should be used to raise the systemic blood pressure only if blood loss has occurred. Clotting factors would be indicated only if coagulopathies were demonstrated and after appropriate fluid resuscitation was initiated.

10. Correct answer—D.

Inadequate intravascular volume associated with septic shock is not related to myocardial dysfunction from depressant factors. Although myocardial dysfunction occurs during septic shock as a result of myocardial depressant factors, this aspect of sepsis is not related to an inadequate volume of blood, but rather inadequate pumping. Vascular endothelial dysfunction causing capillary leakage, abnormal distribution of intravascular volume resulting in venous pooling, and release of endotoxins causing vasodilation all occur in septic shock and result in inadequate intravascular volume.

PEDIATRIC-SPECIFIC ANSWERS

11. Correct answer—C.

When caring for a child suspected of ingesting a toxic agent, the first action that should be taken is to ensure a patent airway and adequate ventilation. Airway, breathing, and circulation (ABCs) are always the first steps to be taken. Administration of activated charcoal to prevent absorption of toxins may be helpful, especially if the toxin is still present in the gastrointestinal tract. Vomiting should be induced to stop exposure to and absorption of the toxic agent only when the agent will not cause additional damage with emesis. The airway must be carefully protected by ensuring an adequate gag reflex and normal levels of consciousness. Whenever possible, the toxic agent should be identified to determine an antidote and/or appropriate treatment, but the first action is always to ensure the ABCs.

12. Correct answer—B.

Narcotic poisoning results in seizures, respiratory depression, hypotension, pinpoint pupils, and decreased level of consciousness. Salycilates predominantly cause a mixed metabolic acidosis and respiratory alkalosis, but not commonly seizures. Methanol causes severe metabolic acidosis, changes in mentation, and visual disturbances, but does not typically cause seizures. Tricyclic antidepressants normally cause electrocardiographic changes such as a widened QRS complex and ventricular tachydysrhythmias.

13. Correct answer—D.

Naloxone is used to reverse narcotic toxicity. Its usefulness in treating clonidine toxicity is controversial. Atropine and pralidoxime are used to treat organophosphate insecticide poisoning. Sodium bicarbonate is used to treat tricyclic antidepressants. Mucomyst (N-acetylcysteine) is used to treat overdoses of acetaminophen.

14. Correct answer—A.

Aliphatic hydrocarbons are low viscosity and the most commonly ingested of all hydrocarbons. Cardiac dysrhythmias are not commonly associated with aliphatic hydrocarbons. They are more commonly associated with aromatic hydrocarbons. Chemical pneumonitis, respiratory arrest, CNS depression, coma, gastrointestinal irritation, and myocardial dysfunction are common manifestations of aliphatic hydrocarbon ingestion.

15. Correct answer—C.

Aspiration of hydrocarbons is most likely to present with dyspnea, wheezing, cyanosis, and pulmonary edema. Fever, infiltrates, and sputum are more commonly associated with infectious processes associated with aspiration of oropharyngeal secretions. Dyspnea, cough, pulmonary edema, and hypoxemia are commonly associated with aspiration of oral secretions or inert fluids.

16. Correct answer—B.

Contraindications to the use of syrup of ipecac include a poor gag reflex, decreased level of consciousness, seizures, and hydrocarbon ingestion. All of these conditions make it difficult for children to protect their own airways and therefore increase the risk of aspiration. Acidosis is not a contraindication.

17. Correct answer—A.

Activated charcoal works by both preventing absorption of toxins from the gastrointestinal tract and enhancing elimination of toxins already absorbed into the bloodstream. Charcoal is able to remove toxins already in the bloodstream because of the diffusion gradient between intravascular toxin levels and the toxin levels within the gut lumen. After absorption into the bloodstream, toxins actually reenter the gut lumen because of a diffusion gradient. When charcoal is present in the gut, it is able to absorb toxins as they reenter the gastrointestinal tract and facilitate elimination. Charcoal doesn't inactivate toxins within the gastrointestinal tract, but rather absorbs them so they cannot enter the bloodstream. Charcoal is not used to promote emesis to eliminate toxins; this is done by administering syrup of ipecac. Charcoal is not used to treat toxic ingestion by neutralizing gastric acid and reducing the hazards of aspiration. Charcoal is also frequently administered with sorbitol to enhance gastrointestinal elimination by creating temporary diarrhea.

18. Correct answer—D.

Ingestion of corrosives is associated with burning in the mouth, stomach, and throat, anxiety, apprehension, white and swollen mucous membranes, violent vomiting, hemoptysis, shock, drooling, and inability to clear or swallow secretions.

19. Correct answer—A.

Serum alcohol levels are expected to peak ½ to 1 hour after ingestion, but can peak as late as 6 hours after ingestion if gastric emptying is delayed.

20. Correct answer—C.

The immediate priority in treating this child is to intubate endotracheally and nasogastrically. Because this young man has an altered level of consciousness that compromises his ability to maintain his own airway, endotracheal or nasotracheal intubation is the highest priority. Nasogastric intubation is also indicated to empty his stomach contents and further help decrease the potential of aspiration. Charcoal is not generally used to absorb any remaining alcohol, but rather is used to treat other toxic ingestions. Inducing vomiting in this child with altered sensorium would be contraindicated as a result of his inability to protect his airway and the threat of aspiration. Naloxone is used to reverse narcotic overdoses, not alcoholic poisoning.

21. Correct answer—B.

Proper administration of charcoal for a toxic ingestion is to administer charcoal within 1 hour of poisoning, but after vomiting has been induced. If charcoal is administered first it can inactivate the emetic and minimize its effectiveness. Inducing vomiting after the administration of charcoal would also be counterproductive because charcoal needs to remain in the gastrointestinal tract to be effective.

22. Correct answer—D.

The nursing diagnostic category most appropriate for the child with an accidental poisoning that occurred at home is high risk for poisoning. Unless alterations are made in the home environment, other children may be at risk, and the affected child may be at risk for a second incident. An important function of the critical care nurse is to assess the home environment with the caregivers and educate them about risk factors and how to alter them for a safer environment. Impaired gas exchange would be relevant only if aspiration occurred or acute respiratory distress syndrome developed. Self-care deficit: feeding is a nursing diagnosis that refers to individuals' ability to feed themselves. Impaired swallowing occurs with certain toxidromes such as corrosives, but not with all.

23. Correct answer—D.

The prognosis for this child is most closely related to the amount of hypoxia suffered. The temperature of the water and the length of submersion are important because they influence the amount of hypoxia suffered. Saltwater versus freshwater drowning is clinically insignificant. Fluid shifts, hemolysis, and electrolyte derangements are unusual in near-drowning victims.

24. Correct answer—A.

Priorities for treating this child will not include maintaining mild hypothermia. Hypothermia may decrease damage to the central nervous system, but it complicates resuscitation because it increases susceptibility to ventricular fibrillation and asystole, impairs the effectiveness of resuscitation drugs, and impairs glucose metabolism as well as oxygen delivery. Improving peripheral perfusion, ensuring adequate glucose stores, and improving cardiac and respiratory function are all priorities in resuscitation of a near-drowning pediatric patient.

25. Correct answer—C.

The critical care nurse would expect to observe signs and symptoms of increased intracranial pressure 48 to 72 hours following the near-drowning incident, but can occur up to 1 week following injury.

26. Correct answer—B.

Approximately ⅓ of pediatric victims have a successful neurological outcome even when admitted to a critical care unit flaccid and comatose following a near-drowning.

27. Correct answer—A.

Syndrome of inappropriate antidiuretic hormone (SIADH) secretion is characterized by an elevated urine sodium level, a decreased serum sodium level, and an elevated urine specific gravity. All these symptoms are characteristic of SIADH when fluid is retained and sodium is wasted. Diabetes insipidus is characterized by fluid losses, dilute urine, decreased urine specific gravity, and hypernatremia. Acute respiratory distress syndrome is not directly related to alterations in electrolytes. Electrolyte shifts associated with saltwater or freshwater near-drowning are actually related to anoxia.

28. Correct answer—B.

Outcome criteria related to cardiac function for a child with thermal injuries within the first 12 hours of injury would not include a cardiac index of 3.5 to 4.5 L/min/m^2 of body surface area. This cardiac index is within normal limits. For a critically ill child with a thermal injury, cardiac index would appropriately be elevated to respond to the shock state that would accompany this injury. Peripheral pulses should be restored and maintained at normal. Intracompartmental pressures should be less than 30 mm Hg to prevent compartmental syndrome, which would threaten the viability of affected tissues and/or limbs. Absence of peripheral paresthesia would be one indicator of adequate peripheral perfusion.

29. Correct answer—D.

Decreased cardiac output related to low central venous pressure (CVP) is not an appropriate nursing diagnosis for this patient because a low CVP is secondary to intravascular hypovolemia and is therefore not a primary factor. Decreased cardiac output related to extravascular fluid shifts and/or insufficient intravascular volume is appropriate because in thermal injuries capillary leakage allows large volumes of fluid to leave the intravascular for the extravascular space. Decreased cardiac output related to myocardial dysfunction occurs in thermal injuries and has been attributed to the release of myocardial-depressant factor and stress induced increases in pulmonary and systemic vascular resistance.

30. Correct answer—A.

Vasodilators would be indicated for this patient if the systemic vascular resistance were elevated and compromising cardiac output by having a high afterload. There must, however, be adequate intravascular volume before vasodilators can be used or hypotension will be worsened. Capillary leakage and fluid remobilization are not affected by the use of vasodilators.

31. Correct answer—B.

After restoring adequate intravascular volume, the nurse would expect the physician to prescribe dobutamine to improve both the function of his heart and his cardiac output. Dobutamine improves cardiac function by its positive inotropic effects. Cardiac output is further enhanced by its peripheral vasodilatory effects that reduce afterload. Nitroprusside would reduce afterload, but not improve the myocardial dysfunction often associated with thermal injuries. Digoxin would not be the drug of choice to improve function and would not be as effective in reducing afterload. Dopamine would be a positive inotrope and help improve myocardial function, but it would also increase afterload by causing an increase in systemic vascular resistance.

32. Correct answer—D.
The nurse would anticipate outcome criteria for a patient with significant thermal injuries to include a normal skin temperature and extremities that are warm to touch. These both indicate adequate peripheral perfusion. Urinary output should be 1.0 cc/kg/hr or greater to indicate adequate renal perfusion. An S_3 heart sound representing a gallop rhythm and a CVP of 18 mm Hg would both be unlikely during the first hours when intravascular volume is depleted.

33. Correct answer—B.
A second-degree burn is also called partial-thickness and involves the entire epidermis and part of the dermis. It is characterized by blisters with the area below where blisters have been removed as pink and sensitive to both touch and temperature. Additionally, second-degree burns are surrounded by edematous tissue. First-degree (superficial) burns affect only the epidermis and are erythematous, painful, edematous, and blanch with pressure. Third-degree burns (full-thickness) affect the entire epidermis and dermis. Eschar is present. There is little pain where third-degree burns are present because nerve endings have been destroyed. Fourth-degree burns involve the epidermis, dermis, subcutaneous tissue, and even muscle, bone, or tendons.

34. Correct answer—C.
The Rule of Nines is not an accurate method for determining the extent of a thermal injury in children, especially those under 4 years of age because children do not have the same proportions of body surface area (BSA) with corresponding body parts. The Lund and Browder method is very accurate and involves a chart that can be consulted to determine affected area by age and burn sites. The palmar method is an estimate by using the child's own palm as 1% of BSA and then estimating burned areas. Calculation of actual BSA affected is the most accurate, but is difficult without computer programs, which are gaining more widespread use.

35. Correct answer—A.
The critical care nurse would be alert for hyperkalemia associated with severe thermal injuries because of the potassium that is released from necrotic cells. Hyponatremia, hypocalcemia, and hypomagnesemia are also frequent electrolyte derangements associated with severe thermal injury when dilution occurs from resuscitation fluids or SIADH.

36. Correct answer—C.
Hypotension is a late sign of inadequate intravascular volume resuscitation in a burn injured patient. Diminished pulses, tachycardia, hypotension, oliguria, low

central venous pressure, acidosis, cold extremities, and poor capillary refill time all occur before hypotension. In infants and children, an increase in systemic vascular resistance accompanies shock states until severe compromise occurs.

37. Correct answer—A.
There are several formulas for calculating fluid administration needs in the burn injured child. The modified Parkland formula is among the most commonly used. Based on this formula, the approximate fluid resuscitation needs of a 10 kg child with a 40% TBSA burn and a BSA of 0.47 m^2 would be 865 cc. The formula for calculation is:

$$(4\ \text{cc/kg/\% TBSA injury}) + (1500\ \text{mL/m}^2\ \text{BSA})$$

38. Correct answer—D.
The first ½ calculated resuscitation volume should be administered over the first 8 hours, and the second ½ of the calculated volume should be administered over the next 16 hours.

39. Correct answer—B.
Hypotonic solutions such as 0.45% normal saline are not appropriate fluids for volume resuscitation in the first 24 hours following a thermal injury because they may lower serum sodium concentrations and increase movement of fluid from the intravascular to the extravascular space. Albumin and 1.5% normal saline are hypertonic solutions that may help keep or return fluid to the intravascular space. Ringer's lactate is an excellent isotonic solution that also helps replace lost electrolytes. Normal saline is another isotonic solution frequently used in fluid resuscitation.

40. Correct answer—A.
Outcome criteria for fluid resuscitation in a burn injured patient would not include administration of the total calculated resuscitation volume. Although the calculated volume is important in determining the patient's fluid volume needs, it is the clinical response with such signs as return of peripheral pulses, warm, pink extremities, and an adequate central venous pressure of 5 mm Hg that indicates the desired outcome has been achieved.

41. Correct answer—C.
In a child with a smoke inhalation injury, oxygen saturation should be measured by cooximetry to be accurate. Pulse oximetry, transcutaneous O_2 monitoring, and calculations based on pH and PaO_2 are inaccurate because they do not exclude carboxyhemoglobin levels associated with carbon monoxide poisoning.

42. Correct answer—D.
Immune dysfunction in children with burn injuries is related to loss of skin integrity, invasive monitoring and therapies, poor lymphocyte function, changes in leukocyte function, circulating burn injury associated toxins, and many antimicrobial agents. Low immunoglobulin levels, which may occur during the first week following injury, are not associated with an increase in infections.

43. Correct answer—B.
Physical examination of this infant's skin would be expected to reveal pale skin with bruising as a result of anemia and thrombocytopenia associated with HUS. Purpuric lesions are more characteristic of meningococcemia. Mottled skin would indicate a shock state, and red blotching would be more indicative of some kind of rash. Ulcerations would not be expected with HUS.

44. Correct answer—A.
Dialysis would be instituted for this child if anuria persisted for 24 hours. Oliguria with evidence of uremia (elevated BUN or creatinine) would also be an indication for dialysis if diuretic therapy and protein restriction were not effective. Hyperkalemia can be treated with insulin and glucose, an exchange resin, or sodium bicarbonate. Only if refractory to these treatments would an elevated potassium require dialysis.

45. Correct answer—C.
Fresh, packed red blood cells would be the preferred blood product to treat anemia in HUS. The concentration of red blood cells that are fresh would be least likely to cause fluid volume overload and improve the hematocrit and hemoglobin. Irradiated red blood cells are indicated only in such conditions as DiGeorge's syndrome where graft-versus-host disease is a potential threat. Whole blood would provide proportionately too much volume and too few red blood cells to effectively treat anemia in the presence of renal dysfunction. Platelets would be important in treating thrombocytopenia, but be of no value in treating anemia.

NEONATAL-SPECIFIC ANSWERS

46. Correct answer—D.
Maternal cocaine use is a high risk factor for congenital cardiac defects, hydrocephalus, meconium aspiration, limb defects, cranial defects, placenta abruptio, hypoxia, genitourinary anomalies, and bowel infarctions.

47. Correct answer—B.
These signs and symptoms are most likely to be a result of narcotic abstinence syndrome. Fetal cocaine exposure results in infants who are jittery, cranky, poor feeders, and unresponsive to cuddling or comforting measures. Fetal alcohol syndrome has characteristic facial, neurologic, behavior, and growth features. (See Table 8-7.) Fetal tobacco syndrome is characterized by symmetric intrauterine growth retardation.

48. Correct answer—A.
This infant would least likely be at risk for developing respiratory distress syndrome. For unknown reasons, perhaps intrauterine stress factors, accelerate lung maturity makes RDS unusual. Skin breakdown is a likely complication related to hyperactivity and poor nutritional status. Malnutrition often began in utero

and feeding difficulties, vomiting, and diarrhea postnatally may further complicate nutritional status. Seizures are a common complication of narcotic abstinence syndrome.

49. Correct answer—C.
In order to reduce irritability in a narcotic addicted neonate, the critical care nurse would reduce eye contact, swaddle the infant tightly, rock the baby, arrange nursing care to minimize stimulation, and verbally comfort the baby.

50. Correct answer—A.
Infants of substance abuse mothers are at risk for HIV infection because of the social factors surrounding drug abuse. Respiratory distress syndrome has a decreased incidence in narcotic exposed infants. Hypoglycemia would be a risk factor as a result of poor nutritional stores and immaturity of hepatic and autonomic systems. Congenital diaphragmatic hernia has no known increased incidence in substance abuse mothers.

51. Correct answer—B.
Heroin has not been associated with congenital anomalies, but has been associated with meconium aspiration, aspiration pneumonia, increased incidence of sudden infant death syndrome, and congenital infections. Cigarettes have been associated with intrauterine growth retardation and an increased risk of congenital malformations. Alcohol has been associated with such congenital anomalies as central nervous system anomalies, facial anomalies, cardiac anomalies, renal anomalies, and skeletal anomalies. Cocaine has been associated with a variety of congenital anomalies of the heart, genitourinary system, limbs, central nervous system, and gastrointestinal system.

52. Correct answer—D.
A neonate with a history of abruptio placentae and suspected maternal substance abuse should be screened for cocaine use, which is associated with this perinatal emergency. Fetal alcohol syndrome is also associated with abruptio placentae.

53. Correct answer—D.
An important nursing intervention when caring for the infant of a mother with substance abuse is to swaddle and rock the baby for comfort measures. Eye contact can increase irritability and stimulation. Physical contact in holding tightly and rocking can help soothe the infant and prevent self-stimulation. Use of water mattresses has been found to be helpful in calming irritable and cranky drug exposed neonates.

54. Correct answer—C.
When working with drug dependent mothers, the critical care nurse should be open and honest and avoid judgmental behavior. Encouraging the mother to consider adoption or foster care will not build an effective nurse-patient relationship.

Looking to a grandparent for a more stable parenting model may be counterproductive because most substance abusing women have come from families with physical or sexual abuse. Few have been in families with positive parenting role models. While HIV risk is increased in infants born of women who have substance abuse problems, testing cannot be ordered without parental consent.

55. Correct answer—B.

Apgar scores alone without the support of clinical examination and findings are not an accurate predictor of the severity of HIE. Categorizing the severity based on Apgar scores cannot be determined. Clinical recovery from HIE cannot be determine by Apgar scores at one and five minutes.

56. Correct answer—D.

Physical examination of an infant with mild hypoxia would be expected to reveal irritability, poor sucking, uninhibited reflexes, sympathetic nervous system overwork, and hyperalertness. Flaccid muscle tone, seizures, increased intracranial pressure, and poor brainstem function are indicative of severe hypoxia. Lethargy, hypotonia, seizures, stupor, and abnormal muscle tone are symptoms of moderate asphyxia.

57. Correct answer—A.

Cardiogenic shock from right and left ventricular dysfunction is a common complication for the infant with hypoxic-ischemic encephalopathy. The kidney is the most commonly affected organ resulting in acute renal failure. Persistent pulmonary hypertension, disseminated intravascular coagulation, and necrotizing enterocolitis are other common complications in organ systems outside the central nervous system.

58. Correct answer—C.

Positive outcomes for cardiac dysfunction related to HIE would include warm, pink extremities, urinary output of 1 mL/kg/hr, and absence of pulmonary edema. These are all indicators of adequate myocardial function and peripheral perfusion. Bounding peripheral pulses are abnormal and most commonly indicate fluid overload or a patent ductus arteriosus.

59. Correct answer—B.

The most important initial nursing measure for the infant with HIE would be to maintain a patent airway, as well as optimize oxygenation and ventilation. Resuscitation and care always begins with airway, breathing, and circulation. Obtaining a compound tomographic scan (CT scan) to evaluate neurologic injury is important, but not an initial priority. Evaluating renal function and assessing for necrotizing enterocolitis are also important, but are not more important initially than respiratory function.

60. Correct answer—A.

It is appropriate for the critical care nurse to share with this infant's parents that generally there are not long-term problems with brain damage of an infant with mild HIE. For the infant with moderate HIE, 15% to 20% will have long-term neurological sequelae. Nearly all infants will have permanent neurological sequelae if they have severe HIE. Brain damage is not related to how long the baby is artificially ventilated.

61. Correct answer—A.
Seizure activity more than 48 hours following birth is usually associated with severe HIE and permanent neurological damage. Hypotonia and little spontaneous movement during the first 24 hours after birth are associated with moderate HIE. Dilation of pupils during the first 24 hours may be seen with mild HIE.

62. Correct answer—B.
This infant is properly classified as small for gestational age (SGA) because of her weight. Her growth pattern is also asymmetrical, with her weight falling below predicted norms but her length and head circumference are within normal limits for her gestational age.

63. Correct answer—D.
As SGA infant is most at risk for hypoglycemia, congenital malformations, asphyxia, polycythemia, persistent pulmonary hypertension, and meconium aspiration. Hyperbilirubinemia, apnea, and respiratory distress syndrome are more common complications with premature appropriate for gestational age (AGA) infants.

64. Correct answer—D.
Hypocalcemia and hypoglycemia are common metabolic imbalances in the infant of a diabetic mother (IDM) who is large for gestational age (LGA). Neither imbalances in sodium nor hypercalcemia are imbalances specifically associated with IDM or LGA.

65. Correct answer—B.
The critical care nurse would recognize an order for administering calcium gluconate 10% 3 mL/kg for hypocalcemia as appropriate. Because LGA IDM neonates are at risk for hypocalcemia, this would be the most appropriate order. Treatments for sodium imbalance would be unexpected.

66. Correct answer—A.
High risk for altered body temperature is the most appropriate nursing diagnosis for this infant. Large for gestational age infants are at high risk for asphyxia as a result of central nervous system trauma, hypoglycemia, and difficulty with thermoregulation. Fluid volume deficit, impaired swallowing, and altered tissue perfusion are not common complications associated with LGA or IDM.

67. Correct answer—C.
This patient's diagnosis is most likely transposition of the great arteries, which is commonly associated with LGA and IDM. Because there may be an intact ventricular septum, an elevated pulmonary pressure and no other anatomical

variances that would cause irregular patterns of blood flow, a murmur may not be present. Transient tachypnea of the newborn would not be expected to result in such severe hypoxemia. Respiratory distress syndrome does not usually present in such immediate distress. Peripheral pulmonary stenosis is a condition where peripheral pulmonary arteries are small and a characteristic murmur is evident, but is not associated with severe cyanosis.

68. Correct answer—A.
A large for gestational age infant is at risk for polycythemia. There is no increased risk for alterations in white blood cell count or platelets. A hemoglobin of 12.7 g/dL is low, and not indicative of polycythemia.

69. Correct answer—D.
Any infant weighing more than the 90th percentile for gestational age is defined as being large for gestational age.

70. Correct answer—A.
Small for gestational age infants who are term or postterm are at risk for hypoglycemia, meconium aspiration, and congenital malformations. Preterm appropriate for gestational age infants are at risk for apnea, hyperbilirubinemia, and hyaline membrane disease.

71. Correct answer—A.
In anticipating home discharge needs, the critical care nurse would identify potential need for home apnea monitoring for the preterm appropriate for gestational age (AGA) infant because of their increased incidence of apnea related to prematurity. Home enteral nutritional therapy, oxygen therapy, and shift nursing care would be dependent on additional individual complications.

72. Correct answer—A.
An appropriate nursing diagnosis related to apnea seen in preterm AGA infants is high risk for ineffective breathing pattern.

73. Correct answer—C.
An examination of the skin that reveals no transparency, no lanugo, no wrinkling, no desquamation, and the underlying blood vessels as difficult to visualize indicates a gestational age of 36 to 37 weeks. As early as 30 to 34 weeks the skin would be more transparent and blood vessels apparent. At 39 to 41 weeks gestation, the subcutaneous tissue decreases resulting in desquamation and wrinkling.

74. Correct answer—B.
After 12 hours, sole creases are not a valid indicator of gestational age as a result of the drying of the skin. Creases first appear on the *anterior* portion of the foot and progress from the toes to the heels with increasing gestational age. Sole creases increase in number and character with increasing gestational age.

75. Correct answer—C.

An infant with a raised areola but without any nodule of palpable breast tissue is estimated to be 34 weeks gestation. A neonate as young as 28 to 30 weeks gestation may not even have any visible areola. Palpable breast tissue does not occur until 36 weeks gestation.

76. Correct answer—B.

An infant who is born at 37 weeks gestation and is plotted to be at the 5th percentile for weight and the 50th percentile for length is correctly classified as an asymmetrically SGA preterm. The infant is preterm because it was born before 38 weeks gestation. The growth is asymmetrical because length and weight are not at the same percentile. Because weight is below the 10th percentile, the infant is classified as small for gestational age.

77. Correct answer—D.

The tests are completely descended into the scrotum at 40 weeks gestation.

78. Correct answer—D.

A major reason for accurately determining gestational age and size for gestational age is to anticipate common complications and initiate treatment early. Assessment of gestational age and size is not generally performed to determine nutritional and metabolic needs. Apnea is not prevented by calculating gestational age.

79. Correct answer—A.

The most important immediate nursing action for an intubated infant with a sudden drop in arterial saturations measured by pulse oximetry would be to check the patency of the endotracheal tube. The first step is always to ensure and maintain a patent airway. Other steps such as suctioning should only be done if assessment reveals a strong likelihood of occlusion such as absence of breath sounds. Increasing the FiO_2 to 1.0 would not be helpful without ensuring the tube is patent. Pulling back the endotracheal tube 1.5 cm would only be indicated if a chest x-ray showed that the tube was in the right bronchus or if breath sounds were absent unilaterally.

80. Correct answer—B.

An ultrasound would be most helpful in determining the amount of placental separation in a placentae abruptio. The complete blood cell count would be helpful in determining the amount of blood loss, but may not always be accurate or helpful immediately. Amniocentesis will not measure the amount of blood between the placenta and uterine wall and offers no information on placental separation. Vaginal examination also will not offer specific or measurable information about the degree of separation.

81. Correct answer—D.

The nurse ensures that the physician is notified immediately when an abruption is suspected and should then take the initial action of inserting a large bore intravenous line. Prepping the abdomen for a cesarean section is necessary, but does not take priority over ensuring an adequate circulating volume in the presence of frank hemorrhage. A Foley catheter is also indicated in the presence of hypovolemia, potential organ hypoperfusion, and renal necrosis associated with abruption, but again is not more important than inserting an IV to ensure adequate circulating volume. Ordering a type and cross match is also important, but does not take priority.

82. Correct answer—C.

A desired outcome in treating a patient with abruptio placentae is urinary output of ≥30 cc/hr. Because hypovolemia leaves the patient at risk for prerenal failure and renal necrosis is associated with abruption, adequate urinary output is critical to her management. Liver dysfunction is not specifically related to abruption. A Couvelaire uterus is an *undesirable* outcome because this is a uterus with muscle fibers full of blood. Finally, seizure activity is not normally expected to be associated with abruption, but rather with pregnancy induced hypertension or eclampsia.

83. Correct answer—B.

The best assessment of fetal well-being during an abruptio placentae would be evaluation of fetal heart rate for decelerations and variability. These are good indicators of fetal well-being and response to stress. The fetal movement count is a gross indicator used primarily in the home by the mother to roughly estimate well-being. A vaginal examination would reveal little information on fetal well-being unless a prolapsed cord was discovered and absence of pulsation was noted. An ultrasound of the abdomen would also offer little specific information on how the fetus was tolerating the abruption.

84. Correct answer—A.

When preparing a patient for an emergency cesarean section following a placentae abruptio, sending a urine for toxicology screen when catheterizing the patient would be indicated because of the high incidence of abruption and cocaine use. Omitting surgical consent because of the urgency of surgery is not indicated unless no responsible next of kin can be located or the mother herself cannot give consent. Obtaining liver function studies with other blood work is not a priority because liver dysfunction is not generally associated with an abruption. Notifying the primary pediatrician should be accomplished as soon as possible but not delay preparing the patient for emergency surgery.

85. Correct answer—D.

A liver palpable 4 cm below costal margin and a total bilirubin 21.5 μmol/L are not expected complications of hypoxic-ischemic encephalopathy (HID) related to abruptio placentae. The critical care nurse must be most alert for signs/symptoms of hypoxic-ischemic encephalopathy listed in the box on p. 390. Urine output <0.5 cc/kg/hr and periorbital edema would be expected with renal involvement, which occurs with approximately 50% of cases. A platelet count of 110,000/mm^3 and oozing from venipuncture sites would also indicate disseminated intravascular coagulation, a frequent complication of HIE. Hypotonia, seizures, and arterial pH 7.10, pO_2 192 torr, pCO_2 16 torr are also indicative of hypoxia with successful cardiopulmonary resuscitation at delivery.

86. Correct answer—A.

The critical care nurse would review cardiac tests such as the echocardiogram and electrocardiogram for right ventricular dilatation when caring for an infant born by emergency caesarean section for prolapsed cord because the neonate would be at risk for persistent fetal circulation or persistent pulmonary hypertension related to the hypoxic event. Left ventricular hypertrophy generally is found in left heart disease that is obstructive such as interrupted aortic arch, coarctation of the aorta, and aortic stenosis. Coronary artery insufficiency is generally associated with anomalous coronary arteries or following arterial switch surgery for transposition of the great arteries. Junctional nodal rhythms are not generally, but may rarely, be associated with hypoxemia. Cardiac dysrhythmias are more common in neonates born of mothers with eclampsia who have been treated with magnesium sulfate.

87. Correct answer—A.

The signs and symptoms of electrolyte disturbance that the critical care nurse would anticipate in caring for an infant born of a mother treated for eclampsia are weakness, lethargy, hypotonia, poor suck, apnea, and hypotension, all of which are indicative of hypermagnesemia. Magnesium sulfate used to treat eclampsia in the mother can cause hypermagnesemia in the neonate. Muscle weakness, peaked T waves on electrocardiogram, and widened QRS complex are indicative of hyperkalemia. Apnea, irritability, twitching, and seizures are indicative of hyponatremia whereas listlessness, irritability, apnea, seizures, and coma are sign of hypernatremia.

88. Correct answer—B.

The critical care nurse would follow the complete blood count carefully in a neonate born of a mother with pregnancy induced hypertension for thrombocytopenia. A decrease in fetal-neonatal platelet count is a side effect of maternal use of hydralazine for hypertension.

CHAPTER 9

Successful Test-Taking Strategies

Certification is an excellent way to achieve professional recognition and advancement in nursing. For pediatric and neonatal critical care nurses, certification is available through the American Association of Critical Care Nurses and the National Certification Corporation. See Table 9-1 for further information about these certification examinations.

There are many tangible benefits to becoming certified in your area of expertise. Your professional advancement may be enhanced and also many hospitals offer a differential to staff nurses who are certified. Unlike going on for an advanced degree, certification allows you to pace your studying and control your schedule more easily. How much you study is an important key to passing a certification exam, but it's not the only key.

Simply studying is not enough to guarantee you'll pass a certification exam. You need to know how to prepare yourself mentally, how to decide on what to study, and most of all, *how to take a test.*

PREPARING FOR THE TEST

Preparing for the test involves more than just sitting down and studying. To prepare yourself, use the following tips to guarantee your success.

Start studying early. Mastery learning is a concept used in elementary education. It's a simple philosophy: that which we do over and over we learn well. If you've ever played a musical instrument, you know that learning a new song is difficult. But repetition, playing the song over and over, plants it in your mind and on your fingers. Soon you're playing the song automatically. Think about how you first struggled to learn drug dosages, but with time and repetition they now come to you automatically. Starting to study early so you can review key material often will make it become second nature to you. You will recall it easily for the test, increase your confidence, and reduce your anxiety. Start studying at least 2 months before the examination.

Table 9-1

Certifications Available to Neonatal and Pediatric Critical Care Nurses

American Association of Critical Care Nurses	National Certification Corporation
Address: 101 Columbia, Aliso Viejo, CA 92656	Address: 645 North Michigan Avenue, Suite 900, Chicago, IL 60611
Phone: 1-800-899-2226	Phone: 1-800-367-5613
Certification granted: CCRN	Certification granted: RNC
Specialty area(s): Pediatric and Neonatal	Specialty area(s): Neonatal

Focus on the outline. The organization offering the examination will provide you with an outline of the most important information. Often this content is weighted so you know for what areas you should study most heavily. For example, on the certification examination for pediatric critical care nurses, only 5% of the questions deal with gastrointestinal problems. This translates to only 16 questions out of 200 on the entire test. When deciding on what topics to spend the most time, this area would *not* rank among the highest priorities.

Practice, practice, practice test questions. For objective and easy scoring, the tests are comprised of multiple choice questions with no essays. You need to practice taking multiple choice exams as much as you need to learn important content.

Don't cram! Trying to learn a great deal of information in a limited time is difficult. You will find it hard to build your confidence and to cover the essential content thoroughly enough to recall and apply it easily. Don't cram the night before the examination. It will only add to your anxiety if you find something you don't know at the last minute. Do something you enjoy the night before to relax and get your mind off the test. One night of studying isn't going to make you pass or fail.

Don't memorize—understand! Whenever possible, don't memorize material, but rather try to understand it. If you memorize the information you run the risk of failing to remember it—or even to remember it correctly. For instance, don't try to memorize all the effects of the sympathetic nervous system, but rather, think of all of the things the body would need to do for "flight or fight." Then you'll easily recall that pupils dilate to see better, heart rate and respiratory rate increase. Blood flow to the gut decreases because it is not essential in an emergency. If you must memorize facts, such as the cranial nerves, make your strategy work. That old pneumonic "On old Olympus towering tops a Finn and German viewed some Hopps" really isn't helpful. It's too hard to remember what each *o* and *t* stands for. A good example is to remember epidural bleeds are arterial (both start with vowels) whereas subdural bleeds are venous (both start with consonants). Carefully read the rationales to the answers in this book, not just the right answer. Understanding the correct answer and why other choices were wrong will help you answer a similar question on the real exam.

STRATEGIES TO USE DURING THE TEST

When the day has come to take the exam, use these tried and true strategies once you begin taking the test. Follow the suggestions below to help you outsmart the test writers.

Be confident! You have prepared well, and you know the material. If you feel insecure, you will easily feel intimidated by questions that are only a little more difficult. Confidence will keep you thinking clearly. When you first open your test booklet, if you see a question you don't know, just skip it and come back later. Begin the test with confidence by answering the easy questions first. You can always spend more time on the hard ones later.

Devise a ritual. Rituals can give you a sense of control in a situation that often makes most people feel out of control. Maybe wearing lucky clothes or carrying a good luck charm will work for you. The key is to believe you have control, even if you need an object to help make this control tangible.

Dress for success. Wear dressy clothes to feel sharp or casual clothes for comfort. Being comfortable physically or in your appearance can help you relax and feel confident. Some people perform best on examinations in suits and high heels. Others do better in casual clothes like blue jeans and sweatshirts.

Get a good night's sleep. Nothing will help you be more relaxed than being well rested. On the night before the test, go to bed early with a favorite book, a cup of hot chocolate, or a good movie. Try to clear your head about tomorrow.

Eat well. Eat well the day of the examination. Stay away from sweets and concentrate on high energy foods such as grains, pasta, and protein. Sugars (such as a doughnut at the sweet shop on the way to the exam) may slow you down.

Guess! These tests do not have a penalty for guessing. By eliminating wrong choices, you increase your odds of guessing correctly.

For example:
Signs and symptoms of inflammation include:
~~A. Ecchymosis, swelling, fever~~
B. Pain, tenderness, swelling
~~C. Purulent drainage, pallor~~
~~D. Cool, puffy, moist~~

Mark on your test booklet. Use the following strategies to highlight important information, eliminate incorrect information, and pick apart questions and answers. You will then be certain you are using your knowledge to find the correct answer and pass your certification exam.

Bring and use highlighters as well as pencils. By using different color highlighters or pens, you can easily and consistently dissect questions and answers. For example, use one color highlighter to mark the diagnosis in each question. Use another color to identify exactly what the question is asking. When you go back over to check questions and answers you can easily pick out key information. More strategies on marking questions and answers are below.

For example:
Jennifer S. is a 2-year-old white female with bronchiolitis who has been admitted to your critical care unit. Which of the following blood gases shows she is in the *early* stages of acute respiratory failure?
A. pH 7.35, $pO_2$65, $pCO_2$60
B. pH 7.40, $pO_2$85, $pCO_2$45
C. pH 7.25, $pO_2$85, $pCO_2$35
D. pH 7.45, $pO_2$70, $pCO_2$32

Write down critical information as you remember it. If you have trouble remembering the normal serum sodium level and it's an important number to know, write it down as soon as you open your test booklet. This will prevent you from going blank later in the exam. Having this information clearly written down will also help you when you are solving higher lever questions that expect you to know more than just numbers.

For example:
Jason L. has been admitted to your pediatric unit because he has developed electrolyte imbalances related to his chronic renal failure. What laboratory values would you most likely see on this patient?
A. Potassium 7.0, creatinine 8.0, hypermagnesemia
B. Potassium 3.0, creatinine 0.8, hypermagnesemia
C. Potassium 5.0, creatinine 1.8, hypermagnesemia
D. Potassium 7.0, creatinine 2.0, hypermagnesemia

Knowing normal values is important in choosing the correct combination of laboratory values for this patient.

RULES FOR DISSECTING QUESTIONS AND ANSWERS

Circle abnormal test results and other values. Circling abnormal test results or other values will help you pick out crucial information quickly.

For example:
Adam Jones is a 4-day-old full term infant who has a bilirubin level of (15mg)/100ml. Based on this, you could expect to find which of the following during your assessment.
A. Straw-colored urine, clay-colored stools
B. Yellow sclera, clear yellow urine
C. Lethargy, dark amber urine
D. Urine with dark flecks, clear sclera

Draw arrows to show whether values given are increased or decreased. Drawing arrows next to any laboratory results will help you pick out correct answers or identify important information in the question.

For example:
Mary J. had a mitral valve replacement 6 months ago and was recently hospitalized with pneumonia. She is taking coumadin to prevent clotting problems associated with her prosthetic valve. Which of the following PT values would be an emergency?
↑ **A.** 20 seconds
— **B.** 18 seconds
↑↑↑ **C.** 36 seconds
↑ **D.** 24 seconds

Eliminate unnecessary information in case studies. Sometimes questions presented as case studies can have a great deal of information, not all of which is important. Crossing out superfluous information can help you focus on the truly significant information.

For example:
Joey P. is a 9-day-old patient who has been admitted to your unit because he was febrile, tachypneic, lethargic, and feeding poorly. ~~His mother states that she had a flu virus during the early part of her pregnancy and never gained weight well.~~ Which of the following diagnostic tests would *not* be helpful in diagnosing sepsis?
A. Culture and sensitivity of cerebrospinal fluid
B. Complete blood count
C. C-reactive protein and erythrocyte sedimentation rate
D. Serum chemistry
The information about the mother's flu and weight gain during pregnancy is not important to the infant's present condition. Her illness was early in her pregnancy and had resolved long before this infant's illness.

Especially note what the question says. Sometimes it's not the correct answer the test is looking for at all. Other times all of the answers except one are correct. Look carefully for the following phrases:

A. "all of the following are true *except* . . . "
B. "which of the following is *incorrect?*. . . "
C. "*should not* . . . "

Note if the question is looking for a right or wrong answer. It's easy to see correct information and select it without realizing the questions was directed at identifying a *wrong* answer.

For example:
In the early period of pulmonary edema, the blood gases would be most likely to show all of the following *except*:
A. a pH of 7.35
B. a pCO_2 of 30
C. a pO_2 of 80
D. a pH of 7.48

Correct and cross out wrong answers. When you are reading over answers, cross out or even correct wrong answers. This makes narrowing your choices much easier.

For example:
Which of the following tests are used to evaluate heparin therapy?
~~**A.** Fibrin split products~~ (used for DIC)
~~**B.** Prothrombin time~~ (used to evaluate coumadin)
C. Partial thromboplastin time
~~**D.** Protamine levels~~ (used to reverse heparin)

Focus on the one very different answer. Sometimes even when you don't know an answer you can pick out the choice that is very different from the others. This is either usually the right answer or a choice that may easily be eliminated.

For example:
All of the following are signs of imminent brain herniation *except*:
A. Increased BP
B. Bradycardia
C. Changes in respiration
D. Partial motor seizures
Seizures are very different from the other three choices, which are all vital signs. *D* is the correct answer.

Cross out answers that are the same things. Look carefully to see if some of your choices really are the same.

For example:
Chvostek's sign can be seen in all of the following *except*:
~~A. Hypocalcemia~~
~~B. Hypomagnesemia~~
~~C. Hyperphosphatemia~~
D. Hyperkalemia
Calcium and magnesium levels usually rise and fall together, whereas phosphate levels move reciprocally. Knowing this, *D* is the only correct choice. *A, B,* and *C* would all result in the same symptoms.

Often the longest answer is the right one. Look carefully at any answer that is longer than the others. Very often, this is the right answer.

For example:
Which of the following assessment findings would you expect in a patient with a small bowel obstruction?
A. Rebound tenderness
B. No stool for 48 hours
C. High-pitched tinkling sounds upon ausculation, diarrhea
D. Absent bowl sounds.

Don't hurry though two-part answers. Whenever answers have two or more parts, read them carefully. At least two will usually begin with correct answers. You must read through to the end to eliminate the wrong answer.

For example:
When caring for a patient who has returned from a cardiac catherterization and has been sedated, it is most critical to observe the patient closely for:
A. Ability to maintain airway and stomach pain
B. Chest and mouth pain
C. Ability to maintain airway and a gag reflex
D. Headache and neck pain
While the first part of *A* and *C* are correct, the second part of *C* is the better answer.

Often "None of the above" or "All of the above" are the correct answers. Whenever you see these phrases, be sure you have carefully evaluated each answer. Usually these phrases clue you into the correct answer.

For example:
Which of the following is often seen in diabetic ketoacidosis?
A. Hyperglycemia
B. Acidemia
C. Hyperkalemia
D. All of the above

Don't change an answer unless you're sure. Usually your first answer is the correct one. Don't change an answer unless you're certain. For instance, unless you reread a question or answer and realize you misread it the first time, changing the answer usually is the wrong choice.

REMEMBER THESE TIPS

Following these tips will help you turn your hard work and expertise into a winning score. Professional recognition and advancement you've worked hard for are yours for the taking. Just a few more tips will put you far on the road to success.

Believe in yourself! You have learned so much to be a nurse, and you have learned so much since you have become a nurse. Believe in yourself and show the world through certification.

Use magical thinking. Visualize yourself taking the test and being calm. When you have some quiet time while you are studying or as you go to sleep at night, picture yourself sitting in a room getting ready to take the certification exam. Now picture yourself as unruffled and confident. Imagine yourself taking the test and being relaxed—and successful.

When taking practice exams or making notes, associate picking up your pencil with relaxation. If text anxiety is your problem, practice relaxation techniques well ahead of time and "anchor" them to something tangible. For example, each time you pick up your pencil to study, close your eyes and take a moment to picture your self relaxing. Imagine a clam, warm light coming from the pencil and flowing through your body soothing you. Soon, each time you pick up your pencil you will automatically relax, including the day of your test!

Study with friends for support, or take the test in a different city! Some people take risks more easily when they are shared. Get other nurses who are interested in taking a certification exam and form a study group. Content is more easily learned when it is divided and shared. You can give each other great moral support and encouragement. When I took the critical care certification exam, however, I actually took it in a different city and didn't tell any of my friends. For me, it was less of a risk and threat if I didn't pass. But by following these tips, I passed with flying colors!

CHAPTER 10

Practice Examinations

Pediatric Sample Test

1. The critical care nurse observes continuous, noisy bubbling in the water seal chamber of the chest tube drainage system. The most appropriate action would be to:
- A. Check the suction tubing for any kinks or clots obstructing drainage
- B. Milk the chest tube gently to remove clots
- C. Raise the tubing between the patient and the collection system to empty stagnant drainage
- D. Clamp tube at insertion site briefly to observe for cessation of bubbling

---

Case Study

A 3.3 kg infant is admitted to the critical care unit and diagnosed with severe dehydration associated with diarrhea. She is irritable, with very dry mucous membranes and no tears with crying. Questions 2 to 4 refer to this case study.

---

2. The top priority in the first minutes of intervention for this patient is:
- A. Establishment of a vascular access
- B. Calculation of mean arterial pressure
- C. Determination of life-threatening electrolyte imbalances
- D. Intubation with assisted ventilation

3. The infant would be expected to also have which of the following clinical signs and symptoms?
- A. Decreased urine specific gravity, cool and pale skin, decreased serum pH, tachycardia
- B. Decreased urine specific gravity, cool and mottled skin, decreased serum pH, hypotension
- C. Increased urine specific gravity, cool and pale skin, increased serum pH, hypertension
- D. Increased urine specific gravity, cool and mottled skin, decreased serum pH, tachycardia

4. Immediate fluid resuscitation for this infant would most likely include:
A. 10 mL bolus of a crystalloid solution given over 3 minutes
B. 35 mL bolus of a crystalloid solution given over 5 minutes
C. 65 mL bolus of a crystalloid solution given over 15 minutes
D. 100 mL bolus of a crystalloid solution given over 1 hour

5. A patient with the following blood gases is admitted to the critical care unit. Which of the following changes in ventilatory therapy would be most likely to improve the blood gases?
pH: 7.31
pO_2: 88 torr
pCO_2: 53 torr
HCO_3^-: 19 mEq/L
A. Increase the FiO_2 by 10%
B. Increase the respiratory rate
C. Decrease the peak inspiratory pressure
D. Increase the inspiratory/expiratory ratio

Case Study

An infant with coarctation of the aorta is admitted to the pediatric unit, where he undergoes a physical examination and diagnostic testing. Tests include echocardiography and cardiac catheterization. Questions 6 and 7 refer to this case study.

---

6. Which signs and symptoms of coarctation would most likely be seen during the physical examination?
A. Bounding femoral pulses and weak brachial pulses
B. Bounding femoral and brachial pulses
C. Weak femoral pulses and absent brachial pulses
D. Weak femoral pulses and strong brachial pulses

7. Before surgery, this infant is likely to be treated with which medication?
A. Dopamine to increase systemic pressure
B. Dobutamine to increase myocardial contraction
C. Sodium bicarbonate to treat acidosis
D. Prostaglandin therapy to open the ductus

8. During the nursing assessment, a 28-hour-old neonate is found to have generalized petechiae and oozing from a heelstick site. The infant is afebrile, sucking well, and is alert and active when awake. There is a maternal history of systemic lupus erythematosus. Blood is drawn for a complete blood count with differential. Some of the results are as follows:

Red blood cell count:	3.8 million/mm^3
Hemoglobin:	12 mg/dL
Hematocrit:	36%
White blood cell count:	6100/mm^3
Platelet count:	10,000/mm^3

Which of the following laboratory values would the nurse also expect to be abnormal?

A. Prothrombin time (PT)
B. Partial thromboplastin time (PTT)
C. Prothrombin consumption test
D. Bleeding time

9. An infant with idiopathic thrombocytopenic purpura (ITP) is found to have a platelet count of 22,000/mm^3, bleeding from heelsticks, and generalized petechiae. Which of the following treatments would have the *highest* priority for this infant?

A. Transfusion of platelets
B. Intravenous immune gamma globulin
C. Heparin therapy
D. Exchange transfusion

Case Study

A 10-year-old boy has been admitted to the intensive care unit following a head injury from a skateboarding accident. He has a urine output of 11 mL/kg/hr, a urine specific gravity of 1.003, a serum osmolality of 326 mOsm/kg, and a serum sodium of 163 mEq/L. Questions 10 to 12 refer to this case study.

---

10. Which of the following signs and symptoms would the critical care nurse expect to find during assessment of this child?

A. Bounding pulses, tachycardia, seizures, cyanosis
B. Stupor, hypertension, mottling of extremities
C. Weak and thready pulse, hypotension, pale extremities
D. Tachycardia, hypertension, thirst, equivocal pulses

11. What would be the most *immediate* priority in treating this patient?

A. Restoration of intravascular fluid volume
B. Administration of dDAVP
C. Administration of anticonvulsant pharmacologic agents
D. Restoration of normal serum sodium levels

12. An appropriate nursing diagnosis for this patient is:
A. Potential for fluid volume excess related to inadequate secretion of antidiuretic hormone
B. Potential for hypothermia related to excess fluid loss
C. Altered tissue perfusion: peripheral related to decreased circulating volume
D. Potential fluid volume deficit related to increased urinary output

13. The critical care nurse observes fluid fluctuations in the water seal chamber during respirations. The most appropriate action in the case of this patient with a chest tube and drainage system would be to:
A. Milk the chest tube gently to remove clots that may have formed
B. Note that the drainage system is functioning properly
C. Immediately observe the patient for respiratory distress
D. Disconnect the system and hand ventilate the patient until the system can be replaced

---

Case Study

A normotensive neonate is admitted to the critical care unit with an increase in serum glucose levels, decreased urinary output after 24 hours of increased output, and respiratory alkalosis. The critical care nurse monitors this infant in compensated shock closely for signs and symptoms of decompensation. Questions 14 to 16 refer to this case study.

---

14. This infant in compensated shock will likely exhibit all of the following signs and symptoms *except*:
A. Bounding upper and lower extremity pulses
B. Increased cardiac output and index
C. Increase in serum glucose levels
D. Compensated metabolic acidosis

15. The critical care nurse knows this neonate with septic shock is most directly at risk for developing which of the following additional conditions?
A. Persistent pulmonary hypertension
B. Aspiration pneumonia
C. Intraventricular bleeding
D. Generalized seizures

16. Which outcome indicates effective management of an infant in uncompensated septic shock?
A. Urinary output of 1 mL/kg/hr
B. Capillary refill of 2.5 seconds
C. Arterial pH of 7.33
D. Cardiac index of 2.3 L/min/m^2

17. A 3-day-old infant is admitted to the critical care unit following acute onset of apparent abdominal pain, distended abdomen, lethargy, hypovolemic shock, and bloody stools. She is diagnosed with a volvulus. Based on this history and diagnosis, the nurse also would expect all of the following signs and symptoms *except*:
A. Bilious vomiting
B. Hematemisis
C. Shock
D. Hypertension

Case Study

A patient is admitted to the critical care unit with a diagnosis of hypoxic-ischemic encephalopathy following a traumatic delivery. Questions 18 to 20 refer to this case study.

---

18. The *first* nursing priority would be to assess:
A. Pupillary reaction
B. Level of consciousness
C. Ability to maintain airway
D. Blood glucose level

19. The critical care nurse would recognize as signs and symptoms of mild hypoxic-ischemic encephalopathy all of the following *except*:
A. Irritability
B. Tachycardia
C. Hyperalertness
D. Hypotonia

20. This infant is intubated and mechanically ventilated. Besides providing optimal oxygenation, which of the following is also a benefit of mechanical ventilation in this type of infant?
A. Reduction of intracranial pressure
B. Prevention of seizure activity
C. Prevention of long-term complications
D. Reduction of hypocarbia

21. Following a cardiac catheterization, the nurse should expect to observe for all of the following *except*:
A. Seizures
B. Decreased pulses distal to the venipuncture site
C. Respiratory distress
D. Hematoma at the venipuncture site

Case Study

A 4-month-old infant is brought to the emergency room with acute abdominal pain manifested by screaming and drawing the knees to the abdomen. His history was negative for any chronic illnesses or other significant health problems. His growth and development appear normal. He had another episode of pain on the way to the emergency room. His latest pain occurred shortly after reaching the emergency room and being put in an examination room. This time he passed a red, currant jelly-like stool.

Questions 22 to 24 refer to this case study.

22. Based on this data, the nurse suspects:
A. Necrotizing enterocolitis
B. Appendicitis
C. Acute volvulus
D. Intussusception

23. Another expected finding upon physical examination would be:
A. Dance sign
B. Kehr's sign
C. Kernig's sign
D. Cullen's sign

24. Indications for surgical correction include all of the following *except*:
A. Signs of perforation
B. Bloody stools
C. Previous episodes of intussusception
D. Abdominal symptoms for more than 48 hours

25. When caring for a child suspected of ingesting a toxic agent, the *first* action should be to:
A. Administer activated charcoal to prevent absorption of toxin
B. Induce vomiting to stop exposure and absorption of the toxic agent
C. Ensure a patent airway and adequate ventilation
D. Identify the toxic agent to determine an antidote and/or treatment

26. Two hours after returning from surgery, the critical care nurse observes a decreased level of responsiveness in her patient. He is breathing spontaneously on room air. Blood gases are obtained and are as follows:

pH:	7.22
pO_2:	90 torr
pCO_2:	63 torr
HCO_3^-:	23 mEq/L
Base excess:	+2

Which of the following actions would be most appropriate based on these findings?

A. Administration of 100% oxygen by facial mask to improve hypoxia
B. Administration of narcotic analgesics to decrease pain and improve deep breathing
C. Administration of sodium bicarbonate to correct acidosis
D. Administration of naloxone to reverse effects of anesthesia

27. An oliguric patient with rising blood urea nitrogen (BUN) and serum creatinine levels has a urine specific gravity of 1.010. His serum and urine osmolalities are both 285 mOsm/L. This patient most likely has:

A. Prerenal failure
B. Postrenal failure
C. Intrarenal failure
D. Hepatorenal failure

28. An intubated and ventilated patient suddenly shows a decrease in the pulse oximetry reading from 95% saturation to 81%. The patient is exhibiting nasal flaring, intercostal retractions, tachypnea, and use of accessory respiratory muscles despite the ventilator showing an adequate tidal volume and absence of peak pressure alarms. Which of the following actions should the critical care nurse do first?

A. Disconnect from the ventilator and manually bag the patient
B. Immediately suction the endotracheal tube
C. Increase the FiO_2 to 100%
D. Auscultate breath sounds

29. Which outcome indicates effective management of an infant with coarctation before surgical correction?

A. Adequate hourly urinary output
B. Active precordium
C. Absence of pleural effusion
D. Decrease in arterial pH level

30. A patient in the critical care unit has a systolic pressure of 80 mm Hg, a diastolic pressure of 52 mm Hg, a pulse rate of 110 beats per minute, a respiratory rate of 30, and an intracranial pressure of 20 mm Hg. What is this patient's cerebral perfusion pressure?

A. 61 mm Hg
B. 41 mm Hg
C. 32 mm Hg
D. 66 mm Hg

31. In right-to-left cardiac shunts, the nursing diagnostic category impaired gas exchange typically is related to:

A. Increased pulmonary blood flow
B. Decreased ventilation to perfusion
C. Decreased pulmonary vascular pressures
D. Decreased pulmonary blood flow

Case Study

Michael was a 3460 g full term infant with a history of meconium stained amniotic fluid noted 2 hours before delivery. He was suctioned at birth and found to have meconium below the cords. Apgar scores were 7 at one minute and 8 at five minutes. He was tachypneic with nasal flaring and expiratory grunting. His pulse oximetry reading on his right finger was 98% saturation whereas the pulse oximetry on his right toe was only 65%. His blood gases by umbilical artery catheter on 80% hood were as follows:

pH: 7.32
pO_2: 72 mm Hg
pCO_2: 40 mm Hg

Questions 32 to 34 refer to this case study.

---

32. Which of the following is the most likely explanation for the differences in pulse oximetry readings between his upper and lower extremities?

A. Coarctation of the aorta
B. Persistent pulmonary hypertension
C. Poor reading on the lower extremity pulse oximeter
D. Poor peripheral circulation related to acidosis

33. After the infant was intubated, what pH level in analyzing the blood gases would the nurse view as the best outcome of ventilatory therapy?

A. 7.35
B. 7.47
C. 7.50
D. 7.67

34. Based on the desired outcome of the pH level in question 33, for what complications would the critical care nurse be alert?
A. Hyponatremia
B. Hypocalcemia
C. Hyperkalemia
D. Hypermagnesemia

35. A 4-year-old child is admitted to the critical care unit with a 2-hour history of drowsiness progressing to seizures at which point his parents immediately called emergency medical services and brought him to the emergency room. He had no previous history of seizures or head injury. The parents deny he was sick before this episode. Toxic ingestion was immediately suspected based on his history and presenting symptoms. Which of the following common toxidromes is most likely to be responsible for this child's presentation?
A. Salycilates
B. Narcotics
C. Methanol
D. Tricyclic antidepressants

36. A nurse observes shakiness in an infant. Which of the following interventions can help identify if this activity is a tremor or a seizure?
A. Stimulate sucking
B. Hold the infant's arms
C. Observe for nystagmus
D. Note change in consciousness

37. After 2 hours of fluid resuscitation for severe DKA, a 14-year-old patient offers each of the following complaints. Which of these would signal the most critical potential complication?
A. Nausea
B. Thirst
C. Incontinence
D. Headache

38. When assessing a newborn or child, the critical care nurse identifies which heart sound as *not* normal?
A. Fixed split of S_2
B. Physiologic split of S_2
C. Systolic murmur
D. An S_3 heart sound

39. An infant was admitted to the critical care unit for meconium aspiration and was intubated on 80% oxygen for the last 3 days. Upon examination, the nurse finds decreased breath sounds over the lung fields, lethargy, restlessness, dyspnea, and an increasing A-a gradient. No increase in secretions, fever, or wheezing are noted. These findings are most consistent with the development of:
A. Pneumonia
B. Foreign body aspiration
C. Oxygen toxicity
D. Airway obstruction

40. Heart sounds such as S_1 and S_2 are typically caused by:
A. Turbulent blood flow
B. The sound of shunting blood
C. Blood crossing valves
D. Closing of valves

Case Study

A female infant was admitted to the critical care unit for perinatal asphyxia and 4 days later developed acute renal failure. She had a prolonged episode of hypotension during her delivery and an immediate resuscitation period. Her urine output has fallen to 0.35 mL/kg for the last 24 hours. Questions 41 and 42 refer to this case study.

---

41. To prevent complications, initial treatment of this infant focusing on her history should include:
A. Fluid bolus of 20 mL/kg of Ringer's lactate
B. 10 mL/kg of packed red blood cells
C. Dopamine 2 to 5 mcg/kg/min
D. Calcium gluconate

42. Which of the following medications would be *least* likely to require an adjustment in dosage for this infant?
A. Gentamicin
B. Digoxin
C. Pancuronium bromide
D. Dobutamine

43. An infant is admitted from the emergency room with supraventricular tachycardia (SVT). Which symptoms would the critical care nurse expect?
A. Poor pulses, hypertension, tachypnea
B. Poor feeding in infants, restlessness, tachypnea
C. Bounding pulses, hypotension, anxiety
D. Restlessness, hypertension, bounding pulses

44. While caring for an intubated and mechanically ventilated patient, the critical care nurse notices sudden, profound cyanosis and bradycardia. She observes asymmetrical chest excursion and decreased amplitude of the QRS complex, and auscultates shifted breath sounds. What immediate action should the critical care nurse take?

A. Elevate the head of the bed and increase the FiO_2 to 1.0
B. Suction the endotracheal tube to remove any obstruction
C. Call for a stat x-ray to check tube placement
D. Begin chest compressions while preparing to administer epinephrine

45. A 10-day-old infant with a history of meconium aspiration has developed disseminated intravascular coagulation. Which of the following therapies would be a priority in treating DIC in this infant?

A. Heparin therapy to reverse diffuse systemic clotting
B. Transfusion of clotting factors to correct depleted levels
C. Aggressive respiratory therapy to correct hypoxemia and acidosis
D. Transfusion of platelets to correct depleted levels

Case Study

A 15-year-old boy is referred to the emergency room by his pediatrician for suspected hepatitis. For the past 2 weeks he has had a decreased appetite, nausea, and fatigue. He reports he has been sleeping poorly. Upon physical examination, the pediatrician found yellowing of the sclera, multiple and diffuse ecchymotic areas, and ascites. He has been admitted to the intensive care unit. Below are some of his admitting data.

Blood pressure:	84/52 mm Hg
Pulse:	112 beats per minute
Respiratory rate:	31 breaths per minute
Temperature:	36.8°C (100.6°F)

Questions 46 to 48 refer to this case study.

---

46. To follow the severity of his liver disease, the critical care nurse would monitor closely all of the following laboratory values *except*:

A. Alanine aminotransferase (ALT)
B. Aspartate aminotransferase (AST)
C. Alkaline phosphatase (ALP)
D. Acid phosphatase (AP)

47. The critical care nurse would question an order for which of the following medications?

A. Diazepam
B. Dobutamine
C. Potassium chloride
D. Amoxicillin

48. Lactulose is ordered for this patient to:
A. Reduce the incidence of esophageal varices
B. Decrease indirect serum bilirubin levels
C. Decrease ammonia levels
D. Reduce bacteria in the colon

49. Aspiration of hydrocarbons is most likely to present with which of the following clinical pictures?
A. Cough, sputum, fever, infiltrates
B. Dyspnea, cough, pulmonary edema, hypoxemia
C. Dyspnea, wheezing, cyanosis, pulmonary edema
D. Fever, wheezing, cough with sputum

50. A 7-year-old boy has been admitted to the critical care unit with his parents at the bedside following a bicycle-motor vehicle accident. As the nurse applies electrocardiogram electrodes to his chest, she explains the purpose and he responds by nodding and looking away. The nurse explains that blood must be drawn and asks his parents to leave the room. He continues to look away and offers no protest as his parents leave. The critical care nurse interprets this behavior as a child who possibly:
A. Is very cooperative and mature for his age
B. Is too frightened to protest
C. Has compromised neurological or cardiopulmonary function
D. Has a poor relationship with his parents

Case Study

A neonate is admitted to the critical care unit appearing pale with retractions, tachypnea, grunting, nasal flaring, and use of accessory muscles. The chest x-ray is described as ground-glass in appearance. Breath sounds by auscultation are decreased. Blood gases are as follows:

pH: 7.30
pO_2: 53 torr
pCO_2: 49 torr
HCO_3^-: 18 mEq/L

Questions 51 and 52 refer to this case study.

---

51. This infant is showing signs and symptoms of:
A. Aspiration pneumonia
B. Persistent pulmonary hypertension
C. Respiratory distress syndrome
D. Bronchopulmonary dysplasia

52. An important factor in the development of respiratory disease in this patient is the pathophysiology of:
A. Decreased surfactant production
B. Decreased 2,3-DPG production
C. Increased surfactant metabolism
D. Increased 2,3-DPG production

53. Postoperative care of a patient who has undergone repair of a tracheoesophageal fistula would include:
A. Deep suctioning to avoid leakage of gastric secretions into the trachea
B. Use of a pacifier to maintain oral stimulation in absence of oral feeds
C. Suctioning only to the end of the endotracheal tube
D. Use of a gastrostomy tube for feeding

54. A 15-year-old boy is a patient following a head injury from a baseball. During the first hours after admission, he sleeps unless awakened, but can be aroused easily and is oriented. The critical care nurse correctly documents this condition as:
A. Semicomatose
B. Lethargy
C. Obtunded
D. Stuporous

55. Beta-blockers, such as propranolol, should *not* be used to treat SVT accompanied by congestive heart failure because:
A. Beta-blockers may decrease cardiac output
B. Beta-blockers can increase circulating catecholamines
C. SVT is refractory to treatment with beta-blockers
D. Cardioversion is the only effective treatment

56. A 15-year-old girl develops SIADH following neurosurgery. Her serum sodium level is 128 mEq/L, serum osmolality is 256 mOsm/L, urine specific gravity is 1.022, and urine output is 1.0 mL/kg/hr. Which of the following would be the treatment of choice?
A. Fluid restriction to 50% of maintenance requirements
B. Administration of 3 mL/kg of 3% NaCl solution
C. Lasix 3 mg/kg
D. Administration of hypertonic saline and diuretics

Case Study

A 3-day-old infant is admitted to the critical care unit with a history of irritability, opisthotonos, stridor, and periods of apnea. Sucking has been poor and the nurse at transfer reveals to the critical care nurse that the neonate has also been difficult to console, and actually quiets better when left lying on his stomach. The critical care nurse's assessment reveals an increased head circumference, decreased gag reflex, and bulging fontannels. The infant is diagnosed with hydrocephalus. Questions 57 and 58 refer to this case study.

---

57. Which of the following signs and symptoms would the critical care nurse recognize as indicating further serious deterioration in the infant's condition?
A. Lethargy
B. Lower extremity spasticity
C. Sluggish pupillary response
D. Emesis

58. The tests most helpful in diagnosing and evaluating hydrocephalus are:
I. Computerized axial tomography
II. Skull x-rays
III. Ultrasound imaging
IV. Magnetic resonance imaging
A. I, II, and III
B. I, II, and IV
C. II and III
D. I and IV

59. Which statement best describes how activated charcoal works?
A. Prevents absorption and enhances elimination of toxins
B. Inactivates toxins within the gastrointestinal tract
C. Promotes emesis to eliminate toxins from the gut
D. Neutralizes gastric acid to reduce hazard of aspiration

60. When caring for an infant with symptomatic congenital heart block, the critical care nurse would question all of the following orders *except*:
A. Digoxin to increase the pumping of the heart
B. Beta-blocking agents to block abnormal impulses
C. Temporary or permanent pacing
D. Electrocardioversion

Case Study

A 4-year-old girl is admitted to the critical care unit with hypovolemic shock and a serum potassium of 2.8 mEq/L related to diarrhea. Questions 61 and 62 refer to this case study.

---

61. Which of the following signs and symptoms related to hypokalemia would the critical care nurse expect to find during an assessment?
A. Weakness, bradycardia, prolonged PR interval
B. Nausea, tented T waves, fatigue
C. Fatigue, weakness, flattened T wave
D. Muscle pain, nausea, wide QRS complex

62. Which of the following pharmacological treatments is indicated for treating this patient?
A. Kayexalate given as an enema or orally
B. Potassium infusion of 15 to 20 mEq/L/hr
C. Potassium replacement by bolus
D. Digoxin for cardiac dysrhythmias

63. Which of the following signs would be important in identifying renal trauma?
A. Turner's sign
B. Cushing's triad
C. Cullen's sign
D. Trousseau's sign

64. An advantage of an intraventricular catheter in monitoring intracranial pressure over other methods includes:
A. Less invasiveness into brain tissue
B. Ability to inject medications
C. Reduced rate of infection
D. Ability to block leakage of CSF

65. Which of the following calculations of fluid therapy is optimal for normovolemic neonate with respiratory distress syndrome who is intubated and mechanically ventilated?
A. 50% of maintenance fluid requirements
B. 75% of maintenance fluid requirements
C. 100% of maintenance fluid requirements
D. 125% of maintenance fluid requirements

66. An afebrile, acyanotic patient returned 12 hours ago from surgical repair of an omphalocele. During suctioning, the critical care nurse observes for the first time thick, clear to white secretions. Which nursing action would be most effective in promoting airway clearance?
A. Assess adequacy of humidification
B. Send sputum for culture and sensitivity
C. Use saline lavage to thin secretions
D. Use sterile suction technique only

Case Study

An infant female patient has critical aortic stenosis. During the past hour, she has developed tachycardia, urinary output of less than 1.0 mL/kg, mottling of the skin, elevation in central venous pressure, increased liver size, and barely palpable pulses.

Questions 67 to 71 refer to this case study.

---

67. Her symptoms are probably the result of:
- A. Hypovolemic shock
- B. Septic shock
- C. Cardiogenic shock
- D. Hemorrhagic shock

68. Which nursing diagnosis is *most* appropriate for this patient?
- A. Ineffective thermoregulation associated with poor perfusion of temperature regulation centers
- B. Impaired gas exchange related to decreased pulmonary flow
- C. Decreased cardiac output related to myocardial dysfunction
- D. Ineffective breathing pattern related to obstructed pulmonary flow

69. The physician may prescribe vasodilators for this patient. These drugs help to improve cardiovascular functions by:
- A. Increasing systemic vascular resistance
- B. Inotropic and chronotropic actions
- C. Decreasing afterload
- D. Improving renal perfusion

70. To decrease the workload on her heart and improve her cardiac output, the nurse would expect the physician to prescribe:
- A. Nitroprusside
- B. Propranolol
- C. Digoxin
- D. Dopamine

71. Which would *not* be considered a positive outcome for her therapy?
- A. Urinary output of 0.5 cc/kg/hr
- B. Resolution of an S_3 heart sound
- C. Warm, dry skin
- D. A rise in arterial oxygen saturation

72. Which symptoms are *not* associated with ingestion of corrosives?
- A. Burning in the mouth, stomach, throat
- B. Anxiety, apprehension
- C. White and swollen mucous membranes
- D. Increased oral secretions and swallowing

73. In caring for the patient with a newly inserted tracheostomy, which of the following is critical to ensure maintenance of the airways?
- A. Snugly secure the ties around the tracheostomy tube so that only a small gauze fits between the tube and the skin
- B. Keep a tracheostomy tube one size smaller at the bedside
- C. Secure the tracheostomy tube with a bow to prevent knotting of the ties
- D. Secure the tie at the side of the neck to provide easy access in emergencies

74. A 10-year-old patient with known portal hypertension suddenly develops acute onset of bright red vomiting. Her blood pressure drops quickly to 88/56. The critical care nurse would anticipate *immediate* intervention to include isotonic intravenous fluid administration and:
A. Vasopressin
B. Dopamine
C. Dobutamine
D. Digoxin

75. Which of the following is the most critical complication immediately following a tracheostomy?
A. Tenacious secretions
B. Infection
C. Speech delays
D. Decannulation

Case Study

An 18-month-old infant is admitted to the PICU following a Fontan procedure for repair of a single ventricle. He is intubated and on a positive pressure ventilator. After the first 16 hours, he begins to develop a decrease in urine output, an increase in his right atrial pressure (RAP), and an increase in his left atrial pressure (LAP). His urine output has decreased to 0.5 mL/hr with an increase in urine sodium and urine osmolality. Questions 76 and 77 refer to this case study.

---

76. The nurse suspects this patient most likely has developed:
A. Chronic renal failure
B. Congestive heart failure
C. Diabetes insipidus (DI)
D. Hypothyroidism

77. Which of the following nursing diagnoses would be the *most* appropriate for this patient?
A. Fluid volume excess
B. Altered tissue perfusion: renal
C. Ineffective breathing pattern
D. Impaired gas exchange

78. Following placement of a ventriculoperitoneal shunt, the critical care nurse would recognize which of the following as a desired outcome?
A. Rapid return to a normal intracranial pressure (ICP)
B. Gag reflex with suctioning
C. Firm, round fontanels
D. Dilated scalp veins

Case Study

A 3-day-old male infant is transferred from the emergency room to the intensive care unit. He was brought in earlier by his parents, who stated that he became extremely blue when he awoke this morning and started crying. He is diagnosed with tetralogy of Fallot and as having had a hypercyanotic, or tet, spell. Questions 79 and 80 refer to this case study.

79. When assessing this baby, what area of the body is *best* for reliably assessing cyanosis?
A. Ear lobes
B. Palms of hands
C. Soles of feet
D. Nail beds

80. If this patient were to remain cyanotic without surgical correction, which finding would the nurse expect to observe in future assessments?
A. Anemia
B. Clubbed fingers
C. Obesity
D. Thick, coarse hair

81. A 5-year-old boy is admitted after being involved in a motor vehicle accident in which he did not wear a seat belt. He is complaining of numbness and tingling in his legs and feet, and has decreased sensation. His x-rays are normal and show no evidence of fractures or other abnormalities. The critical care nurse plans care to include:
A. Removing the cervical collar
B. Discontinuing log rolling to turn the patient
C. Administration of antianxiety medications
D. Continuation of spinal cord protective measures

82. Following complaints of headache, unexplained emesis, blurring vision, and change in ability to perform daily physical activities, a 13-year-old girl is admitted to the critical care unit with a diagnosis of astrocytoma. Following the initiation of antineoplastic therapy, the critical care nurse observes the patient closely for all of the following *except*:
A. Sepsis
B. Increased intracranial pressure
C. Hydrocephalus
D. Intraventricular hemorrhage

83. A 15-year-old boy is admitted to the critical care unit with a diagnosis of acute alcohol toxicity. He is unconscious and responding only to noxious stimuli. His friends report a 3-hour drinking binge that began 4 hours ago and stopped just 1 hour before admission to the unit. Serum alcohol levels in this child can be expected to peak:

A. ½ to 1 hour after ingestion
B. Up to 12 hours after ingestion
C. Up to 8 hours after ingestion
D. ¼ to ½ hour after ingestion

84. Which of the following represents appropriate postoperative management of chest tubes in the infant who has undergone repair of a congenital diaphragmatic hernia?

A. Chest tube on affected side to water seal
B. Chest tube on unaffected side to water seal
C. Chest tube on affected side to low suction
D. Chest tube on unaffected side to low suction

85. An infant with a history of polyhydramnios is noted soon after birth to have copious oral secretions. The critical care nurse recognizes which of the following conditions as the most likely cause of these symptoms:

A. Down syndrome
B. Cleft lip
C. Tracheoesophageal fistula
D. Fulminant pulmonary edema

86. A lumbar puncture is ordered for a full term infant with decreased level of responsiveness, irritability, hyperventilation, and seizure activity 1 hour before the test. The results were as follows:

Cerebrospinal fluid pressure:	normal
White blood cell count:	4 cells/mm^3
Red blood cell count:	0 cells/mm^3
Protein:	53 mg/dL
Glucose:	54 mg/dL

Which of the following diagnoses is *most* likely based on these findings?

A. Encephalopathy
B. Viral meningitis
C. Bacterial meningitis
D. Intraventricular hemorrhage

87. A 10-year-old child was admitted to the critical care unit after being hit by a car. She complains of needing to void, but she appears unable. Physical examination reveals an easily palpable and full bladder. The next action the critical care nurse should take is to:

A. Immediately catheterize the patient to minimize bladder damage
B. Inspect the urinary meatus for blood before catheterization
C. Delay catheterization until a renal ultrasound can be completed
D. Gently crede the bladder to assist in voiding

88. For cyanotic lesions such as tetralogy of Fallot that cause decreased pulmonary blood, an early palliative intervention before final correction may include:
A. Pulmonary artery banding
B. Systemic-to-pulmonary shunt
C. Aortoplasty
D. Intubation and oxygen therapy

Case Study

Over the last 4 hours of caring for a septic patient, the nurse notes the oozing of blood from the intravenous sites and the development of petechiae over the trunk. Blood is drawn for testing. Some of the results are as follows:

Platelet count:	121,000/mm^3
Erythrocyte count:	3.8 million/mm^3
Hematocrit:	36%
Partial thromboplastin time:	41 seconds
Prothrombin time:	18 seconds
Fibrinogen level:	140 mg/dL

Questions 89 and 90 refer to this case study.

---

89. Based on these results and the patient's history, the nurse recognizes the patient is most at risk for:
A. Idiopathic thrombocytopenic purpura
B. Disseminated intravascular coagulation
C. Aplastic anemia
D. Nonimmune hemolytic anemia

90. The nurse would expect this patient's treatment plan to potentially include all of the following therapies *except*:
A. Administration of platelets
B. Infusion of fresh frozen plasma
C. Intravenous antibiotics
D. Prothrombin complex concentrates

Case Study

A 26-hour-old neonate is admitted to the critical care unit with hypotension, cold and mottled skin, bradycardia, and a pH of 7.21. A lumbar tap reveals increased pressure, white blood cell count of 4 cell/mm^3, glucose of 55 mg/dL, and erythrocytes at 518 cells/mm^3. Questions 91 to 93 refer to this case study.

---

91. The assessment findings and results of the diagnostic tests suggest which neurological problem?
A. Hydrocephalus
B. Intraventricular hemorrhage
C. Intracerebral hematoma
D. Encephalitis

92. What diagnostic test would be *least* helpful in diagnosing this condition?
A. Ultrasonography
B. Skull x-rays
C. Magnetic resonance imaging
D. Computerized axial tomography

93. Which of the following interventions would be the *greatest* priority?
A. Correcting the acidosis
B. Sending cultures on the CSF
C. Initiating fluid and vasopressor support
D. Typing and cross matching for blood products

94. What condition do the following blood gas results indicate?

pH:	7.33
pO_2:	72 torr
pCO_2:	30 torr
HCO_3^-:	14 mEq/L
SaO_2:	89%

A. Respiratory acidosis
B. Respiratory alkalosis
C. Metabolic acidosis
D. Metabolic alkalosis

95. Positive patient outcomes in treating hypovolemic shock would *not* include:
A. Sunken fontannels
B. Central venous pressure of 8 mm Hg
C. Warm, dry skin
D. Pulmonary artery wedge pressure of 12 mm Hg

96. A patient's peak inspiratory pressures have increased steadily over the last 24 hours. This can indicate an/a:
A. Increase in lung compliance
B. Decrease in lung compliance
C. Improvement in lung disease
D. Decrease in oxygen requirements

97. A 6-year-old victim of a pedestrian-motor vehicle accident has shown no neurological deficits in his extremities during the 2 hours since his admission to the critical care unit. When planning his care, the critical care nurse writes nursing orders to continue with complete neurological assessments every hour. The *best* reason for this action is:

A. All the diagnostic tests have not been completed to rule out neurological injuries
B. Onset of neurological manifestations of injury are often delayed in children
C. Neurological assessments for sensation and pain are often unreliable in children of this age group
D. Neurological assessments are a poor indicator of neurological function and injury

98. For the child in hypovolemic shock from gastrointestinal fluid losses, which is the preferred intravenous fluid to maximally increase the intravascular volume?

A. Dextrose 5% in water
B. 0.45% normal saline solution
C. 0.9% normal saline solution
D. 7% normal saline solution

99. The critical care nurse carefully assesses a patient with hemorrhagic shock requiring multiple transfusions for which electrolyte imbalance?

A. Hypernatremia
B. Hypokalemia
C. Hypophosphatemia
D. Hypocalcemia

100. After endotracheal intubation, the critical care nurse notes decreased pulse oximetry readings, absent breath sounds and excursion in the left chest, and high peak pressure alarms on the ventilator. The critical care nurse suspects the patient has a:

A. Left pulmonary embolus
B. Pneumothorax
C. Pneumomediastinum
D. Right bronchial intubation

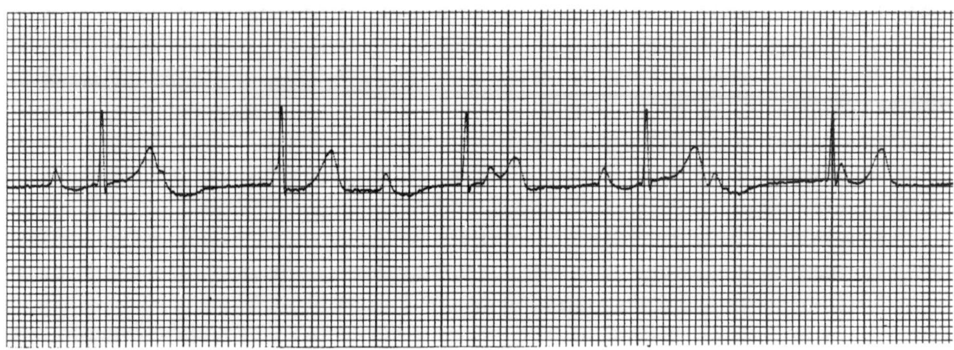

(From Hazinski, 1992.)

101. The critical care patient's monitor suddenly presents the rhythm shown above. Which treatment would the physician *most* likely prescribe?

A. Vagal maneuvers
B. Verapamil
C. Atropine
D. Isuprel

102. Which of the following is an optimal level of PEEP? A level that:

A. Maintains the PaO_2 >85 torr
B. Decreases lung compliance
C. Achieves the highest pO_2
D. Reduces intrapulmonary shunting

103. Prostaglandin E_1 therapy would most likely be helpful in treating which defect during the neonatal period?

A. Pulmonary atresia
B. Atrioventricular canal
C. Truncus arteriosus
D. Patent ductus arteriosus

104. An infant has been admitted to the critical care unit with a history of poor growth and feeding. Her current assessment findings include heart rate of 188 beats/minute, respiratory rate of 76 breaths/minute, nasal flaring, rales, and differential cyanosis. The most likely cause of these symptoms is:

A. Persistent pulmonary hypertension
B. Transient tachypnea of the newborn
C. Coarctation of the aorta
D. Diaphragmatic hernia

105. A neonate is found at birth to be severely tachypneic (rate of 115), with severe sternal retractions, nasal flaring, central cyanosis, and largely absent breath sounds. A chest x-ray demonstrates bowel located in the chest, an underdeveloped left lung, and the appearance of dextrocardia. The critical care nurse recognizes these symptoms as most consistent with:
A. Pneumothorax
B. Diaphragmatic hernia
C. Respiratory distress syndrome
D. Meconium aspiration

106. Following a motor vehicle accident, a child complains of right upper quadrant pain. A chest x-ray reveals a right pleural effusion. The critical care nurse also suspects:
A. Pulmonary infarction
B. Liver trauma
C. Splenic rupture
D. Lacerated kidney

107. For the patient on prostaglandin E_1 with a ductal-dependent lesion, which assessment finding would be a priority for the critical care nurse?
A. Presence of peripheral pulses
B. Presence of fixed, split S_2
C. Continuous murmur at base of the heart
D. Continuous murmur at apex of the heart

108. A postoperative open-heart patient has the following clinical findings: cardiac index of 2.8 L/min/m^2, systemic vascular resistance of 2780 dynes, a sodium level of 141 mEq/L, and a calcium level of 8.1 mg/dL. The most appropriate pharmacologic management would be:
A. Calcium chloride 10% at 20 mg/kg
B. Dobutamine at 0.5 mg/kg/min
C. Calcium gluconate at 100 ml/kg
D. Dopamine at 3 mcg/kg/min

109. A patient is diagnosed with tetralogy of Fallot and intubated for acute acidosis and hypoxemia. She is on room air, pressure support, and a rate of 26 breaths/minute. She also is started on prostaglandin E_1 at 0.5 mcg/kg/min. Her physical examination reveals clear, bilateral breath sounds. At the end of her assessment, the critical care nurse notices a sudden drop in the pulse oximeter from 85% to 78%. The most important *immediate* nursing action would be to:
A. Check the patency of the endotracheal tube
B. Increase the FiO_2 to 0.3
C. Suction aggressively for a mucous plug
D. Assess the patency of the prostaglandin E_1 infusion

110. Postoperative ventilatory management of a 3200 g neonate with a congenital diaphragmatic hernia includes mechanical ventilation with:

A. Peak inspiratory pressure of 30 cm H_2O
B. Tidal volume of 80 cc
C. Positive end expiratory pressure of 10 cm H_2O
D. Tidal volume of 30 cc

111. The nurse documents the following vital signs for a postoperative open-heart patient whose extremities are cold, femoral pulses are weak, and pedal pulses are absent: blood pressure of 53/28 mm Hg, heart rate of 195 beats/minute, urinary output of 0.03 ml/kg/hr, right atrium (RA) pressure of 8 mm Hg, and a pulmonary capillary wedge pressure of 15 mm Hg. The drug of choice for treating this patient would be:

A. Dobutamine at 20 mcg/kg/min
B. Epinephrine at 0.01 mcg/kg/min
C. Amrinone at 10 mcg/kg/min
D. Isuprel at 0.05 mcg/kg/min

112. Increasing the inspiratory/expiratory ratio through mechanical ventilation has which of the following therapeutic benefits?

A. Improves refractory hypercarbia
B. Decreases bronchospasm
C. Recruits atelectatic lung areas
D. Decreases oxygen toxicity

113. Proper administration of charcoal for a toxic ingestion is:

A. Administer charcoal immediately, then induce vomiting
B. Administer charcoal within 1 hour of poisoning after vomiting is induced
C. Administer charcoal after emetic to absorb toxin and remaining emetic
D. Administer charcoal within 1 hour of poisoning before vomiting is induced

114. When treating a critically ill patient with a bleeding disorder, which of the following does the nurse need to be aware is not contained in fresh frozen plasma?

A. Factor VIII
B. Platelets
C. Fibrinogen
D. Thrombin

Case Study

A patient has been transferred to the critical care unit following repair of a ventricular septal defect. Questions 115 and 116 refer to this case study.

---

115. Which finding does *not* indicate that this patient still has a leak in the patch repair?
A. Systolic murmur
B. Mottling
C. Congestive heart failure
D. Tachypnea

116. Which test would be *most* helpful in diagnosing a residual ventricular septal defect?
A. Electrocardiogram
B. Echocardiogram
C. Chest x-ray
D. Computed tomography scan

117. Rejection of liver transplants commonly occurs:
A. At the first day
B. Between the fourth and tenth days
C. At 1 month
D. Between 4 and 8 weeks

118. Over time, a ventricular septal defect will cause which finding?
A. Ventricular hypertrophy
B. Decreased pulmonary blood flow
C. Systemic hypertension
D. Arteriovenous malformations

119. Administering 100% oxygen at rapid ventilatory rates to the infant suspected of having persistent pulmonary hypertension of the newborn is helpful in:
A. Improving PaO_2 as a result of recruitment of lung areas
B. Improving PaO_2 by dilating pulmonary vessels
C. Confirming the diagnosis because the PaO_2 is not improved
D. Improving refractory hypercarbia

120. An infant returns to the critical care unit following placement of a ventriculoperitoneal (VP) shunt. Which of the following positions are optimal for the infant?
I. Supine with the head aligned straight
II. Prone with the head turned to the unaffected side
III. On the affected side
IV. On the unaffected side
A. I or IV
B. I or II
C. I or III
D. II or IV

Case Study

A 7-year-old boy is brought to the hospital with respiratory distress and is diagnosed with croup. Questions 121 and 122 refer to this case study.

121. Which of the following clinical findings do not characterize croup?
- A. Rales and crackles
- B. Dyspnea and stridor
- C. Hoarseness or husky voice
- D. Cough and "barking"

122. The ventilation/perfusion ($\dot{V}/\dot{Q}$) mismatch observed in this child would be related to:
- A. Decreased perfusion as a result of capillary leak
- B. Decreased ventilation as a result of airway obstruction
- C. Decreased ventilation as a result of air trapping
- D. Decreased perfusion related to decreased cardiac output

123. Patients with asplenia syndrome are at an increased risk for:
- A. Hemorrhage
- B. Infections
- C. Hemolysis
- D. Thrombocytopenia

Case Study

An 8-month-old male child has severe congestive heart failure related to a ventricular septal defect. Questions 124 to 126 refer to this case study.

124. The nurse would expect this patient to have all of the following signs and symptoms of congestive heart failure *except*:
- A. Increased urinary output
- B. Decreased cardiac output
- C. Hepatomegaly
- D. Cardiomegaly

125. An adrenergic response to congestive heart failure is typically manifested by:
- A. Polyuria
- B. Warm, dry skin
- C. Tachycardia
- D. Poor feeding

126. A positive outcome of this patient's care management would include:
A. Increase in liver size
B. Urinary output of 0.5 mL/kg/hr
C. Presence of adventitious breath sounds
D. Decrease in pulmonary pressures

127. For the child with suspected epiglottitis, which of the following potential orders would the critical care nurse best defer until an x-ray is obtained?
A. Listening to breath sounds
B. Starting humidified oxygen
C. Obtaining a urine sample
D. Drawing arterial blood gases

128. Which of the following nursing interventions would the critical care nurse find *least* helpful in monitoring for complications in an infant following surgical placement of a VP shunt?
A. Measurement of abdominal girth
B. Measurement of head circumference
C. Measurement of chest circumference
D. Measurement of emesis

129. A 12-year-old child with cystic fibrosis is admitted to the pediatric intensive care unit with severe hemoptysis, a blood pressure of 88/40, a sinus rate of 118, respiratory rate of 22, a capillary refill time of 4 seconds, 2+ femoral pulses, and equivocal bilateral dorsalis pedis pulses. A central line is placed and volume expanders are infused at a rate of 20 ml/kg. The blood pressure following 30 minutes of fluid resuscitation is 86/38, the heart rate is 122, and the respiratory rate is 22. The nurse can anticipate which of the following to be initiated immediately:
A. Placement of indwelling arterial and pulmonary catheters
B. Initiation of amrinone at 5 mcg/kg/min
C. Administration of whole blood at 30 mL/kg
D. Initiation of a dopamine drip at 5 mcg/kg/min

130. In a patient with severe neutropenia, which of the following would be signs and symptoms of wound infection?
A. An increase in white blood cell count, fever
B. Irritability, hypothermia, anorexia
C. Fever, purulent drainage
D. Erythema, tenderness, exudate

Case Study

A patient was admitted to the critical care unit after being brought to the emergency department by her mother, who reported that her daughter demonstrated poor feeding for the past 36 hours, rapid breathing, decreased level of activity, and fewer wet diapers. Physical assessment showed moderate sinus tachycardia, increased liver size, rales, and a gallop rhythm. Laboratory results showed decreased serum osmolality and slightly decreased hematocrit and blood urea nitrogen levels. Questions 131 to 134 refer to this case study.

131. The most likely cause of her symptoms is:

A. Hypovolemic shock
B. Acute renal failure
C. Pneumonia
D. Congestive heart failure

132. The first action the nurse should take for this patient is to:

A. Begin oxygen therapy at ½ liter flow
B. Assess airway, adequacy of respirations, peripheral pulses
C. Monitor cardiac rhythm
D. Draw blood for baseline arterial blood gas levels

133. Which diagnostic test would be most helpful in confirming her diagnosis?

A. Magnetic resonance imaging
B. Electrocardiogram
C. Echocardiogram
D. Stress testing

134. A desired outcome in treating this patient includes:

A. Liver palpable <2 to 3 cm below costal margin
B. Increased arterial blood pressure
C. Negative cultures of pulmonary secretions
D. Normal serum creatinine levels

135. All of the following may be desired patient outcomes for an 8-year-old child with diabetes insipidus *except*:

A. Heart rate of 95 beats per minute at rest
B. Central venous pressure (CVP) of 12 mm Hg
C. Blood pressure of 110/60
D. Blood urea nitrogen (BUN) level of 15 mg/dL

Case Study

A 3-year-old child is admitted to the critical care unit after a near-drowning episode. She is flaccid and comatose. According to the emergency medical technician at the scene, she was severely bradycardic and apneic whey they arrived, but the parents were doing rescue breathing. They immediately intubated her, administered atropine, and had a good response. Questions 136 to 138 refer to this case study.

136. The prognosis for this child is most closely related to:
A. Temperature of the water
B. Length of submersion time
C. Saltwater vs. freshwater drowning
D. Extent of hypoxia suffered

137. Priorities for treating this child will focus on all of the following *except*:
A. Maintaining mild hypothermia
B. Improving peripheral perfusion
C. Ensuring adequate glucose stores
D. Improving cardiac function

138. The critical care nurse would expect to observe signs and symptoms of increased intracranial pressure after how many hours in this child?
A. 12 to 24
B. 24 to 48
C. 48 to 72
D. 72 to 96

139. A 16-year-old boy develops a decrease in urine output 5 days following renal transplantation. Which of the following signs and symptoms will help confirm a diagnosis of renal transplant rejection rather than a diagnosis of acute tubular necrosis?
A. Weight gain, rise in blood urea nitrogen, abdominal tenderness
B. Weight gain, rise in serum creatinine and blood urea nitrogen
C. Elevated serum potassium, flank pain, generalized edema
D. Anorexia, nausea, decreased white blood cell function

140. In a patient with pulmonary hemorrhage, which of the following will assist in restoring functional residual capacity and minimize FiO_2 requirements?
A. Increasing the tidal volume
B. Using positive end expiratory pressure
C. Increasing the respiratory rate
D. Decreasing the inspiratory/expiratory ratio

141. A patient is admitted to the critical care unit 2 weeks after repair of a ventricular septal defect with the following clinical findings: temperature of 83.6°C (103.8°F), white blood cell count of 14,500/cm^3, erythrocyte sedimentation rate (ESR) of 61 mm/hr, nasal flaring, pleural effusion, and decreased activity tolerance. The most likely cause of these symptoms is:

A. Viral pneumonia
B. Pericarditis
C. Postpericardiotomy syndrome
D. Respiratory syncytial virus

142. During the care of an infant, the critical care nurse notes eye rolling and profuse diaphoresis accompanied by tachycardia. The nurse suspects the infant may be:

A. Experiencing a rapid increase in intracranial pressure
B. Exhibiting seizure activity
C. In supraventricular tachycardia
D. Hypoglycemic

143. A 9-year-old male patient is brought to the critical care unit in status asthmaticus. He has a productive cough that raises thick, white, tenacious secretions. Wheezing is audible without a stethoscope. Dyspnea is apparent from nasal flaring, tachypnea, and use of accessory respiratory muscles. While admitting the patient, the nurse observes decreased wheezing and increasing lethargy. Which of the following immediate actions would be most appropriate?

A. Continue to observe the patient as his condition improves
B. Prepare for immediate intubation
C. Prepare for chest tube insertion
D. Begin an epinephrine infusion

144. A 14-year-old boy is diagnosed with acute respiratory failure secondary to pulmonary trauma from a pedestrian accident. He is intubated and placed on a mechanical ventilator. In order to minimize multisystem organ failure, which of the following treatments would be most effective?

A. Maintain a hematocrit greater than 40% to increase oxygen delivery
B. Maintain PaO_2 greater than 90% to minimize hypoxemia
C. Maintain low normal cardiac index to decrease cardiac work
D. Increase the FiO_2 to 1.0 to maximize oxygen delivery

Case Study

An 8-year-old child, now being admitted to the intensive care unit, was diagnosed at birth with congenital heart block. Recently, she collapsed during play and was unable to maintain a pulse rate greater than 40 beats/minute. She has a temporary pacemaker in place and is waiting for insertion of a permanent pacemaker. Questions 145 and 146 refer to this case study.

---

145. Where would this patient's pacing catheter be positioned if it were inserted percutaneously?
A. Left ventricle
B. Right ventricle
C. Touching the sinoatrial node
D. Distal to the atrioventricular node

146. The critical care nurse does *not* need to observe for which complication once her transvenous leads are placed?
A. Hemorrhage
B. Cardiac perforation
C. Hiccups
D. Seizures

147. Which of the following is critical during aerosol therapy to meet the ventilatory demands of an acute asthma attack?
A. Maintain an FiO_2 >0.4
B. Ensure adequate oxygen flow
C. Perform chest physiotherapy to clear secretions
D. Monitor terbutaline levels

148. The goal of treatment in status asthmaticus includes all of the following *except*:
A. Increased oxygen delivery
B. Improved ventilation
C. Increased residual volume
D. Decreased airway obstruction

149. An 8-year-old child is admitted to the pediatric intensive care unit (PICU) with a history of a fever, skin rash, proteinuria, cervical lymphadenitis, and erythema as well as pain of the hands and feet. His laboratory findings included elevations in his C-reactive protein and erythrocyte sedimentation rate. For which complication should the critical care nurse be alert?
A. Myocarditis
B. Endocarditis
C. Hepatitis
D. Glomerulonephritis

150. The critical care nurse observes a patient apparently beginning seizure activity. After assessing the airway, the *immediate* priority should be to:
A. Insert an artificial airway
B. Restrain the extremities to protect from injury
C. Observe the seizure activity
D. Administer diazepam

151. The critical care nurse would question an order for which of the following immunosuppressive drugs in the first day following renal transplantation?
A. Cyclosporin
B. Azathioprine
C. Prednisone
D. Cyclophosphamide

152. When caring for a 10-year-old patient with a pulmonary artery catheter, the critical care nurse notices that the diastolic pressure suddenly drops from 10 mm Hg to 2 mm Hg. Which of the following is the most likely cause?
A. Migration of the catheter tip
B. Balloon rupture in the pulmonary artery
C. Clot formation at the catheter tip
D. Blood in the transducer

153. A 10-year-old child is admitted to the critical care unit with premature ventricular complexes, nonspecific ST segment changes, and a decrease in QRS and T wave voltage. Clinically, the child has decreased peripheral pulses, urinary output of 0.8 mL/kg/hr, and a gallop rhythm. An echocardiogram has ruled out structural heart disease, but identified the presence of pericardial effusion and decreased ventricular motion. The parents state that the child had flulike symptoms for approximately the last 5 days. The most likely cause of these findings is:
A. Hypertrophic cardiomyopathy
B. Myocarditis
C. Endocarditis
D. Kawasaki's disease

154. Head circumference on an infant should be measured:
A. Directly over the orbits
B. Around the tragus of the ears
C. Above the supraorbital ridges
D. Over the base of the skull

155. When caring for a near-drowning victim, the critical care nurse observes an elevated urine sodium level (>120 mEq/L), a serum sodium level of 122 mEq/L, and a urine specific gravity of 1.044. The nurse suspects this patient is developing:
A. Syndrome of inappropriate antidiuretic hormone secretion
B. Diabetes insipidus
C. Acute respiratory distress syndrome
D. Electrolyte shifts related to saltwater near-drowning

156. A 14-year-old girl is brought to the hospital following a motor vehicle-bicycle accident. She is complaining of chest pain exacerbated by inspiration and has shallow respirations. Upon close observation, the critical care nurse notices paradoxical respirations. These are most likely because of a:

A. Pneumothorax
B. Hemothorax
C. Flail chest
D. Fractured rib

157. In administering aerosol bronchodilators, the critical care nurse observes for all of the following side effects *except*:

A. Bradycardia
B. Restlessness
C. Nausea
D. Dysrhythmias

158. An 18-month-old girl is brought to the emergency room 1 week after being discharged following a Fontan procedure. She has cyanosis, mottled extremities, decreased urine output, listlessness, dyspnea, and a blood pressure of 42/36 mm Hg. The critical care nurse can expect to *immediately* assist with:

A. Insertion of a pulmonary artery catheter
B. Pericardiocentesis
C. Pleural tap
D. Insertion of a central venous line

159. A child with Kawasaki's disease is complaining of chest pain unrelieved by positioning or other independent nursing interventions. Which intervention is a priority for the critical care nurse?

A. Administering prescribed analgesics after further pain assessment
B. Obtaining a 12-lead electrocardiogram (ECG) and assessing for ST segment changes
C. Administering gamma globulin to decrease inflammation
D. Preparing the child for pericardiocentesis

160. Which of the following foreign body aspirants will be readily visible on chest x-ray, facilitating diagnosis?

A. Popcorn
B. Hot dog
C. Paper clip
D. Pencil eraser

161. Normal serum levels of aminophylline are:

A. 5 to 10 mcg/mL
B. 10 to 20 mcg/mL
C. 20 to 30 mcg/mL
D. 25 to 35 mcg/mL

162. The hypoxia associated with asthma is a result of:
A. Ventilation/perfusion mismatch
B. Hypoventilation
C. Left-to-right shunting
D. Increased oxygen demands

Case Study

A 6-year-old child has been admitted to the PICU with a sickle cell crisis. The history includes six prior PICU admissions for sickle cell disease. Initial assessment reveals a nonpalpable spleen, hepatomegaly, fever, abdominal pain, and mild hematuria. Questions 163 and 164 refer to this case study.

---

163. For which of the following is this patient at the greatest risk?
A. Infection
B. Respiratory distress syndrome
C. Disseminated intravascular coagulation
D. Consumptive coagulopathy

164. Eight hours after admission this child develops left-sided weakness and a dilated, sluggishly reactive right pupil. The critical care nurse should *first* prepare the child for:
A. Blood transfusion
B. CAT scan to diagnose the neurological deficit
C. Administration of streptokinase or TPA
D. Administration of heparin

165. Barbiturates may be used to treat increased intracranial pressure because their *primary* effect is to:
A. Promote an oncotic diuresis
B. Decrease metabolic demand
C. Decrease muscular activity
D. Relieve pain

166. Beta-agonists are used to treat asthma. These are most often administered:
A. Orally
B. Intravenously
C. Intramuscularly
D. By aerosol

167. A 6-year-old patient returns from the operating room after having undergone a Fontan procedure for a single ventricle. He has a wedge pressure of 18 mm Hg, right ventricular pressure of 38/12 mm Hg, cardiac index of 2.8 L/min/m^2, and heart rate of 185 beats/minute. Which drug will most likely improve his cardiovascular function?
A. Dopamine
B. Nitroprusside
C. Epinephrine
D. Amrinone

168. For which condition should the nurse slow or stop an amrinone infusion and notify the physician?
A. Increased pulmonary capillary wedge pressure
B. Decreased cardiac output
C. Cardiac dysrhythmia
D. Increased right ventricular filling pressure

169. Which of the following medications used to treat asthma is not given by aerosol?
A. Epinephrine
B. Isoproterenol
C. Atropine
D. Aminophylline

170. When morphine sulfate is used to sedate and/or relieve pain in a patient with increased intracranial pressure, to what would the critical care nurse be particularly alert?
A. Level of consciousness
B. Depth of respirations
C. Pupillary response
D. Tachycardia

171. A 3-year-old girl was brought to the emergency department after her mother said she swallowed a coin. Her respiratory rate is 50 breaths/minute, her blood pressure is 96/60, and her pulse rate is 130 beats/minute. She appears anxious, is clinging to her mother, and has difficulty cooperating with the examination. An intermittent nonproductive cough and sternal retractions as well as use of accessory muscles to breath are noted during the examination. As the critical care nurse is examining her, she becomes quiet and her respiratory rate slows to 16. The nurse recognizes this as:
A. Possible resolution of the obstruction
B. Adaptation to the hospital setting
C. Impending respiratory arrest
D. Development of pneumothorax

172. The critical care nurse recognizes as possible complications following foreign body airway obstruction all of the following *except*:
A. Infection
B. Obstruction
C. Hoarseness
D. Cyanosis

Case Study

A 7-year-old boy is admitted to the critical care unit with thermal injuries covering 40% of his body surface area acquired in a bedroom fire where he was playing with matches and his clothes caught on fire. Questions 173 to 177 refer to this case study.

173. Outcome criteria related to cardiac function within the first 12 hours of injury would include all of the following *except*:
A. Peripheral pulses: 3+
B. Cardiac index of 3.5 to 4.5 L/min/m^2 of body surface area
C. Intracompartmental pressures <30 mm Hg
D. Absence of peripheral paresthesia

174. All of the following nursing diagnosis for cardiac function are appropriate for this patient *except*:
A. Decreased cardiac output related to extravascular fluid shift
B. Decreased cardiac output related to myocardial dysfunction
C. Decreased cardiac output related to insufficient intravascular volume
D. Decreased cardiac output related to low central venous pressure

175. The physician may prescribe vasodilators for this patient. What would be an indication for their use?
A. The systemic vascular resistance is elevated
B. The intravascular volume is elevated
C. Capillary leakage is creating significant third-spacing of fluid
D. The fluid remobilization period has begun

176. After restoring adequate intravascular volume, the nurse would expect the physician to prescribe which medication to improve the function of his heart and improve his cardiac output?
A. Nitroprusside
B. Dobutamine
C. Digoxin
D. Dopamine

177. The nurse would anticipate outcome criteria during the first 12 hours for a patient with significant thermal injuries to include:
A. Urinary output of 0.5 cc/kg/hr
B. Resolution of an S_3 heart sound
C. A central venous pressure of 18 mmHg
D. Normal skin temperature

178. Which of the following is contraindicated in all posttransplant liver patients?
A. Saline instillation before suctioning
B. Heparinized flush solutions
C. Irrigation of the nasogastric tube
D. Rectal temperatures

179. When caring for a child who has an end-tidal CO_2 monitoring ($P_{ET}CO_2$) device in place, the critical care nurse notices the reading rapidly falling to near 0 levels. This is most likely due to:
A. Mucous plug in the endotracheal tube
B. Migration of the endotracheal tube into the right bronchus
C. Falling PaO_2 levels
D. Hypoventilation

180. An 8-month-old infant was admitted to the intensive care unit with clear nasal discharge, a respiratory rate of 56, cough, temperature of 100.4°F (38°C), poor feeding, and dyspnea. Examination of the pulmonary system revealed subcostal retractions, nasal flaring, and use of accessory muscles to breath. Crackles, wheezes, and decreased breath sounds were auscultated on admission. The chest x-ray showed hyperinflated lungs as well as atelectatic areas. The critical care nurse suspects the patient has:
A. Bacterial pneumonia
B. Bronchiolitis
C. Aspiration pneumonia
D. Bronchopulmonary dysplasia

181. An infant is brought to the critical care unit for uncontrolled seizure activity. The pharmacological treatment of choice would be:
A. Diazepam 0.5 mg/kg
B. Phenobarbital 20 mg/kg
C. Phenytoin 5 mg/kg
D. Dextrose 200 mg/kg

182. When administering blood to a 12-year-old patient with internal hemorrhaging, the critical care nurse notes the patient has a temperature of 101.1°F (38.4°C), nausea, vomiting, headache, and shaking chills. Which of the following actions would the critical care nurse do *first*?

A. Administer antihistamines to counteract the allergic reaction and observe for dyspnea
B. Insert a Foley catheter to obtain a urine sample for hematuria and measure output
C. Slow the transfusion to a keep open rate and notify the physician
D. Stop the transfusion immediately, keep the IV patent, and notify the physician

183. When examining a child who may have epiglottitis, the critical care nurse would avoid all of the following *except*:

A. Administration of humidified oxygen before blood gas analysis
B. Examining the throat looking for the possibility of overlooked foreign body obstruction
C. Drawing blood gases to evaluate respiratory failure
D. Asking the parents to leave because the child is clinging too much to them to be examined

---

Case Study

A 14-year-old boy is admitted to the pediatric intensive care unit following a pedestrian accident. He has known chest trauma as evidenced by bruising over the sternum and tenderness over the third, fourth, and fifth ribs, left midclavicular line.

Questions 184 to 186 refer to this case study.

---

184. In assessing for a pneumothorax, the critical care nurse would look for:

A. Distant breath sounds, change in pitch, tracheal deviation to the right
B. Hyperresonant breath sounds, crackles, midline trachea
C. Distant breath sounds, change in pitch, tracheal deviation to the left
D. Hyperresonant breath sounds, stridor, midline trachea

185. When the critical care nurse performs a full respiratory assessment, the patient is found to have complaints of chest pain, coarse breath sounds, and a slightly increased respiratory rate accompanied by nasal flaring. There is no use of accessory muscles. The nurse suspects this patient most likely has:

A. Hemothorax
B. Rib fracture
C. Chylothorax
D. Lung contusion

186. Twelve hours after admission to the unit, the patient begins to be somewhat combative and very restless. An emergent examination reveals a gradually decreasing blood pressure over the last 90 minutes to 88/78, jugular vein distension, and cold, pale extremities with weak and thready peripheral pulses. The critical care nurse prepares to *immediately* assist with:
A. Tapping the pleural space
B. Pericardiocentesis
C. Insertion of a chest tube
D. Rapid infusion of colloids

Case Study

A 16-hour-old female infant is admitted to the critical care unit. Her diagnostic workup includes the following information.

pH:	7.21
pO_2:	41 torr
pCO_2:	35 torr
Base deficit:	–8
Blood arterial pressure:	52/43 mm Hg

The tentative diagnosis is sepsis. She received 30 cc/kg of fluids during resuscitative efforts in the emergency room. Questions 187 and 188 refer to this case study.

---

187. Based on these assessment findings, the critical care nurse recognizes that this infant is *most likely* also at risk for developing:
A. Intraventricular hemorrhage
B. Seizures
C. Hydrocephalus
D. Meningitis

188. The *immediate* nursing priority upon admission to the critical care unit would be to:
A. Administer diuretic therapy for fluid overload
B. Administer sodium bicarbonate to correct acidosis
C. Begin vasopressive support to improve perfusion
D. Administer diuretics to decrease intracranial pressure

189. A child with aspiration pneumonia from hydrocarbons would be expected to present with:
A. Severe dyspnea, wheezing, cardiac dysrhythmias, somnolence
B. Fever, irritability, tachycardia, cough
C. Seizures, frothy sputum, cough, fever
D. Acute agitation, nasal flaring, sternal retractions, fever

190. An 11-month-old child with bronchopulmonary dysplasia is most likely to be at risk for developing:
A. Aspiration pneumonia
B. Pneumothorax
C. Bronchiolitis
D. Pulmonary hemorrhage

191. Values obtained by monitoring of end-tidal CO_2 ($P_{ET}CO_2$) in patients without lung disease reflect all of the following *except*:
A. Alveolar pCO_2
B. $PaCO_2$
C. Serum CO_2
D. Exhaled CO_2

192. When changing a dressing on a child with a large thermal injury, the nurse notes that the wound area has blisters and the area below where blisters have been removed is pink and sensitive to both touch and temperature. The area is also edematous. Based on this information, the nurse classifies this injury as:
A. First degree
B. Second degree
C. Third degree
D. Fourth degree

193. A mixed venous blood gas sample is drawn from a pulmonary artery catheter. The critical care nurse interprets the results of the mixed venous pO_2 of 38 mm Hg as indicating:
A. Hypoxia and probable shock
B. Adequate peripheral perfusion
C. Hypoventilation and hypoxia
D. Respiratory acidosis

194. Hypoxic-ischemic encephalopathy is usually accompanied by all of the following *except*:
A. Renal dysfunction
B. Necrotizing enterocolitis
C. Metabolic acidosis
D. Hydrocephalus

195. A 9-year-old boy with respiratory distress syndrome has a fiberoptic pulmonary artery catheter in place to measure continuous mixed venous oxygen saturation (SvO_2). A value of 55% would most likely indicate:
A. Decreased oxygen delivery
B. Decreased oxygen demand
C. Optimal oxygen balance
D. Decreased hemoglobin levels

196. The critical care nurse would be alert to which of the following electrolyte and metabolic derangements associated with severe thermal injuries?
A. Hyperkalemia
B. Hypernatremia
C. Hypercalcemia
D. Hypermagnesemia

197. Which of the following symptoms would the critical care nurse recognize as a common sequelae of hypoxic-ischemic encephalopathy?
A. SIADH
B. Nonketotic hyperglycemia
C. Cardiomyopathy
D. Bronchopulmonary dysplasia

198. Which of the following is a *late* sign of inadequate intravascular volume resuscitation in a burn injured patient?
A. Diminished pulses
B. Tachycardia
C. Hypotension
D. Oliguria

Case Study

A 10 kg child is calculated to have a total BSA of 0.47 m^2. This child has a 40% BSA thermal injury. Questions 199 and 200 refer to this case study.

---

199. What would be the approximate fluid resuscitation needs of this child?
A. 865 cc
B. 565 cc
C. 1000 cc
D. 300 cc

200. Which of the following is *not* an appropriate fluid for volume resuscitation in the first 24 hours following a thermal injury?
A. Albumin
B. 0.45% normal saline
C. Ringer's lactate
D. 1.5% normal saline

Pediatric Test Answers

1. D
2. A
3. D
4. C
5. B
6. D
7. D
8. D
9. B
10. C
11. A
12. C
13. B
14. D
15. A
16. A
17. D
18. C
19. D
20. A
21. A
22. D
23. A
24. B
25. C
26. D
27. C
28. D
29. A
30. B
31. D
32. B
33. C
34. B
35. B
36. A
37. D
38. A
39. C
40. D
41. C
42. D
43. B
44. A
45. C
46. D
47. A
48. C
49. C
50. C
51. C
52. A
53. C
54. C
55. A
56. A
57. D
58. D
59. A
60. C
61. C
62. B
63. A
64. B
65. B
66. A
67. C
68. C
69. C
70. A
71. A
72. D
73. B
74. A
75. D
76. B
77. A
78. B
79. A
80. B
81. D
82. D
83. A
84. A

85. C
86. A
87. B
88. B
89. B
90. D
91. B
92. B
93. C
94. C
95. A
96. B
97. B
98. C
99. D
100. D
101. C
102. D
103. A
104. C
105. B
106. B
107. C
108. A
109. D
110. D
111. B
112. C
113. B
114. B
115. B
116. B
117. B
118. A
119. B
120. A
121. A
122. B
123. B
124. A
125. C
126. D
127. D
128. C
129. A
130. B
131. D
132. B
133. C
134. A
135. B
136. D
137. A
138. C
139. A
140. B
141. C
142. B
143. B
144. B
145. B
146. D
147. B
148. C
149. A
150. C
151. A
152. A
153. B
154. C
155. A
156. C
157. A
158. B
159. B
160. C
161. B
162. A
163. A
164. A
165. B
166. D
167. D
168. C
169. D
170. B
171. C
172. D
173. B
174. D
175. A
176. B

177. D
178. B
179. A
180. B
181. B
182. D
183. A
184. A
185. D
186. B
187. A
188. C
189. A
190. C
191. C
192. B
193. B
194. D
195. A
196. A
197. A
198. C
199. A
200. B

SCORING YOUR EXAMINATION

Below 65% (less than 130 correct answers):
You are not in the passing range yet. Keep studying. Evaluate where your weaknesses are, but keep reviewing all the material. Don't try to cram; just study whenever you can and review, review, review. This will help you master the material.

65% to 75% (130 to 150 correct answers):
You are barely above the passing mark of 65% or 130 correct answers. Keep studying! Try to pinpoint the body systems or types of questions causing you the most difficulty and focus your attention on these areas.

75% to 85% (150 to 170 correct answers):
You are doing very well! Keep reviewing to continue to master the material, but relax and increase your confidence. Review the test-taking strategies in Chapter 9 again to eliminate any factor that nerves or anxiety may have on your final score.

85% to 100% (170 to 200 correct answers):
What a terrific job! Keep reviewing the material to keep it fresh. Congratulations!

Neonatal Sample Test

1. A normotensive neonate is admitted to the critical care unit with an increase in serum glucose levels, decreased urinary output after 24 hours of increased output, and respiratory alkalosis. The critical care nurse monitors this infant in compensated shock closely for signs and symptoms of decompensation. The critical care nurse knows this neonate with septic shock is most directly at risk for developing which of the following additional conditions?
   A. Persistent pulmonary hypertension
   B. Aspiration pneumonia
   C. Intraventricular bleeding
   D. Generalized seizures

2. Which is the primary cause of cardiac arrest in infants?
   A. Congestive heart failure
   B. Cardiac arrhythmias
   C. Respiratory problems
   D. Trauma

3. The critical care nurse observes continuous, noisy bubbling in the water seal chamber of the chest tube drainage system. The most appropriate action would be to:
   A. Check the suction tubing for any kinks or clots obstructing drainage
   B. Milk the chest tube gently to remove clots
   C. Raise the tubing between the patient and the collection system to empty stagnant drainage
   D. Clamp tube at insertion site briefly to observe for cessation of bubbling

4. An infant with the following blood gases is admitted to the critical care unit. Which of the following changes in ventilatory therapy would be most likely to improve the blood gases?
   pH: 7.31
   pO_2: 88 torr
   pCO_2: 53 torr
   HCO_3: 19 mEq/L
   A. Increase the FiO_2 by 10%
   B. Increase the respiratory rate
   C. Decrease the peak inspiratory pressure
   D. Increase the inspiratory/expiratory ratio

Case Study

An infant with coarctation of the aorta is admitted to the pediatric unit, where he undergoes a physical examination and diagnostic testing. Tests include echocardiography and cardiac catheterization. Questions 5 to 7 refer to this case study.

---

5. Which signs and symptoms of coarctation would most likely be seen during the physical examination?
   A. Bounding femoral pulses, weak brachial pulses
   B. Bounding femoral and brachial pulses
   C. Weak femoral pulses, absent brachial pulses
   D. Weak femoral pulses, strong brachial pulses

6. Before surgery, this infant is likely to be treated with which medication?
   A. Dopamine to increase systemic pressure
   B. Dobutamine to increase myocardial contraction
   C. Sodium bicarbonate to treat acidosis
   D. Diuretic therapy to treat congestive failure

7. Which outcome indicates effective management of this infant with coarctation before surgical correction?
   A. Adequate hourly urinary output
   B. Active precordium
   C. Absence of pleural effusion
   D. Decrease in arterial pH level

8. In anticipating home discharge needs, the critical care nurse would identify potential need for which of the following for the preterm appropriate for gestational age (AGA) infant?
   A. Home apnea monitoring
   B. Home enteral nutritional therapy
   C. Home oxygen therapy
   D. Home shift nursing care

9. Which outcome indicates effective management of an infant in uncompensated septic shock?
   A. Urinary output of 1 mL/kg/hr
   B. Capillary refill of 2.5 seconds
   C. Arterial pH of 7.33
   D. Cardiac index of 2.3 L/min/m^2

10. A 24-hour-old 4 kg neonate is admitted to the critical care unit with a diagnosis of infantile polycystic disease. Infantile polycystic kidney disease is characterized by which of the following laboratory tests?
   A. Hyperkalemia, hypocalcemia, hyperphosphatemia, acidosis
   B. Hypokalemia, hypocalcemia, hyperphosphatemia, acidosis
   C. Hyperkalemia, hypercalcemia, hypophosphatemia, alkalosis
   D. Hypokalemia, hypercalcemia, hypophosphatemia, alkalosis

11. Which of the following assessment findings in an infant is *not* indicative of an increase in intracranial pressure?
A. Lethargy
B. Bulging fontanels
C. Hypotension
D. Tachycardia

12. The critical care nurse observes fluid fluctuations in the water seal chamber during respirations. The most appropriate action in the care of this patient with a chest tube and drainage system would be to:
A. Milk the chest tube gently to remove clots that may have formed
B. Note that the drainage system is functioning properly
C. Immediately observe the patient for respiratory distress
D. Disconnect the system and hand ventilate the patient until the system can be replaced

13. Two hours after returning from surgery, the critical care nurse observes a decreased level of responsiveness in the neonate she is caring for. He is breathing spontaneously on room air. Blood gases are obtained and are as follows:

pH:	7.22
pO_2:	90 torr
pCO_2:	63 torr
HCO_3^-:	23 mEq/L
Base Excess:	+2

Which of the following actions would be *most* appropriate based on these findings?
A. Administration of 100% oxygen by facial mask to improve hypoxia
B. Administration of narcotic analgesics to decrease pain and improve deep breathing
C. Administration of sodium bicarbonate to correct acidosis
D. Administration of naloxone to reverse effects of anesthesia

14. The nurse is *least* likely to effectively assess for fluid overload in an infant in which area?
A. Periorbital
B. Sacral
C. Supraclavicular
D. Pedal

15. Which heart sound would a critical care nurse recognize and report as *not* normal in an infant?
A. Fixed split of S_2
B. Physiologic split of S_2
C. Systolic murmur
D. An S_3 heart sound

16. Which of the following complications would the critical care nurse suspect in the care of a neonate with an omphalocele?
A. Hypothermia
B. Fluid overload
C. Arrhythmias
D. Cyanosis

17. An intubated and ventilated infant suddenly shows a decrease in the pulse oximetry reading from 95% saturation to 81%. The patient is exhibiting nasal flaring, intercostal retractions, tachypnea, and use of accessory respiratory muscles despite the ventilator showing an adequate tidal volume and absence of peak pressure alarms. Which of the following actions should the critical care nurse do *first*?
A. Disconnect from the ventilator and manually bag the patient
B. Immediately suction the endotracheal tube
C. Increase the FiO_2 to 100%
D. Auscultate breath sounds

18. Which of the following ventilators is most effective for an infant?
A. Pressure cycled
B. Volume cycled
C. Time cycled
D. Negative pressure

19. When planning home discharge, an appropriate nursing diagnosis for complications related to posterior apneic episodes would be:
A. High risk for ineffective breathing pattern
B. Nutritional, altered: less than body requirements
C. Impaired gas exchange
D. Caregiver role strain

20. Which of the following tests is *most* helpful in determining Rh hemolytic disease in the newborn?
A. Total bilirubin level
B. Indirect Coomb's test
C. Hemoglobin
D. Indirect bilirubin level

21. In distributive shock, the nursing diagnostic category fluid volume deficit is related to all of the following factors *except*:
A. Vascular endothelial dysfunction and leakage
B. Abnormal distribution of intravascular volume
C. Release of endotoxins causing vasodilation
D. Myocardial dysfunction from depressant factors

22. An infant admitted to the NICU for hypoglycemia has been stabilized on intravenous glucose infusions. Which of the following principles will guide the critical care nurse's interventions when discontinuing IV glucose therapy? After blood glucose levels have stabilized,

A. The infusion may be discontinued
B. The infusion rate may be decreased by 75%
C. The infusion may be slowly weaned
D. The solution may be replaced by normal saline

23. Which statement about S_3 heart sounds in infants and children is *not* true?

A. May be a normal finding
B. May indicate aortic stenosis
C. May precede the development of rales
D. May indicate poor ventricular function

24. Which statement best describes a major difference between fetal and postnatal circulation?

A. The foramen ovale opens after birth to allow more blood flow to the lungs
B. Pulmonary vascular resistance is higher than systemic vascular resistance in the fetus
C. The ductus arteriosus becomes patent after birth to allow diversion of blood from high pulmonary pressure
D. The foramen ovale closes so no blood mixing occurs in the ventricles

25. In counseling the family of a neonate with extrophy of the bladder, the most appropriate statement for the critical nurse to share would be:

A. "Most of the infants have a great deal of trouble with bed wetting and bladder control as they get older."
B. "These children can achieve normal bladder control with surgery that involves six stages."
C. "Most infants can achieve good bladder control with surgery and medical therapy."
D. "Your infant will probably have surgery to correct this condition within the first week of life."

Case Study

Michael was a 3460 g full term infant with a history of meconium stained amniotic fluid noted 2 hours before delivery. He was suctioned at birth and found to have meconium below the cords. Apgar scores were 7 at one minute and 8 at five minutes. He was tachypneic with nasal flaring and expiratory grunting. His pulse oximetry reading on his right finger was 98% saturation whereas the pulse oximetry on his right toe was only 65%. His blood gases by umbilical artery catheter on 80% hood were as follows:

pH: 7.32
pO_2: 72 mm Hg
pCO_2: 40 mm Hg

Questions 26 to 28 refer to this case study.

---

26. Which of the following is the most likely explanation for the differences in pulse oximetry readings between his upper and lower extremities?
A. Coarctation of the aorta
B. Persistent pulmonary hypertension
C. Poor reading on the lower extremity pulse oximeter
D. Poor peripheral circulation related to acidosis

27. After the infant was intubated, what pH level in analyzing the blood gases would the nurse view as the best outcome of ventilatory therapy?
A. 7.35
B. 7.47
C. 7.50
D. 7.67

28. Based on the desired outcome of the pH level in question 27, for what complications would the critical care nurse be alert?
A. Hyponatremia
B. Hypocalcemia
C. Hyperkalemia
D. Hypermagnesemia

29. Which compensatory mechanism is used by infants to increase cardiac output?
A. Increased stroke volume
B. Decreased afterload
C. Increased heart rate
D. Increased preload

Case Study

A patient is admitted to the critical care unit with a diagnosis of hypoxic-ischemic encephalopathy following a traumatic delivery. Questions 30 to 32 refer to this case study.

---

30. The *first* nursing priority would be to assess:
A. Pupillary reaction
B. Level of consciousness
C. Ability to maintain airway
D. Blood glucose level

31. The critical care nurse would recognize as signs and symptoms of mild hypoxic-ischemic encephalopathy all of the following *except*:
A. Irritability
B. Tachycardia
C. Hyperalertness
D. Hypotonia

32. This infant is intubated and mechanically ventilated. Besides providing optimal oxygenation, which of the following is also a benefit of mechanical ventilation in this type of infant?
A. Reduction of intracranial pressure
B. Prevention of seizure activity
C. Prevention of long-term complications
D. Reduction of hypocarbia

33. Which of the following nursing diagnoses would be *most* appropriate for the neonate who has undergone surgical correction for an omphalocele?
A. High risk for infection
B. Ineffective airway clearance
C. Diarrhea
D. Hypothermia

34. Maternal cocaine use is a high risk factor for all of the following complications *except*:
A. Congenital cardiac defects
B. Hydrocephalus
C. Meconium aspiration
D. Placenta previa

35. All of the following are possible complications of Rh incompatibility in the newborn *except*:
A. Hydrops fetalis
B. Brain damage
C. Hepatic failure
D. Shock

36. The critical care nurse's care of the neonate with extrophy of the bladder would include:
A. Covering the exposed bladder with petroleum gauze
B. Use of a sterile cord clamp on the umbilical cord
C. Insertion of an indwelling urinary catheter
D. Using a clear, occlusive dressing to cover the bladder

Case Study

An infant female patient has critical aortic stenosis. During the past hour, she has developed tachycardia, urinary output of less than 0.5 ml/kg, mottling of the skin, elevation in central venous pressure, increased liver size, and barely palpable pulses.

Questions 37 to 41 refer to this case study.

---

37. Her symptoms are probably the result of:
A. Hypovolemic shock
B. Septic shock
C. Cardiogenic shock
D. Hemorrhagic shock

38. Which nursing diagnosis is most appropriate for this patient?
A. Ineffective thermoregulation associated with poor perfusion of temperature regulation centers
B. Impaired gas exchange related to decreased pulmonary flow
C. Decreased cardiac output related to myocardial dysfunction
D. Ineffective breathing pattern related to obstructed pulmonary flow

39. The physician may prescribe digoxin for this patient. These drugs help to improve cardiovascular function by:
A. Increasing systemic vascular resistance
B. Inotropic actions
C. Decreasing afterload
D. Improving renal perfusion

40. To improve her cardiac output, the nurse would expect the physician to prescribe:
A. Nitroprusside
B. Prostaglandin
C. Digoxin
D. Dopamine

41. Which would *not* be considered a positive outcome for her therapy?
A. Urinary output of 0.5 cc/kg/hr
B. Resolution of an S_3 heart sound
C. Warm, dry skin
D. A rise in arterial oxygen saturation

42. Which of the following would the critical care nurse recognize as the earliest sign of impending respiratory problems?
A. Tachypnea
B. Grunting
C. Nasal flaring
D. Intercostal retractions

Case Study

A 35-week small for gestational age (SGA) infant is admitted to the NICU. Twelve hours after birth she is tachypneic, has temperature lability, sweating, sneezing, tremors, and a poor cry. She is a poor feeder and has slept little. Questions 43 to 46 refer to this case study.

---

43. These signs and symptoms are most likely to be a result of:
A. Maternal cocaine use
B. Narcotic abstinence syndrome
C. Fetal alcohol syndrome
D. Fetal tobacco syndrome

44. This infant would *least* likely be at risk for which of the following?
A. Respiratory distress syndrome
B. Skin breakdown
C. Malnutrition
D. Seizures

45. In order to reduce irritability in the neonate, the critical care nurse would:
A. Position the infant prone
B. Cover the hands with mittens
C. Reduce eye contact
D. Minimize verbal stimuli

46. The critical care nurse recognizes that this infant is also at risk for:
A. HIV infection
B. Respiratory distress syndrome
C. Hyperglycemia
D. Congenital diaphragmatic hernia

47. A full term 2450 g infant of a diabetic mother (IDM) is admitted to the neonatal intensive care unit (NICU) for observation following low glucose levels. To which of the following signs and symptoms would the critical care nurse be alert as a possible complication in caring for an IDM?
A. Chvostek's sign
B. Cullen's sign
C. Kehr's sign
D. Cushing's sign

Case Study

A small infant admitted to the neonatal intensive care unit weights 1400 g and is 42 cm in length. Physical examination is performed to help determine gestational age. Questions 48 to 50 refer to this case study.

---

48. Examination of the skin reveals no transparency, no lanugo, and the underlying blood vessels are difficult to visualize. There is no visible wrinkling or desquamation. Based on this information, the critical care nurse estimates the gestational age at:
A. 30 to 32 weeks
B. 33 to 34 weeks
C. 36 to 37 weeks
D. 39 to 41 weeks

49. Which of the following statements is important when the nurse assesses sole creases for estimation of gestational age?
A. Creases first appear on the posterior portion of the foot
B. After 12 hours, sole creases are not a valid indicator
C. Creases first appear on the heel and progress to the toes
D. Sole creases diminish with increasing gestational age

50. An infant with a raised areola but without any nodule of palpable breast tissue is estimated to be what gestational age?
A. 28 weeks
B. 30 weeks
C. 34 weeks
D. 40 weeks

51. An infant is born at 37 weeks gestation and is plotted to be at the 5th percentile for weight and the 50th percentile for length. This neonate is correctly classified as:
A. Symmetrically AGA preterm
B. Asymmetrically SGA preterm
C. Symmetrically SGA preterm
D. Asymmetrically AGA preterm

52. An infant was admitted to the critical care unit for meconium aspiration and was intubated on 80% oxygen for the last 3 days. Upon examination, the nurse finds decreased breath sounds over the lung fields, lethargy, restlessness, dyspnea, and an increasing A-a gradient. No increase in secretions, fever, or wheezing is noted. These findings are most consistent with the development of:
A. Pneumonia
B. Foreign body aspiration
C. Oxygen toxicity
D. Airway obstruction

53. Which of the following is important in obtaining a history of an infant with congenital cardiac disease?
A. Family history of coronary heart disease
B. Mother's cholesterol intake during pregnancy
C. Maternal allergies
D. Fetal exposure to medications or alcohol

54. In assessing an infant with congestive heart failure, the nurse would use the bell of the stethoscope to best hear:
B. S_3 and S_4 heart sounds
B. High-pitched murmurs
C. Stenotic valves
D. An ejection click

55. Which diagnostic test would be most helpful in documenting blood flow through a patent ductus arteriosus?
A. Chest x-ray
B. Magnetic resonance imaging
C. Doppler echocardiography
D. Electrocardiogram

56. All of the following would be helpful in promoting airway clearance *except*:
A. Restricting fluids to minimize formation of secretions
B. Suctioning airway
C. Providing humidification
D. Cupping and postural drainage

57. Which of the following is an indication for an exchange transfusion to treat Rh incompatibility in the full term newborn?
A. Indirect bilirubin level greater than 20 mg/dL
B. Cord hemoglobin of 14 g/dL
C. Total bilirubin level greater than 20 mg/dL
D. Positive direct Coomb's test

Case Study

A neonate is admitted to the critical care unit directly from the delivery room in respiratory distress. He is small for his gestational age. Physical examination reveals low set ears, widely spaced eyes, large hands, and bowed legs. The labor and delivery room nurse reports a perinatal history of oligohydramnios. Questions 58 to 60 refer to this case study.

---

58. The most likely cause of these findings is:
A. Polycystic kidney disease
B. Turner's syndrome
C. Potter's syndrome
D. Hydronephrosis

59. The most likely cause of this neonate's respiratory distress is
A. Bronchiolitis
B. Pneumothorax
C. Aspiration
D. Tracheoesophageal fistula

60. Interventions for this infant would most likely be planned to:
A. Increase urinary output
B. Decrease metabolic acidosis
C. Provide comfort measures
D. Maximize nutritional status

61. While caring for an intubated and mechanically ventilated infant, the critical care nurse notices sudden, profound cyanosis and bradycardia. She observes asymmetrical chest excursion and decreased amplitude of the QRS complex, and auscultates shifted breath sounds. What *immediate* action should the critical care nurse take?
A. Elevate head of bed and increase the FiO_2 to 1.0
B. Suction endotracheal tube to remove any obstruction
C. Call for stat x-ray to check tube placement
D. Begin chest compressions while preparing to administer epinephrine

62. Prostaglandin E_1 therapy would most likely be helpful in treating which defect during the neonatal period?
A. Pulmonary atresia
B. Atrioventricular canal
C. Truncus arteriosus
D. Patent ductus arteriosus

63. Which finding is most common in infants with digoxin toxicity?
A. Nausea and vomiting
B. Diarrhea
C. Seizures
D. Lethargy

64. Which of the following abused substances is *least* likely to cause congenital anomalies?
A. Alcohol
B. Heroin
C. Cocaine
D. Cigarettes

65. The incidence of patent ductus arteriosus is related to:
A. Birth weight and length
B. Size for gestational age
C. Gestational age and birth weight
D. Mechanical ventilation

66. At what gestational age are the testes completely descended into the scrotum?
A. 30 weeks
B. 33 weeks
C. 36 weeks
D. 40 weeks

67. A neonate with hypoplastic left heart syndrome has the following blood gases: pH of 7.2, PCO_2 of 55 torr, PO_2 of 40 torr, oxygen saturation of 75%, and a base deficit of –6. Which ventilatory therapy is most appropriate?
A. FiO_2 of 0.4
B. FiO_2 of 0.6
C. FiO_2 of 0.2
D. FiO_2 of 1.0

68. Phenylketonuria requires dietary restrictions that may include:
A. Low iron formulas
B. Breast milk
C. Soy-based formula
D. Lactose-free formulas

69. A shunt study on a cyanotic infant found that the PaO_2 has changed little at 51 torr after 10 minutes of oxygenation at an FiO_2 of 1.0. Based on the results of this test, the infant's cyanosis is most likely caused by which condition?
A. Tetralogy of Fallot
B. Meconium aspiration
C. Respiratory distress syndrome
D. Atrioventricular canal

70. Neonates are inefficient at increasing cardiac output because of immature development of:
A. Parasympathetic innervation of the heart
B. Sympathetic innervation of the heart
C. Great vessel size
D. Aortic valve

71. All of the following are related to the development of bronchopulmonary dysplasia *except*:
A. Patent ductus arteriosus
B. High inspired oxygen levels
C. Positive pressure ventilation
D. Negative pressure ventilation

72. A neonate is admitted to the critical care unit following unexplained seizure activity. In planning this newborn's treatment, the critical care nurse recognizes the *highest* priority is given to:
A. Correcting metabolic imbalances
B. Administering prophylactic anticonvulsant therapy
C. Obtaining an EEG to identify focal site
D. Obtaining a lumbar puncture to rule out meningitis

73. Which of the following medications are *not* used to treat bronchopulmonary dysplasia?
A. Diuretics
B. Beta-blockers
C. Vasodilators
D. Corticosteroids

74. Factors that are responsible for failure to thrive in a neonate with a congenital heart defect include all of the following *except*:
A. Increased basal metabolic rate
B. Respiratory distress
C. Catecholamine depletion
D. Decreased caloric intake

75. Which drug should be used with caution in the neonate with severe tetralogy of Fallot?
A. Propranolol
B. Digoxin
C. Furosemide
D. Prostaglandin E_1

76. A neonate with a history of abruptio placentae and suspected maternal substance abuse should be screened for which of the following substances?
A. Marijuana
B. Amphetamines
C. Heroin
D. Cocaine

77. A neonate estimated to be about 30 weeks gestation is in the neonatal intensive care unit. She has a respiratory rate of 78 breaths/minute, a heart rate of 170 beats/minute, and the presence of calf, palmar, and plantar pulses. The critical care nurse recognizes these clinical findings as consistent with:
A. Premature closure of the ductus arteriosus
B. A large ventricular septal defect
C. Total anomalous venous return
D. Patent ductus arterious

78. Patients experiencing respiratory distress related to increased pulmonary blood flow and elevated pulmonary pressures should be positioned with their head elevated to:
A. Increase peripheral perfusion
B. Increase vital capacity
C. Decrease the work of breathing
D. Increase cardiac output

Case Study

During the care of a 2-day-old newborn the critical care nurse notes that there are decreased bowel sounds and abdominal distension. The baby also appears to be more lethargic. Further examination reveals a gradual decrease in urine output over the last 12 hours, and the neonate's most recent stool tested positive for occult blood. The Apgar scores of this baby were 2 at one minute and 5 at five minutes. There had been some meconium aspiration that required suctioning and resuscitative effort in the delivery room. Questions 79 to 81 refer to this case study.

79. Based on the birth history and present signs and symptoms, the nurse suspects:
A. Respiratory distress syndrome
B. Diaphragmatic hernia
C. Hirschsprung's disease
D. Necrotizing enterocolitis

80. Other clinical signs and symptoms of this condition may include:
A. Increased gastric residuals, jaundice, bradycardia
B. Ileus, tachycardia, cyanosis, bright red vomitus
C. Current jelly-like stools, dehydration, bowel obstruction
D. Bright red rectal bleeding, jaundice, hypotension

81. After establishing that the baby is maintaining her airway well and her respiratory status is adequate, the *first* priority in caring for this infant would be:
A. Stop oral feedings and begin continuous tube feedings
B. Assess for infection by taking an accurate rectal temperature
C. Stop all feedings and put in an intravenous line for fluids
D. Test any gastric secretions for occult blood

82. A major reason for accurately determining gestational age and size for gestational age is to:
A. Assess nutritional needs
B. Prevent apnea
C. Determine metabolic needs
D. Predict common complications

83. An infant has been admitted to the critical care unit with a history of poor growth and feeding. Her current assessment findings include heart rate of 188 beats/minute, respiratory rate of 76 breaths/minute, nasal flaring, rales, and differential cyanosis. The most likely cause of these symptoms is:
A. Persistent pulmonary hypertension
B. Transient tachypnea of the newborn
C. Coarctation of the aorta
D. Diaphragmatic hernia

84. An important nursing intervention when caring for the infant of a mother with substance abuse is:
A. Ample eye contact to promote bonding
B. Minimal physical contact to avoid overstimulation
C. Use of firm mattresses to promote sense of security
D. Swaddling and rocking for comfort measures

Case Study

A neonate is admitted to the critical care unit appearing pale with retractions, tachypnea, grunting, nasal flaring, and use of accessory muscles. The chest x-ray is described as ground-glass in appearance. Breath sounds by auscultation are decreased. Blood gases are as follows:

pH: 7.30
pO_2: 53 torr
pCO_2: 49 torr
HCO_3^-: 18 mEq/L

Questions 85 and 86 refer to this case study.

---

85. This infant is showing signs and symptoms of:
A. Aspiration pneumonia
B. Persistent pulmonary hypertension
C. Respiratory distress syndrome
D. Bronchopulmonary dysplasia

86. An important factor in the development of respiratory disease in this patient is the pathophysiology of:
A. Decreased surfactant production
B. Decreased 2,3-DPG production
C. Increased surfactant metabolism
D. Increased 2,3-DPG production

87. Which of the following findings would indicate proper endotracheal tube placement immediately after intubation?
A. Presence of breath sounds over the upper left quadrant
B. Bronchial breath sounds over the trachea
C. Good excursion of the right chest during ventilation
D. Bilateral chest expansion with manual ventilation

88. Which diagnostic test would be most helpful in documenting blood flow through a patent ductus arteriosus?
A. Chest x-ray
B. Magnetic resonance imaging
C. Doppler echocardiography
D. Electrocardiogram

89. A neonate is determined to be small for gestational age and 34 weeks gestation. She has been intubated for hypoxia and apnea. She is on an FiO_2 of 0.8, pressure support, and a rate of 30 breaths/minute. Her physical examination reveals clear, bilateral breath sounds. At the end of her assessment, however, the critical care nurse notices a sudden drop in the pulse oximeter from 95% to 78%. The most important *immediate* nursing action would be to:
A. Check the patency of the endotracheal tube
B. Increase the FiO_2 to 1.0
C. Suction aggressively for a mucous plug
D. Pull back the endotracheal tube 1.5 cm

90. When working with drug dependent mothers, the critical care nurse should:
A. Encourage the mother to consider adoption or foster care
B. Look to a grandparent for a more stable parenting model
C. Be open and honest and avoid judgmental behavior
D. Order testing for HIV for the neonate

91. An umbilical vein catheter can be used to monitor:
A. Arterial blood pressure
B. Central venous pressure
C. Left atrial pressure
D. Left ventricular filling pressure

Case Study

A neonate is admitted to the NICU directly from the delivery room because he is bradycardic, hypothermic, and shows poor reflex activity. He is admitted with a tentative diagnosis of congenital hypothyroidism. Questions 92 and 93 refer to this case study.

---

92. During the admission assessment, the critical care nurse would anticipate all of the following findings *except*:
A. Thin, patchy hair pattern
B. Narrow pulse pressure
C. Abdominal distension
D. Cold, dry skin

93. Laboratory findings to confirm the diagnosis in this neonate would be:
A. Elevated protein bound iodine
B. High free thyroxine levels
C. Low T_4 and high TSH levels
D. Increased thyroxine levels

94. Grunting is often observed with respiratory distress. This breathing technique:
A. Increases vital capacity to decrease hypoxemia
B. Increases end expiratory pressure to promote gas exchange
C. Decreases large airway obstruction to decrease air trapping
D. Decreases the work of breathing to decrease oxygen demands

95. Which of the following nursing interventions will produce a more reliable peripheral measurement of the hematocrit?
A. Placing a blood pressure cuff around the upper arm, inflating to the systolic pressure, and waiting 1 minute
B. Placing the extremity in a dependent position to encourage venous engorgement
C. Wrapping the extremity in a warm pack to increase circulation to the area
D. Manually milking the extremity to encourage arterial flow and venous congestion

96. Infants in respiratory distress need to be positioned with their heads elevated about 30 degrees to:
A. Increase lung volume
B. Decrease work of breathing
C. Prevent aspiration
D. Decrease oxygen consumption

97. Atropine should not be used routinely during intubation to prevent vagal bradydysrhythmias because it may:
A. Cause laryngospasms and airway obstruction
B. Increase hypoxia by decreasing respiratory drive and chest wall excursion
C. Mask bradydysrhythmias from hypoxia associated with intubation
D. Increase the risk of aspiration as a result of increased production of secretions

98. Which of the following would be *most* helpful in determining the amount of placental separation in a placentae abruptio?
A. Complete blood cell count
B. Ultrasound
C. Amniocentesis
D. Vaginal examination

99. Postoperative care of a patient who has undergone repair of a tracheoesophageal fistula would include:
A. Deep suctioning to avoid leakage of gastric secretions into the trachea
B. Use of a pacifier to maintain oral stimulation in absence of oral feeds
C. Suctioning only to the end of the endotracheal tube
D. Use of a gastrostomy tube for feeding

Case Study

An infant is admitted to the neonatal intensive care unit following meconium aspiration with a diagnosis of hypoxic-ischemic encephalopathy (HIE). Initial Apgar scores were 4 at one minute and 6 at five minutes. Questions 100 to 103 refer to this case study.

100. The final Apgar score:
A. Represents severe distress
B. Does not accurately predict severity of HIE
C. Indicates mild to moderate HIE
D. Suggests clinical recovery

101. Physical examination of an infant with mild hypoxia would be expected to reveal:
A. Flaccid muscle tone, seizures, increased intracranial pressure
B. Poor brainstem function, convulsions, poor muscle tone
C. Lethargy, hypotonia, seizures, stupor
D. Irritability, poor sucking, uninhibited reflexes

102. Which of the following are common complications in other organ systems for the infant with hypoxic-ischemic encephalopathy?
A. Cardiogenic shock
B. Hyperbilirubinemia
C. Urinary retention
D. Pulmonary hypoplasia

103. A positive outcome for cardiac dysfunction related to HIE would include all of the following *except*:
A. Warm, pink extremities
B. Urinary output of 1 mL/kg/hr
C. Bounding peripheral pulses
D. Absence of pulmonary edema

104. A mother during labor suddenly complains of sharp, continuous pain in her abdomen. The nurses's assessment reveals a rigid and tender abdomen, decreased blood pressure, tachycardia, and diaphoresis. The nurse assures her that the physician is immediately notified and should take what *initial* action?
A. Prep the abdomen
B. Insert a Foley catheter
C. Order a type and cross match
D. Insert a large bore intravenous line

105. The most important initial nursing measure for the infant with HIE would be to:
A. Obtain a computed tomographic scan (CT scan) to evaluate neurologic injury
B. Maintain a patent airway, optimize oxygenation and ventilation
C. Evaluate renal function by monitoring urinary output closely
D. Assess for necrotizing enterocolitis by monitoring for occult blood in stool

106. Which of the following calculations of fluid therapy is optimal for a normovolemic neonate with respiratory distress syndrome who is intubated and mechanically ventilated?
A. 50% of maintenance fluid requirements
B. 75% of maintenance fluid requirements
C. 100% of maintenance fluid requirements
D. 125% of maintenance fluid requirements

107. An afebrile, acyanotic patient returned 12 hours ago from surgical repair of an omphalocele. During suctioning, the critical care nurse observes for the first time thick, clear to white secretions. Which nursing action would be most effective in promoting airway clearance?
A. Assess adequacy of humidification
B. Send sputum for culture and sensitivity
C. Use saline lavage to thin secretions
D. Use sterile suction technique only

108. A desired outcome in treating a patient with abruptio placentae is:
A. Liver palpable <2 to 3 cm below costal margin
B. Evidence of a Couvelaire uterus
C. Urinary output of ≥30 cc/hr
D. Absence of seizure activity

Case Study

A 3-day-old infant is admitted to the critical care unit with a history of irritability, opisthotonos, stridor, and periods of apnea. Sucking has been poor and the nurse at transfer reveals to the critical care nurse that the neonate has also been difficult to console, and actually quiets better when left lying on his stomach. The critical care nurse's assessment reveals an increased head circumference, decreased gag reflex, and bulging fontannels. The infant is diagnosed with hydrocephalus. Questions 109 to 111 refer to this case study.

---

109. Which of the following signs and symptoms would the critical care nurse recognize as indicating further serious deterioration in the infant's condition?
A. Lethargy
B. Lower extremity spasticity
C. Sluggish pupillary response
D. Emesis

110. Following placement of a ventriculoperitoneal (VP) shunt, the critical care nurse would recognize which of the following as a desired outcome?
A. Rapid return to a normal intracranial pressure (ICP)
B. Gag reflex with suctioning
C. Firm, round fontannels
D. Dilated scalp veins

111. Which of the following is *not* a likely potential complication of a ventriculoperitoneal shunt?
A. Subdural hematoma
B. Peritonitis
C. Intraventricular hemorrhage
D. Meningitis

112. Which of the following represents effective postoperative management of chest tubes in the infant who has undergone repair of a congenital diaphragmatic hernia?
A. Chest tube on affected side to water seal
B. Chest tube on unaffected side to water seal
C. Chest tube on affected side to low suction
D. Chest tube on unaffected side to low suction

113. The critical care nurse is caring for a patient receiving total parenteral nutrition through a central venous line. When there are 15 cc of solution left in the bottle that is hanging, the nurse discovers that the pharmacy has not brought the next bottle to the unit yet. Which action should the nurse take next?
A. Slow the infusion rate on the remaining 15 cc
B. Follow this bottle with normal saline and monitor serum glucoses carefully
C. Hang a 10% dextrose solution when the first bottle has infused, and monitor blood glucoses
D. Flush the line with heparin when the solution has infused to prevent clotting while the new bottle is prepared

114. An infant with a history of polyhydramnios is noted soon after birth to have copious oral secretions. The critical care nurse recognizes which of the following conditions as the most likely cause of these symptoms:
A. Down syndrome
B. Cleft lip
C. Tracheoesophageal fistula
D. Fulminant pulmonary edema

115. After endotracheal intubation, the critical care nurse notes decreased pulse oximetry readings, absent breath sounds and excursion in the left chest, and high peak pressure alarms on the ventilator. The critical care nurse suspects the patient has a:

A. Left pulmonary embolus
B. Pneumothorax
C. Pneumomediastinum
D. Right bronchial intubation

116. Which of the following parameters increases with bronchopulmonary dysplasia?

A. Functional residual capacity
B. Vital capacity
C. Tidal volume
D. Lung compliance

117. Apnea of prematurity is primarily caused by:

A. Underdevelopment of primary and accessory respiratory muscles
B. Ineffective central nervous system response to increased pCO_2
C. Decreased surfactant metabolism resulting in respiratory insufficiency
D. Failure to clear fluid from lungs in the immediate neonatal period

118. A neonate is found at birth to be severely tachypneic (rate of 115), with severe sternal retractions, nasal flaring, central cyanosis, and largely absent breath sounds. A chest x-ray demonstrates bowel located in the chest, an underdeveloped left lung, and the appearance of dextrocardia. The critical care nurse recognizes these symptoms as most consistent with:

A. Pneumothorax
B. Diaphragmatic hernia
C. Respiratory distress syndrome
D. Meconium aspiration

119. Postoperative ventilatory management of a 3200 g neonate with congenital diaphragmatic hernia includes mechanical ventilation with:

A. Peak inspiratory pressure of 30 cm H_2O
B. Tidal volume of 80 cc
C. Positive end expiratory pressure of 10 cm H_2O
D. Tidal volume of 30 cc

120. A nurse is caring for a mother who just experienced abruptio placentae. After ensuring her airway, breathing, and circulation were stable, attention turned to assessing fetal well-being. The best assessment of fetal well-being would be which of the following?

A. Fetal movement count
B. Evaluation of fetal heart rate
C. Vaginal examination
D. Ultrasound of the abdomen

121. An infant suspected of having duodenal atresia is noted to pass a small amount of light-colored stool from his rectum. The nurse knows this:
A. Rules out a diagnosis of duodenal atresia
B. Is not normal meconium and is consistent with duodenal atresia
C. Makes a diagnosis of intussusception more likely
D. Is more consistent with necrotizing enterocolitis

122. Administering 100% oxygen at rapid ventilatory rates to the infant suspected of having persistent pulmonary hypertension of the newborn is helpful in:
A. Improving PaO_2 as a result of recruitment of lung areas
B. Improving PaO_2 by dilating pulmonary vessels
C. Confirming the diagnosis because the PaO_2 is not improved
D. Improving refractory hypercarbia

123. An infant with persistent pulmonary hypertension and a patent ductus arteriosus is at risk for developing:
A. Ascites
B. Pleural effusion
C. Pulmonary hemorrhage
D. Hepatomegaly

124. Which of the interventions listed below would be the *highest* priority when preparing a patient for an emergency cesarean section following a placentae abruptio?
A. Sending a urine for toxicology screen when catheterizing
B. Omitting surgical consent because of the urgency of surgery
C. Obtaining liver function studies with other blood work
D. Notifying the primary pediatrician

125. A neonate has an indirect bilirubin level of 21 mg/dL at 26 hours of age, an increased reticulocyte count, and microspherocytes and spherocytes seen in his peripheral blood smear. The infant is diagnosed with ABO hemolytic disease. Which of the following interventions should receive the *highest* priority?
A. Transfuse the infant 15 mg/kg of whole blood
B. Administer ferrous sulfate 6 mg/kg/day
C. Infuse 2 mL/kg of packed red blood cells
D. Prepare for an exchange transfusion

126. Which of the following is not associated with the development of idiopathic respiratory distress syndrome (IRDS)?
A. Lecithin/sphingomyelin (L/S) ratio of 3:1
B. Prematurity
C. Persistent fetal circulation
D. Low birth weight

127. Which of the following infants is at greatest risk for developing transient tachypnea of the newborn (TTN)?
A. A spontaneous vaginal delivery: 36 weeks gestation
B. A cesarean section delivery: 41 weeks gestation
C. An induced vaginal delivery: 43 weeks gestation
D. A vaginal delivery with epidural anesthesia: 38 weeks gestation

128. In order to mobilize secretions in the posterior upper right lobe, the critical care nurse would position an infant in:
A. Right side elevated 45 degrees and prone
B. Left side elevated 45 degrees and prone
C. Right side elevated 45 degrees and supine
D. Left side elevated 45 degrees and supine

129. The critical care nurse would review cardiac tests such as the echocardiogram and electrocardiogram for which of the following conditions when caring for an infant born by emergency cesarean section for prolapsed cord?
A. Right ventricular dilatation
B. Left ventricular hypertrophy
C. Coronary artery insufficiency
D. Junctional nodal rhythms

130. Which of the following signs and symptoms of electrolyte disturbance would the critical care nurse anticipate in caring for an infant born of a mother treated for eclampsia?
A. Weakness, lethargy, hypotonia, poor suck, apnea, hypotension
B. Muscle weakness, peaked T-waves on electrocardiogram, widened QRS complex
C. Apnea, irritability, twitching, seizures
D. Listlessness, irritability, apnea, seizures, coma

131. Which of the following is proper suctioning of the neonate who does not have an artificial airway?
A. Perform chest physiotherapy, suction the nasopharyngeal airway, then suction the mouth
B. Suction the mouth, suction the nasopharyngeal airway, then perform chest physiotherapy
C. Suction the mouth, perform chest physiotherapy, then suction the nasopharyngeal airway
D. Perform chest physiotherapy, suction the mouth, then suction the nasopharyngeal airway

132. High frequency ventilation is helpful in reducing barotrauma by:
A. Using large tidal volumes delivered at low pressures
B. Using large tidal volumes delivered at reduced peak inspiratory pressures
C. Using small tidal volumes delivered at the mean airway pressure
D. Using normal tidal volumes delivered at low pressures

133. A premature infant was just intubated for apnea of 30 seconds unresponsive to tactile stimulation and manual ventilation. When auscultating breath sounds, the critical care nurse hears good breath sounds in the right chest, but absent breath sounds on the left. Which of the following is the best *immediate* action?

A. Continue to advance tube until breath sounds are heard bilaterally
B. Remove tube and manually ventilate until the infant can be reintubated
C. Call for stat x-ray and continue to manually ventilate the infant
D. Pull tube back slowly until breath sounds are heard bilaterally

134. A premature infant on long-term ventilatory therapy requiring high positive pressure support to achieve an adequate tidal volume develops an air leak accompanied by severe respiratory distress. Which of the following interventions would the critical care nurse anticipate first in treating this infant?

A. Immediate reduction of pressure support
B. Atropine to treat bradycardia
C. Lower the head of the bed
D. Needle aspiration of air

135. Bronchopulmonary dysplasia is least likely to be associated with which of the following?

A. High FiO_2 administration
B. Hypovolemia
C. Infection
D. Prematurity

136. All of the following are factors associated with the development of necrotizing enterocolitis in the preterm infant *except*:

A. Breast milk
B. Early feedings
C. Low birth weight
D. Respiratory distress syndrome

137. An infant of 30 weeks gestation exhibits periods of apnea lasting 5 to 10 seconds and periods of breathing of 10 to 15 seconds. What is the most likely cause of this pattern?

A. Periodic breathing
B. Apnea of prematurity
C. Transient tachypnea
D. Apneustic breathing

138. At admission to the neonatal intensive care unit, the critical care nurse observes acrocyanosis. The best action for the nurse to take next would be:

A. Administer ¼ liter flow of oxygen by nasal cannula
B. Place the infant in 30% oxygen hood
C. Suction mouth and nose
D. Observe for central cyanosis

139. For which of the following is an infant of 32 weeks gestation at the *least* risk?
A. Persistent pulmonary hypertension
B. Patent ductus arteriosus
C. Apnea of prematurity
D. Hypoglycemia

140. Which of the following tests would not help identify a metabolic cause of apnea in a premature infant?
A. Arterial blood gases
B. Ionized calcium level
C. Serum magnesium level
D. Complete blood count

141. When parents are used as directed donors for their neonates, which of the following statements is most advisable to avoid serious adverse effects?
A. All parentally donated blood should be irradiated
B. Fathers may donate platelets but not red cells
C. Mothers can safely donate plasma but not red cells
D. Fathers may donate red cells only

142. Increasing the respiratory rate in an intubated infant with persistent pulmonary hypertension has which of the following effects:
A. Decreases pCO_2, causes vasodilation of the pulmonary vessels, decreases right-to-left shunting
B. Increases pO_2, causes vasodilation of the pulmonary vessels, decreases right-to-left shunting
C. Increases pCO_2, causes vasodilation of the systemic vessels, decreases left-to-right shunting
D. Increases pO_2, causes vasodilation of the systemic vessels, decreases left-to-right shunting

143. An infant in respiratory distress will assume which of the following positions when possible?
A. Fetal position
B. Sniffing position
C. Knee-chest position
D. Neck flexion position

144. A premature infant is receiving 30% oxygen via hood. In order to monitor the effectiveness of therapy and prevent complications related to oxygen therapy, which of the following is required?
A. Arterial blood gases once a shift
B. Continuous SvO_2 monitoring
C. Ongoing assessment for cyanosis
D. Continuous pulse oximetry monitoring

145. Which of the following statements is most appropriate for the critical care nurse to share with the parents of an infant with mild HIE?

A. "Generally there are no long-term problems with brain damage."
B. "Between two and four infants out of ten will have long-term brain damage."
C. "Nearly all infants will have permanent brain damage."
D. "Brain damage depends upon how long the baby is artificially ventilated."

146. Infants at risk for developing pulmonary hemorrhage include all of the following *except*:

A. Asphyxia
B. Sepsis
C. Low birth weight
D. Oxygen toxicity

147. In a neonate who manifests jaundice within the first 24 hours of life, which of the following is most likely responsible for the hyperbilirubinemia?

A. Sepsis
B. Isoimmunization
C. Physiologic jaundice
D. Breast milk jaundice

148. Dehydration in the neonate with an omphalocele develops *primarily* because of:

A. Third-spacing of fluid
B. Large amounts of watery stools
C. Nasogastric suctioning
D. Evaporative losses

149. A lumbar puncture is ordered for a full term infant with a decreased level of responsiveness, irritability, hyperventilation, and seizure activity 1 hour before the test. The results were as follows:

CSF pressure:	normal
White blood cell count:	4 cells/mm^3
Red blood cell count:	0 cells/mm^3
Protein:	53 mg/dL
Glucose:	54 mg/dL

Which of the following diagnoses is *most likely* based on these findings?

A. Encephalopathy
B. Viral meningitis
C. Bacterial meningitis
D. Intraventricular hemorrhage

150. A 3-day-old infant is diagnosed with acute respiratory failure secondary to apnea of prematurity. In order to minimize multisystem organ failure, which of the following treatments would be most effective?

A. Maintain a hematocrit greater than 40% to increase oxygen delivery
B. Maintain PaO_2 greater than 90% to minimize hypoxemia
C. Maintain low normal cardiac index to decrease cardiac work
D. Increase stimulation to avoid apneic episodes

151. An infant with aspiration pneumonia from oral secretions would be expected to increase their oxygen consumption as a result of which of the following clinical conditions?

A. Fever
B. Seizures
C. Shivering
D. Decreased pO_2

Case Study

A new born full term infant is admitted to the neonatal intensive care unit in septic shock. The infant appears pale, with weak femoral and brachial pulses, a heart rate of 200, and a respiratory rate of 70 with nasal flaring and retractions. The infant is electively intubated based on clinical evaluation of the work of breathing as well as blood gases. Questions 152 and 153 refer to this case study.

---

152. At suctioning, the nurse notes large amounts of bright red blood in the catheter. Which of the following is most likely the cause of bleeding?

A. Trauma from intubation
B. Pulmonary hemorrhage
C. Pulmonary hemosiderosis
D. Trauma related to suctioning

153. Initial treatment of this infant would include fluid resuscitation to achieve a CVP of:

A. 10 cm H_2O
B. 5 cm H_2O
C. 15 cm H_2O
D. 2 cm H_2O

154. A perinatal history consistent with a diagnosis of duodenal atresia includes:

A. Meconium staining
B. Polyhydramnios
C. Preterm labor
D. Metabolic acidosis

Case Study

At birth, an infant is noted to have severe respiratory distress, pronounced heart sounds in the right chest, and a scaphoid abdomen. Questions 155 to 157 refer to this case study.

---

155. The infant is judged to need immediate ventilatory assistance. Which of the following would be contraindicated?
A. Ventilation with a bag and mask
B. Intubation and mechanical ventilation at high rates
C. Intubation and mechanical ventilation at low pressures
D. Mechanical ventilation with paralysis

156. All of the following are priorities for the critical care nurse to monitor in this infant *except*:
A. Preductal saturations
B. Postductal saturations
C. Arterial blood gases
D. Capillary blood gases

157. Additional immediate interventions for this infant include the placement of a nasogastric tube. This is important because it:
A. Provides a route for feeding
B. Prevents aspiration
C. Decreases compression of lungs
D. Decreases shunting

158. Most preterm infants demonstrate which mechanism of apnea?
A. Central apnea
B. Obstructive apnea
C. Neural apnea
D. Mixed apnea

159. All of the following are risk factors related to apnea of preterm infants *except*:
A. Feeding
B. Nasogastric intubation
C. Infection
D. Periodic breathing

160. Which of the following feedings is preferred for an infant whose bowel function has returned following necrotizing enterocolitis?
A. Full strength soy formula
B. Hyperosmolar feedings to increase caloric intake
C. Low osmotic feedings
D. Full strength milk-based formula

161. A 32-week gestation infant is in a 30% oxygen hood and has been noted to have periods of apnea. When the critical care nurse responds to the apnea alarm, the infant is found to have a heart rate of 72 and slight circumoral cyanosis. The first intervention the nurse should do is:
A. Gently stimulate the infant by touch
B. Make a loud noise by clapping or banging
C. Ventilate the infant with a mask and bag
D. Prepare for intubation

162. In assessing an infant with HIE, the critical care nurse recognizes which of the following findings as likely indicating persistent and permanent neurological dysfunction?
A. Seizure activity more than 48 hours following birth
B. Hypotonia 24 hours after birth
C. Dilation of pupils during the first 24 hours
D. Little spontaneous movement during the first 12 hours

163. During feedings, a 33-week gestation infant is noted to have periods of apnea. Which of the following is not a probable cause?
A. Poor coordination of sucking and swallowing
B. Swallowing of air during feeding
C. Gastroesophageal reflux
D. Flexion of the neck during feedings

164. Which of the following positions aids in improving ventilation/perfusion matching?
A. Prone
B. Supine
C. Left lateral
D. Knee-chest

165. A preterm infant is being treated with a methylxanthine for apnea. Which of the following are not toxic or side effects of these drugs?
A. Hypotension and tachycardia
B. Paradoxical apnea
C. Exacerbation of poor nutritional status
D. Seizures

166. Theophylline would be used with caution in an infant with which of the following conditions?
A. Hypovolemia
B. Apnea of prematurity
C. Central apnea
D. Congenital heart block

167. Preterm infants are prone to intraventricular hemorrhages because they:
- **A.** Frequently have clotting disorders
- **B.** Are more likely to receive trauma to the head during delivery
- **C.** Have more vascularization in the ventricular areas
- **D.** Have higher intracranial pressures

Case Study

A 1550 g female infant is born at 38 weeks gestation. She is 46 cm in length and has a head circumference of 32 cm. Questions 168 and 169 refer to this case study.

---

168. This infant is properly classified as:
- **A.** Appropriate for gestational age (AGA)
- **B.** Small for gestational age (SGA)
- **C.** Large for gestational age (LGA)
- **D.** Symmetrically growth retarded

169. For what complication is this infant at greatest risk in the first 8 to 12 hours after birth?
- **A.** Hyperbilirubinemia
- **B.** Apnea
- **C.** Respiratory distress syndrome
- **D.** Hypoglycemia

170. Continuous positive airway pressure (CPAP) is a respiratory therapy often used to treat apnea in newborns. For which of the following types of apnea is CPAP not effective?
- **A.** Obstructive apnea
- **B.** Mixed apnea
- **C.** Apnea of prematurity
- **D.** Central apnea

171. Which of the following provides the best information about the adequacy of tidal volume for a mechanically ventilated infant?
- **A.** A calculated tidal volume of 10 cc/kg
- **B.** A peak inspiratory pressure of 18 cm H_2O
- **C.** Adequate chest wall movement
- **D.** A PaO_2 of greater than 90 mm Hg

172. For neonates who require intubation, high pressures, and high FiO_2, oxygenation should be monitored by:

A. Arterial blood gases at least every 2 to 4 hours and continuous pulse oximetry
B. Arterial blood gases as least every hour and continuous transcutaneous oxygen monitoring
C. Preductal and postductal arterial blood gas sampling every 6 hours and transcutaneous oxygen monitoring
D. Umbilical arterial and venous blood gas sampling every 8 hours and continuous pulse oximetry

173. When observing the infant with hyperbilirubinemia, the critical care nurse would be most concerned with which of the following findings?

A. Dermal icterus
B. Irritable cry
C. Increased urine output
D. Loose stools

174. Use of an umbilical artery catheter has been associated with all of the following *except*:

A. Necrotizing enterocolitis
B. Embolic incidents
C. Hypertension
D. Intracranial hemorrhages

175. Which of the following do *not* increase oxygen consumption in the neonate?

A. Hypothermia
B. Sepsis
C. Fever
D. Chemical paralysis

176. For which of the following conditions would intralipids be contraindicated?

A. Platelet count of 80,000/mm^3
B. Hematocrit of 28%
C. Sodium of 150 mEq/L
D. Negative occult stools

Case Study

The critical care nurse is caring for an infant of a diabetic mother (IDM) who is large for gestational age (LGA). The cardiac monitor is showing abnormal heart rhythms. Questions 177 to 179 refer to this case study.

---

177. Which of the following electrolyte imbalances, which can cause dysrhythmias, is most common in an IDM who is LGA?
A. Hypernatremia
B. Hyponatremia
C. Hypercalcemia
D. Hypocalcemia

178. Which of the following orders would the critical care nurse recognize as appropriate for this patient?
A. Monitor serum calcium—elevated levels usually normalize without treatment
B. Administer calcium gluconate 10% 3 mL/kg for hypocalcemia
C. Restrict fluids and improve ventilation to normalize hyponatremia
D. Restrict sodium in IV fluids, sodium bicarbonate, and other medications

179. Which nursing diagnosis is appropriate for this infant?
A. High risk for altered body temperature
B. Fluid volume deficit
C. Impaired swallowing
D. Altered tissue perfusion

180. Which of the following natural compensatory mechanisms in infants mimics the therapeutic use of continuous distending pressure?
A. Nasal flaring
B. Grunting
C. Use of accessory muscles
D. Tachypnea

181. Which of the following replacement therapies is the most appropriate for a neonate undergoing exchange transfusion for Rh hemolytic disease?
A. Freshly donated red blood cells
B. Banked red blood cells
C. Albumin
D. 10% dextrose solution

182. Which of the following signs would the nurse look for as an adverse response to the use of positive end expiratory pressure in an infant undergoing mechanical ventilation?
A. Decreased chest wall movement
B. Decreased peripheral pulses
C. Decreased breath sounds over the left lung field
D. Increased right-to-left shunting

183. When analyzing blood gases, which of the following findings would the nurse recognize as a problem associated with the use of positive end expiratory pressure?
A. Increase in pCO_2
B. Decrease in pO_2
C. Increase in pH
D. Decrease in arterial saturation

184. A term neonate has been diagnosed with persistent pulmonary hypertension. Treatment includes intubation and mechanical ventilation with high ventilatory rates. Despite mechanical ventilation, oxygenation remains inadequate and right-to-left shunting is significant. Which of the following would the nurse anticipate being used next to improve oxygenation and decrease shunting?
A. Further increase ventilatory rate
B. Sedation and paralysis
C. Increase the FiO_2 and tidal volume
D. Decrease the respiratory rate

185. Which of the following may be helpful in preventing atelectasis after extubation following prolonged mechanical ventilatory support?
A. Nasal CPAP
B. Racemic epinephrine
C. Aminophylline
D. Caffeine

186. A 28 week gestation infant was intubated and mechanically ventilated for 2 weeks for respiratory distress syndrome. Despite aggressive respiratory management, the neonate's need for an FiO_2 of 0.6 and pressures of 36/6 were constant and progress in weaning was poor. What diagnostic test would be indicated to rule out another commonly associated pathology?
A. Echocardiogram
B. Electrocardiogram
C. Renal ultrasound
D. Liver enzyme tests

187. In preterm infants, the most common source of bleeding in an intraventricular hemorrhage is the:
A. Choroid plexus
B. Arachnoid villae
C. Germinal matrix
D. Meningeal artery

188. Which of the following would be used to help medically close a patent ductus arteriosus?
A. Prostaglandin E_1 at 0.05 to 0.1 mcg/kg/min
B. Prostaglandin E_1 at 0.05 to 0.1 mcg/kg dose
C. Indomethacin 0.1 to 0.3 mg/kg dose
D. Indomethacin 0.1 to 0.3 mg/kg/min

189. A neonate with congenital bilateral choanal atresia should also have which of the following diagnostic tests?
A. Liver function tests
B. Echocardiogram
C. Renal ultrasound
D. Barium swallow

190. A full term infant weighing 9720 g is admitted to the critical care unit with cyanosis, metabolic acidosis, and hypoxemia. No murmur is auscultated. This patient's pulse oximetry reading at admission is 75% on 100% oxygen after being intubated in the delivery room. Which of the following diagnoses is most likely?
A. Transient tachypnea of the newborn
B. Respiratory distress syndrome
C. Transposition of the great arteries
D. Peripheral pulmonary stenosis

191. A 10-hour-old 4.2 kg infant of a diabetic mother is observed to be lethargic, have poor muscle tone, and feeding poorly. The *first* action the critical care nurse should take is:
A. Perform a heelstick and measure the glucose level by reagent strip
B. Administer 4 mL of 25% dextrose solution
C. Send a serum sample to the laboratory for determination of the serum glucose level
D. Increase the intravenous infusion of 5% dextrose solution to 25 mL/hr

192. Which of the following therapies is most effective in reducing the development of chronic lung diseases and bronchopulmonary dysplasia in neonates?
A. FiO_2 >0.5 to reduce hypoxemia
B. PEEP levels of 8 to 10 cm H_2O to prevent airway collapse
C. Maintenance fluid therapy of 150 mL/kg/day to prevent tenacious secretions and airway obstruction
D. Indomethacin therapy to close a patent ductus arteriosus

193. What abnormal laboratory results would the critical care nurse anticipate in an LGA infant?
A. Hematocrit: 65%
B. White blood cell count: 26,000/mm^3
C. Hemoglobin: 12.7 g/dL
D. Platelets: 100,000/mm^3

194. To monitor for complications in an infant following surgical repair of gastroschisis, the critical care nurse would look for arterial blood gases that had an elevation in:
A. pO_2
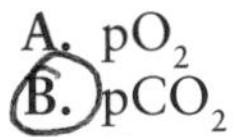
B. pCO_2
C. Base excess
D. pH

195. Nutritional support is critical in infants with bronchopulmonary dysplasia for all of the following reasons *except*:
- A. There is an increase in oxygen consumption
- B. To prevent fractures
- C. To prevent infection
- D. To increase metabolic demand

196. Orders for phototherapy have just been written on a neonate with hyperbilirubinemia. The critical care nurse should prepare the infant by:
- A. Removing all clothing except the diaper to protect the genital area
- B. Removing all clothing including the diaper to maximally expose the skin
- C. Removing all clothing except the diaper and a small shirt to prevent hypothermia
- D. Removing all clothing except a stocking cap to prevent heat loss

197. Neonatal seizures related to pyridoxine deficiency are related to a deficiency in:
- A. Vitamin C
- B. Iron
- C. Magnesium
- D. Vitamin B_6

198. Which of the following defines large for gestational age?
- A. A postterm infant weighing more than the 75th percentile
- B. A preterm infant weighing more than the 10th percentile
- C. A term infant weighing more than the 50th percentile for gestational age
- D. Any infant weighing more than the 90th percentile for gestational age

199. Pneumatosis intestinalis is the hallmark of which condition?
- A. Volvulus
- B. Necrotizing enterocolitis
- C. Hirschsprung's disease
- D. Tracheoesophageal fistula

200. Small for gestational age infants who are term are at risk for which of the following:
- A. Hypoglycemia, meconium aspiration, congenital malformations
- B. Apnea, hyperbilirubinemia, hyaline membrane disease
- C. Congenital malformations, hyperbilirubinemia, hyperglycemia
- D. Meconium aspiration, apnea, hyaline membrane disease

Neonatal Test Answers

1. A
2. C
3. D
4. B
5. D
6. D
7. A
8. A
9. A
10. A
11. C
12. B
13. D
14. D
15. A
16. A
17. D
18. A
19. A
20. D
21. D
22. C
23. B
24. B
25. C
26. B
27. C
28. B
29. C
30. C
31. D
32. A
33. A
34. D
35. C
36. D
37. C
38. C
39. B
40. B
41. A
42. A
43. B
44. A
45. C
46. A
47. A
48. C
49. B
50. C
51. B
52. C
53. D
54. A
55. C
56. A
57. A
58. C
59. B
60. C
61. A
62. A
63. D
64. B
65. C
66. D
67. C
68. B
69. A
70. B
71. D
72. A
73. B
74. C
75. B
76. D
77. D
78. B
79. D
80. A
81. C
82. D
83. C
84. D

85. C
86. A
87. D
88. C
89. A
90. C
91. B
92. A
93. C
94. B
95. C
96. A
97. C
98. B
99. C
100. B
101. D
102. A
103. C
104. D
105. B
106. B
107. A
108. C
109. D
110. B
111. C
112. A
113. C
114. C
115. D
116. A
117. B
118. B
119. D
120. B
121. B
122. B
123. C
124. A
125. D
126. A
127. B
128. A
129. A
130. A
131. D
132. C
133. D
134. D
135. B
136. A
137. A
138. D
139. A
140. D
141. A
142. A
143. B
144. D
145. A
146. D
147. B
148. A
149. A
150. B
151. A
152. B
153. A
154. B
155. A
156. D
157. C
158. D
159. D
160. C
161. C
162. A
163. B
164. A
165. B
166. A
167. C
168. B
169. D
170. D
171. C
172. A
173. B
174. D
175. D
176. A

177. D
178. B
179. A
180. B
181. A
182. B
183. A
184. B
185. A
186. A
187. C
188. C
189. B
190. C
191. A
192. D
193. A
194. B
195. D
196. B
197. D
198. D
199. B
200. A

SCORING YOUR EXAMINATION

Below 65% (less than 130 correct answers):
You are not in the passing range yet. Keep studying. Evaluate where your weaknesses are, but keep reviewing all the material. Don't try to cram; just study whenever you can and review, review, review. This will help you master the material.

65% to 75% (130 to 150 correct answers):
You are barely above the passing mark of 65% or 130 correct answers. Keep studying! Try to pinpoint the body system or types of questions causing you the most difficulty and focus your attention on these areas.

75% to 85% (150 to 170 correct answers):
You are doing very well! Keep reviewing to continue to master the material, but relax and increase your confidence. Review the test-taking strategies in Chapter 9 again to eliminate any factor that nerves or anxiety may have on your final score.

85% to 100% (170 to 200 correct answers):
What a terrific job! Keep reviewing the material to keep it fresh. Congratulations!

Bibliography

CARDIOVASCULAR

Alspach JG: *Core curriculum for critical care nursing,* ed 4, Philadelphia, 1991, WB Saunders Co.

Baker A: Acquired heart disease in infants and children, *Crit Care Nurs Clin North Am* 6(1):175-186, 1994.

Beachy P, Deacon J: *Core curriculum for neonatal intensive care nursing,* Philadelphia, 1992, WB Saunders Co.

Blumer JL, editor: *A practical guide to pediatric intensive care,* St Louis, 1990, Mosby.

Brown PA, Blayney F, Brown CA, Evans KG: *Quick reference to pediatric intensive care nursing,* Rockville, MD, 1989, Aspen Publishers, Inc.

Czerwinski SJ: Complications of pediatric trauma, *Crit Care Nurs Clin North Am* 3(3):479-489, 1991.

Dickenson CM: Thoracic trauma in children, *Crit Care Nurs Clin North Am* 3(3):423-443, 1991.

Elixson EM: Hemodynamic monitoring modalities in pediatric cardiac surgical patients, *Crit Care Nurs Clin North Am* 1(2):263-274, 1989.

Fanaroff AA, Martin RJ, editors: *Neonatal-perinatal medicine: diseases of the fetus and infant,* ed 5, St Louis, 1990, Mosby.

Fink BW: *Congenital heart disease; a deductive approach to its diagnosis,* ed 3, St Louis, 1991, Mosby.

Foldy SM, Gorman JB: Perioperative nursing care for congenital cardiac defects, *Crit Care Nurs Clin North Am* 1(2):231-244, 1989.

Fuhrman BP, Zimmerman JJ, editors: *Pediatric critical care,* St Louis, 1992, Mosby.

Gerraughty AB: Caring for patients with lesions obstructing systemic blood flow, *Crit Care Nurs Clin North Am* 1(2):231-244, 1989.

Hazinski MF, editor: *Nursing care of the critically ill child,* ed 2, St Louis, 1992, Mosby.

Jensen C, Hill CS: Mechanical support for congestive heart failure in infants and children, *Crit Care Nurs Clin North Am* 6(1):165-174, 1994.

Johnston J: Cardiac transplantation in early infancy, *Crit Care Nurs Clin North Am* 4(3):521-526, 1992.

Josker J, Maciejewski M, Cousins M: Advanced case studies in hemodynamic monitoring, *Crit Care Nurs Clin North Am* 6(1):187-197, 1994.
Klaus MH, Fanaroff AA, editors: *Care of the high-risk neonate,* ed 4, Philadelphia, 1993, WB Saunders Co.
Kulik LA: Caring for patients with lesions decreasing pulmonary flow, *Crit Care Nurs Clin North Am* 1(2):215-230, 1989.
Long WA, editor: *Fetal and neonatal cardiology,* Philadelphia, 1990, WB Saunders Co.
Merenstein GB, Gardner SL, editors: *Handbook of neonatal intensive care,* ed 2, St Louis, 1989, Mosby.
Moloney-Harmon P: Initial assessment and stabilization of the critically injured child, *Crit Care Nurs Clin North Am* 3(3):399-410, 1991.
Noonan DM, Koster NK, White-Traut R: Nursing considerations for the neonate awaiting heart transplantation for the hypoplastic left heart syndrome, *J Pediatr Nurs,* 6(5):322-330, 1991.
Norris MKG, House MA: *Organ and tissue transplantation: nursing care from procurement through rehabilitation,* Philadelphia, 1991, FA Davis Co.
Norris MKG, Roland J-MA: Perioperative management of pulmonary circulation in children with congenital cardiac defects, *ACAN Clin Issues Crit Care Nurs* 5(3):255-262, 1994.
Sigardson-Poor KM, Haggerty LM: *Nursing care of the transplant recipient,* Philadelphia, 1990, WB Saunders Co.
Thelan LA, Davie JK, Urden L, Lough ME: *Critical care nursing: diagnosis and management,* ed 2, St Louis, 1994, Mosby.
Wong DL: *Whaley and Wong's nursing care of infants and children,* ed 5, St Louis, 1995, Mosby.

PULMONARY

Alspach JG: *Core curriculum for critical care nursing,* ed 4, Philadelphia, 1991, WB Saunders Co.
Battista MA, Carlo WA: Differential diagnosis of acute respiratory distress in the neonate, *Neonat Resp Diseases* 2(3):1-4, 9-11, 1992.
Beachy P, Deacon J: *Core curriculum for neonatal intensive care nursing,* Philadelphia, 1992, WB Saunders Co.
Blumer JL, editor: *A practical guide to pediatric intensive care,* St Louis, 1990, Mosby.
Brown PA, Playney F, Brown CA, Evans KG: *Quick reference to pediatric intensive care nursing,* Rockville, MD, 1989, Aspen Publishers, Inc.
Cunningham K, Paes BA, Symington A: Pulmonary interstitial emphysema: a review, *Neonat Netw* 11(5):7-15, 1992.
Czerwinski SJ: Complications of pediatric trauma, *Crit Care Nurs Clin North Am* 3(3):479-489, 1991.
Dickenson CM: Thoracic trauma in children, *Crit Care Nurs Clin North Am* 3(3):423-443, 1991.
Fanaroff AA, Martin RJ, editors: *Neonatal-perinatal medicine: diseases of the fetus and infant,* ed 5, St Louis, 1990, Mosby.
Fuhrman BP, Zimmerman JJ, editors: *Pediatric critical care,* St Louis, 1992, Mosby.
Green J: Recognizing epiglottitis, *Nursing 92,* 22(8):33, 1992.
Grisemer AN: Apnea of prematurity: current management and nursing implications, *Pediatr Nurs* 16(6):606-611, 1990.
Gomberg SM: Mistaken identity: is it epiglottitis or croup? *Pediatr Nurs* 16(6):567-570, 1990.
Grobman DW, Foley MM: Surfactant replacement therapy in newborns with hyaline membrane disease, *Crit Care Nurs Clin North Am* 4(3):515-520, 1992.

Harris J, Culp S, Nicolayson R, Waterman C, Whitehorn SL: Respiratory syncytial virus: a pediatric nursing plan of care, *J Pediatr Nurs* 7(2):128-132, 1992.
Hazinski MF, editor: *Nursing care of the critically ill child,* ed 2, St Louis, 1992, Mosby.
Klaus MH, Fanaroff AA, editors: *Care of the high-risk neonate,* ed 4, Philadelphia, 1993, WB Saunders Co.
Merenstein GB, Gardner SL, editors: *Handbook of neonatal intensive care,* ed 2, St Louis, 1989, Mosby.
Moynihan PJ, King R: Caring for patients with lesions increasing pulmonary blood flow, *Crit Care Nurs Clin North Am* 1(2):195-214, 1989.
Myrer ML: New trends in neonatal mechanical ventilation, *Crit Care Nurs Clin North Am* 4(3):507-514, 1992.
Palmisano JM, Martin JM, Krauzowicz BA, Truman KH, Meliones JN: Effects of supplemental oxygen administration in an infant with pulmonary artery hypertension, *Heart Lung* 19(6):627-630, 1990.
Thelan LA, Davie JK, Urden LD, Lough ME: *Critical care nursing: diagnosis and management,* ed 2, St Louis, 1994, Mosby.
Wong DL: *Whaley and Wong's nursing care of infants and children,* ed 5, St Louis, 1995, Mosby.

ENDOCRINE

Alspach JG: *Core curriculum for critical care nursing,* ed 4, Philadelphia, 1991, WB Saunders Co.
Beachey P, Deacon J: *Core curriculum for neonatal intensive care nursing,* Philadelphia, 1992, WB Saunders Co.
Blumer JL, editor: *A practical guide to pediatric intensive care,* St Louis, 1990, Mosby.
Fanaroff AA, Martin RJ, editors: *Neonatal-perinatal medicine: diseases of the fetus and infant,* ed 5, St Louis, 1990, Mosby.
Fuhrman BP, Zimmerman JJ, editors: *Pediatric critical care,* St Louis, 1992, Mosby.
Hazinski MF, editor: *Nursing care of the critically ill child,* ed 2, St Louis, 1992, Mosby.
Klaus MH, Fanaroff AA, editors: *Care of the high-risk neonate,* ed 4, Philadelphia, 1993, WB Saunders Co.
Merenstein GB, Gardner SL, editors: *Handbook of neonatal intensive care,* ed 2, St Louis, 1989, Mosby.
Wong DL: *Whaley and Wong's nursing care of infants and children,* ed 5, St Louis, 1995, Mosby.

HEMATOLOGY/IMMUNOLOGY

Alspach JG: *Core curriculum for critical care nursing,* ed 4, Philadelphia, 1991, WB Saunders Co.
Beachy P, Deacon J: *Core curriculum for neonatal intensive care nursing,* Philadelphia, 1992, WB Saunders Co.
Blumer JL, editor: *A practical guide to pediatric intensive care,* St Louis, 1990, Mosby.
Brown PA, Playney F, Brown CA, Evans KG: *Quick reference to pediatric intensive care nursing,* Rockville, MD, 1989, Aspen Publishers, Inc.
Czarniecki L, Dillman P: Pediatric HIV/AIDS, *Crit Care Nurs Clin North Am* 4(3):447-456, 1992.
Fanaroff AA, Martin RJ, editors: *Neonatal-perinatal medicine: diseases of the fetus and infant,* ed 5, St Louis, 1990, Mosby.
Fuhrman BP, Zimmerman JJ, editors: *Pediatric critical care,* St Louis, 1992, Mosby.
Hazinski MF, editor: *Nursing care of the critically ill child,* ed 2, St Louis, 1992, Mosby.
Klaus MH, Fanaroff AA, editors: *Care of the high-risk neonate,* ed 4, Philadelphia, 1993, WB Saunders Co.

Lewis A: *Nursing care of the person with AIDS/ARC,* Rockville, MD, 1988, Aspen Publishers, Inc.
Merenstein GB, Gardner SL, editors: *Handbook of neonatal intensive care,* ed 2, St Louis, 1989, Mosby.
Moon MW: Pediatric HIV/AIDS, *Crit Care Nurs Clin North Am* 4(3):457-465, 1992.
Wong DL: *Whaley and Wong's nursing care of infants and children,* ed 5, St Louis, 1995, Mosby.

NEUROLOGY

Alspach JG: *Core curriculum for critical care nursing,* ed 4, Philadelphia, 1991, WB Saunders Co.
Beachy P, Deacon J: *Core curriculum for neonatal intensive care nursing,* Philadelphia, 1992, WB Saunders Co.
Blumer JL, editor: *A practical guide to pediatric intensive care,* St Louis, 1990, Mosby.
Brown PA, Blayney F, Brown CA, Evans KG: *Quick reference to pediatric intensive care nursing,* Rockville, MD, 1989, Aspen Publishers, Inc.
Fanaroff AA, Martin RJ, editors: *Neonatal-perinatal medicine: diseases of the fetus and infant,* ed 5, St Louis, 1990, Mosby.
Fuhrman BP, Zimmerman JJ, editors: *Pediatric critical care,* St Louis, 1992, Mosby.
Hazinski MF, editor: *Nursing care of the critically ill child,* ed 2, St Louis, 1992, Mosby.
Klaus MH, Fanaroff AA, editors: *Care of the high-risk neonate,* ed 4, Philadelphia, 1993, WB Saunders Co.
Merenstein GB, Gardner SL, editors: *Handbook of neonatal intensive care,* ed 2, St Louis, 1989, Mosby.
Squires LA: Neonatal seizures, *Crit Care Nurs Clin North Am* 4(3):495-506, 1992.
Vernon-Levett P: Head injuries in children, *Crit Care Nurs Clin North Am* 3(3):411-422, 1991.
Wong DL: *Whaley and Wong's nursing care of infants and children,* ed 5, St Louis, 1995, Mosby.

GASTROINTESTINAL

Alspach JG: *Core curriculum for critical care nursing,* ed 4, Philadelphia, 1991, WB Saunders Co.
Beachy P, Deacon J: *Core curriculum for neonatal intensive care nursing,* Philadelphia, 1992, WB Saunders Co.
Blumer JL, editor: *A practical guide to pediatric intensive care,* St Louis, 1990, Mosby.
Brown PA, Playney F, Brown CA, Evans KG: *Quick reference to pediatric intensive care nursing,* Rockville, MD, 1989, Aspen Publishers, Inc.
Fanaroff AA, Martin RJ, editors: *Neonatal-perinatal medicine: diseases of the fetus and infant,* ed 5, St Louis, 1990, Mosby.
Fuhrman BP, Zimmerman JJ, editors: *Pediatric critical care,* St Louis, 1992, Mosby.
Hazinski MF, editor: *Nursing care of the critically ill child,* ed 2, St Louis, 1992, Mosby.
Klaus MH, Fanaroff AA, editors: *Care of the high-risk neonate,* ed 4, Philadelphia, 1993, WB Saunders Co.
Lebet RM: Abdominal and genitourinary trauma in children, *Crit Care Nurs Clin North Am* 3(3):433-444, 1991.
Merenstein GB, Gardner SL, editors: *Handbook of neonatal intensive care,* ed 2, St Louis, 1989, Mosby.
Sterling CE, Jolley SG, Besser AS, Matteson-Kane M: Nursing responsibility in the diagnosis, care, and treatment of the child with gastroesophageal reflux, *J Pediatr Nurs* 6(5):331-336, 1991.
Wong DL: *Whaley and Wong's nursing care of infants and children,* ed 5, St Louis, 1995, Mosby.

RENAL

Alspach JG: *Core curriculum for critical care nursing,* ed 4, Philadelphia, 1991, WB Saunders Co.
Beachy P, Deacon J: *Core curriculum for neonatal intensive care nursing,* Philadelphia, 1992, WB Saunders Co.
Blumer JL, editor: *A practical guide to pediatric intensive care,* St Louis, 1990, Mosby.
Brown PA, Blayney F, Brown CA, Evans KG: *Quick reference to pediatric intensive care nursing,* Rockville, MD, 1989, Aspen Publishers, Inc.
Fanaroff AA, Martin RJ, editors: *Neonatal-perinatal medicine: diseases of the fetus and infant,* ed 5, St Louis, 1990, Mosby.
Fuhrman BP, Zimmerman JJ, editors: *Pediatric critical care,* St Louis, 1992, Mosby.
Hazinski MF, editor: *Nursing care of the critically ill child,* ed 2, St Louis, 1992, Mosby.
Klaus MH, Fanaroff AA, editors: *Care of the high-risk neonate,* ed 4, Philadelphia, 1993, WB Saunders Co.
Merenstein GB, Gardner SL, editors: *Handbook of neonatal intensive care,* ed 2, St Louis, 1989, Mosby.
Wong DL: *Whaley and Wong's nursing care of infants and children,* ed 5, St Louis, 1995, Mosby.

MULTISYSTEM

Alspach JG: *Core curriculum for critical care nursing,* ed 4, Philadelphia, 1991, WB Saunders Co.
Beachy P, Deacon J: *Core curriculum for neonatal intensive care nursing,* Philadelphia, 1993, WB Saunders Co.
Blumer JL, editor: *A practical guide to pediatric intensive care,* St Louis, 1990, Mosby.
Brown PA, Blayney F, Brown CA, Evans KG: *Quick reference to pediatric intensive care nursing,* Rockville, MD, 1989, Aspen Publishers, Inc.
Campbell LS, Campbell JD: Musculoskeletal trauma in children, *Crit Care Nurs Clin North Am* 3(3):445-457, 1991.
Fanaroff AA, Martin RJ, editors: *Neonatal-perinatal medicine: diseases of the fetus and infant,* ed 5, St Louis, 1990, Mosby.
Fuhrman BP, Zimmerman JJ, editors: *Pediatric critical care,* St Louis, 1992, Mosby
Hazinski MF, editor: *Nursing care of the critically ill child,* ed 2, St Louis, 1992, Mosby.
Kenner C, Hetteberg C: Nursing challenges in the care of very low birth weight infants (<1,000 grams), *AACN Clin Issues Crit Care Nurs* 5(3):231-241, 1994.
Klaus MH, Fanaroff AA, editors: *Care of the high-risk neonate,* ed 4, Philadelphia, 1993, WB Saunders Co.
Merenstein GB, Gardner SL, editors: *Handbook of neonatal intensive care,* ed 2, St Louis, 1989, Mosby.
Thompson DG: Consequences of perinatal asphyxia, *AACN Clin Issues Crit Care Nurs* 5(3):242-245.
Wong DL: *Whaley and Wong's nursing care of infants and children,* St Louis, 1995, Mosby.

TEST-TAKING STRATEGIES

Gaedeke MK: Test taking strategies, *Nursing '95,* October 1995.

Index

R

S

T